An Introduction to Statistics in Early Phase Trials

AN INTRODUCTION TO STATISTICS IN EARLY PHASE TRIALS

STEVEN A. JULIOUS
Medical Statistics Group, School of Health and Related Research, University of Sheffield, UK

SAY BENG TAN
Singapore Clinical Research Institute and Duke-NUS Graduate Medical School, Singapore

DAVID MACHIN
University of Leicester and University of Sheffield, UK

WILEY-BLACKWELL
A John Wiley & Sons, Ltd., Publication

This edition first published 2010

Wiley-Blackwell is an imprint of John Wiley & Sons, formed by the merger of Wiley's global Scientific, Technical and Medical business with Blackwell Publishing.

Registered office
John Wiley & Sons Ltd, The Atrium, Southern Gate, Chichester, West Sussex, PO19 8SQ, UK

Other Editorial Offices
9600 Garsington Road, Oxford, OX4 2DQ, UK
111 River Street, Hoboken, NJ 07030-5774, USA

For details of our global editorial offices, for customer services and for information about how to apply for permission to reuse the copyright material in this book please see our website at www.wiley.com/wiley-blackwell

Library of Congress Cataloguing-in-Publication Data

Julious, Steven A.
An introduction to statistics in early phase trials / Steven Julious, David Machin, Say Beng Tan.
p. ; cm.
Includes bibliographical references and index.
ISBN 978-0-470-05985-2
1. Drugs—Testing—Statistical methods. 2. Clinical trials—Statistical methods.
I. Tan, Say Beng. II. Machin, David, 1939- III. Title.
[DNLM: 1. Clinical Trials, Phase I as Topic—methods. 2. Biometry—methods.
3. Clinical Trials, Phase II as Topic—methods. 4. Models, Statistical.
5. Statistics as Topic—methods. WA 950 J94i 2010]
RM301.27.J85 2010
615′.19012—dc22

2009033763

ISBN: 978-0-470-05985-2

A catalogue record for this book is available from the British Library.

Set in 10.5/12.5 Times by Integra Software Services Pvt. Ltd, Pondicherry, India.

First Impression 2010

MIX
Paper from responsible sources
FSC® C013604
FSC www.fsc.org

Contents

1 Early Phase Trials

1.1 INTRODUCTION

Trials conducted in the early phases of the molecule-to-marketplace clinical development paradigm take compounds from first time into man through to the start of the pivotal clinical trial programme. These early phases could be considered to be the learning and explaining phases. They are learning as by definition there is no experience of the compound in man when starting these studies and many important factors relevant to a compound's development will need to be quantified. They are explaining as early trials help to describe the properties of the compound, inputting to its rationale.

Although it is only in late-phase development that definitive proof can be obtained, early phase studies are important as they inform some of the most important decisions in a clinical programme, such as the most appropriate dose to carry forward, and the posology. They also contribute to important factors such the inclusion/exclusion criteria for a compound with respect to late-phase protocols' populations (or labelling). For the inclusion/exclusion criteria, without sufficient enabling studies these may be so tight as to make recruitment rates impracticably slow.

By definition in early drug development there is little information available when designing trials, and resource is often constrained both financially and in terms of populations available to recruit. These factors can have a major impact on the design and conduct of the trials, with innovative and adaptive designs often being applied as a way of overcoming the restrictions. However, in early phase trials, what is lacking in resource can, in part, be made up for by increased control, for example the trialists themselves control the rate of recruitment in a healthy volunteer study. In addition, early trials often are more tightly controlled with respect to more restricted populations from smaller pools of specialist centres. This can positively benefit statistical variability, enabling smaller signals to be detected from these smaller studies.

1.2 DEFINITIONS OF THE PHASES OF EARLY DEVELOPMENT

The naive view of the phases of clinical development is that they follow a chronological ordering of the form described in Figure 1.1a. In this ordering the distinct phases are like batons in a relay race. Initially a compound is picked up in a preclinical setting by

An Introduction to Statistics in Early Phase Trials Steven A. Julious, Say Beng Tan and David Machin

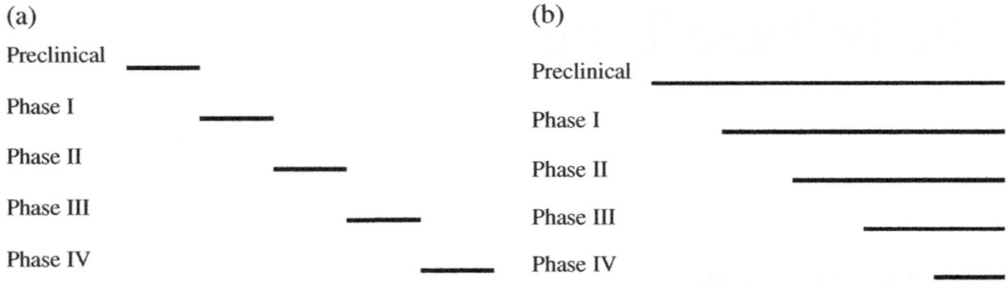

Figure 1.1 Perception of the phases of drug development.

researchers, where work is undertaken until a point is reached when it can be handed on to Phase I. Phase I researchers then take on the baton and run with it until they can hand it on to Phase II and so on.

The ordering of the phases is better described in Figure 1.1b. Here what actually happens in clinical development is that the minimum body of work is done in each phase before the compound progresses to the next phase. The consequence is that much of what would be considered early phase trials actually takes place when a compound is late in development. This minimum body of work is usually referred to as critical-path activities. Hence, where Figure 1.1a can be considered to be accurate is that it figuratively describes these critical-path studies.

The International Conference on Harmonisation of Technical Requirements for Registration of Pharmaceuticals for Human Use (ICH) Topic E8 gives a detailed description of the phases of development (ICH, 1998a), while the Food and Drug Administration (FDA, 2006a) defines the critical path and what we learn along the way as follows:

> At the start of the Critical Path, developers form hypotheses about performance characteristics such as safety, biological or mechanical action, and biocompatibility. They then seek to evaluate and confirm these hypotheses using in vitro, animal, and human testing. Once uncertainty about benefits and risks of a product has been reduced to an acceptable level, the product may be approved for marketing—if the benefits outweigh the risks. The great challenge in development lies in predicting a potential product's performance as early as possible with the greatest degree of certainty.

With this definition, in terms of studies necessary for filing registration, all studies fall along the critical path. However, it can be argued that critical-path studies are just those that drive the development timelines and must be done prior to the start of subsequent activities. Studies that can be done in parallel with other activities, that is, that must be done but not before some pre-prescribed critical path task, are termed non-critical path. As an aside, in this context given that much preclinical work happens when a compound is actually in clinical development there is an argument that 'phase 0' as opposed to 'preclinical' may be a more accurate nomenclature.

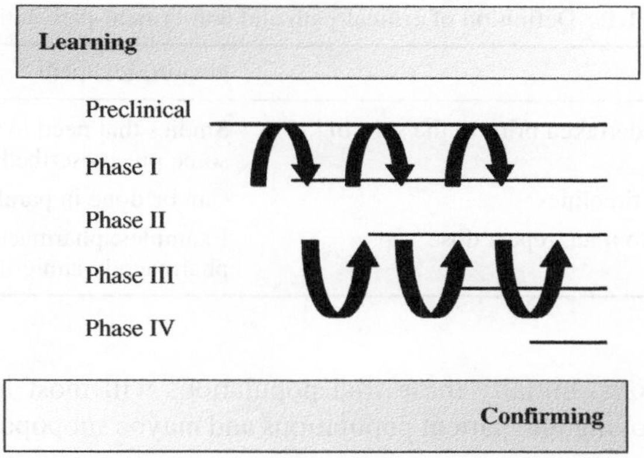

Figure 1.2 Interweaving of the phases of drug development.

For a given compound, therefore, activities in a clinical plan may look like Figure 1.2, moving between learning and confirming, and where critical-path activities preclinically may be triggered by activities in Phase I and vice versa. A compound may also move along the different phases according to different indications or populations for which it may be being targeted.

Due to the wide variety of work undertaken in early phase development, generic definition of the early phases is not really possible. Simply it can be said that Phase I is performed in healthy volunteers and is the phase where safety and tolerability are assessed, while Phase II is undertaken in patients and is the phase where the first assessment of efficacy is made. However, things are not as simple as these definitions imply. In therapeutic areas such as oncology, Phase I may be undertaken in patients, while for certain areas, the size and scale of Phase II may resemble Phase III for other areas.

In truth what can be stated is that a compound must go first time into man (FTIM), and that some time after this study the pivotal Phase III programme must start. From the point of the start of FTIM to the start of the pivotal Phase III programme we can define as early phase development (in addition of course to the early phase work being undertaken in parallel to Phase III).

Subsequent chapters will detail the different types of early phase trials.

1.3 CLINICAL DEVELOPMENT PLANS

When taking a compound from molecule to marketplace it could be argued that the vast majority of studies would fall under the banner of early phase. This greater number of studies equates to a greater variety of types of studies that can be undertaken, from routine 'bleed them and feed them' type studies – for example studies to assess drug or food interactions – through to innovative designs. The trials themselves are undertaken in a

Table 1.1 Definition of critical-path and non-critical-path activities

Critical path	Non-critical path
Studies that must be undertaken prior to the start of subsequent activities	Studies that need to be done but not before some pre-prescribed critical path task
Drive the development timelines	Can be done in parallel
Examples: first time into man; repeat dose study	Examples: pharmacokinetic- or pharmacodynamic-interaction studies

number of populations. Initially these trial populations will most likely be of healthy volunteers before moving into patient populations and maybe subpopulations within these patient populations.

To coordinate all these activities a clinical development plan (CDP) needs to be drafted. This document will be needed to help coordinate the activities, critical path and non-critical path, required for development. The focus initially will be on the critical-path activities, as defined in Table 1.1, as these will determine timelines, whilst non-critical-path activities could be completed in parallel.

Examples of critical-path studies are the first-time-in-man study (which obviously must be done), maybe followed by the repeat-dose study for a chronic intervention. Obviously a compound must be shown to be safe and tolerable in a single-dose study before it can be given in a repeat-dose study. Other studies may follow in sequential order to these.

Examples of non-critical-path activities could be studies to investigate possible pharmacokinetic interaction or pharmacodynamic interactions. These may not fall on the critical path but would need to be done prior to the start of the pivotal programme, as without them the protocol inclusion criteria would be affected and as a consequence the rate of recruitment. Figure 1.3 gives an illustration of how a clinical development plan may be summarized.

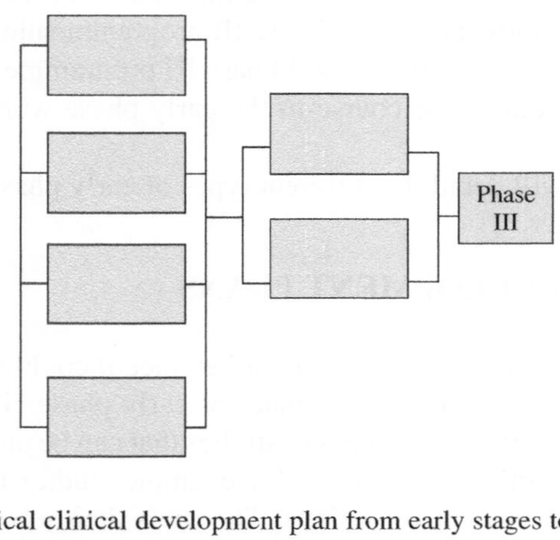

Figure 1.3 Typical clinical development plan from early stages to start of Phase III.

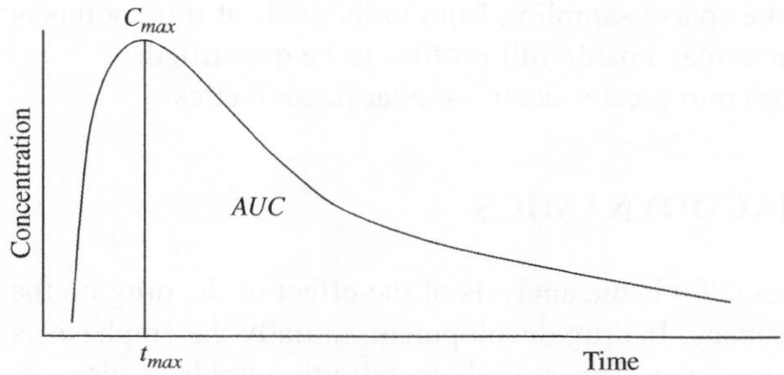

Figure 1.4 Example of an individual extravascular pharmacokinetic profile.

1.4 PHARMACOKINETICS

A main aim of many early phase studies is to assess the pharmacokinetic (PK) activity of a given compound. This is often referred to as analysing the effect of the body on the drug. This is achieved by the derivation of a concentration–time profile for each individual given the compound. Figure 1.4 gives an illustrative example of a hypothetical extravascular pharmacokinetic profile (to be discussed in more detail in Chapter 2).

In truth an analysis of the full pharmacokinetic profile is not usually undertaken but instead appropriate summary statistics are used to assess the pharmacokinetics. This assessment is usually performed by determining the extent and rate of absorption, using the AUC (area under the concentration curve) to assess the extent of absorption and the C_{max} (maximum concentration) to assess the rate of absorption (see Figure 1.4).

Other summary measures that could be used include time to maximum concentration (t_{max}) and the time taken for the apparent terminal plasma concentration to fall by one half (half-life, $t_{½}$). This half-life is often used to determine the dose schedule for a given compound. A short half-life will require regular dosing, whilst a longer half-life will require less-frequent dosing

Once appropriate pharmacokinetic summary parameters are derived for each individual, then inferences across subjects in the study may be drawn through descriptive statistics (for a given dose). Initially only single doses will be given to assess the pharmacokinetics, which if shown to be tolerable will lead to repeat dosing and repeat-dose pharmacokinetics (depending on the indication). However, the single-dose pharmacokinetics is key information, as from these data it is possible, under certain assumptions, to predict the repeat-dose profiles.

Usually, in the very early stages of development, full pharmacokinetic profiles are collected on a tightly controlled, relatively small number of healthy volunteers, in studies which have a main aim of assessing these profiles. For studies later in development, pharmacokinetic information may be obtained on a patient population but it may no longer be a main aim for the individual study – indeed it may now be a substudy to the main study. For such studies, instead of taking full profiles on individuals, sparser pharmacokinetic sampling may be performed. However, these data could be obtained on a larger sample size, and the sparse sampling from individuals at time points across the pharmacokinetic time frame may enable full profiles to be quantified.

Chapter 2 will go into greater detail on pharmacokinetics.

1.5 PHARMACODYNAMICS

Pharmacodynamics (PD) is the analysis of the effect of the drug on the body in terms of both safety and efficacy. In drug development, initially the emphasis is on safety, before moving onto efficacy later. This simplistic definition holds as, depending on indication, studies are conducted initially just in healthy volunteers (to assess safety and tolerability) before moving into patients later (to assess efficacy). However, it is a little too simplistic, as efficacy can be assessed to a degree in healthy volunteers, whilst it could be argued that only in later, and larger, patient trials can safety truly be assessed.

Similarly to pharmacokinetics, pharmacodynamic responses, such as those from efficacy outcomes, biomarker data or a surrogate endpoint in early trials, can be summarized through statistics such as the pharmacodynamic half-life. This half-life could in turn be used to determine dosing schedule.

In addition to assessing the pharmacodynamics and pharmacokinetics independently, PK/PD modelling can be undertaken – which again may inform decisions on dosing schedule. Figure 1.5 gives an illustration of what an indirect response may look like when linking pharmacodynamics with pharmacokinetics for a single dose. The loop (termed a hysteresis loop) indicates how the same level of drug could illicit different responses, dependent on the time relative to dose that the response was assessed. Here you need to know time as well as concentration to be able to predict the effect.

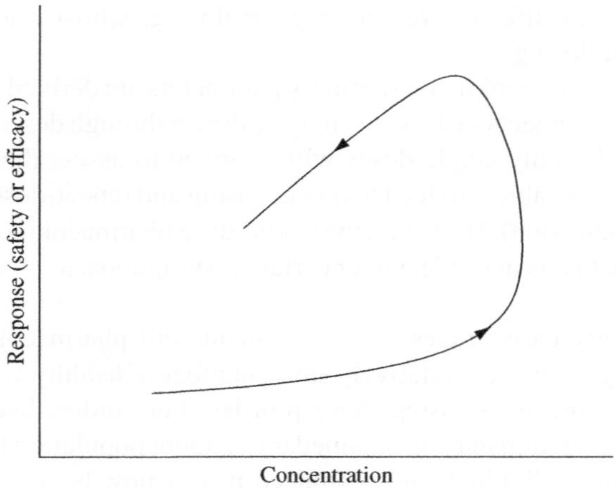

Figure 1.5 Indirect relationship between response and pharmacokinetics for a single dose.

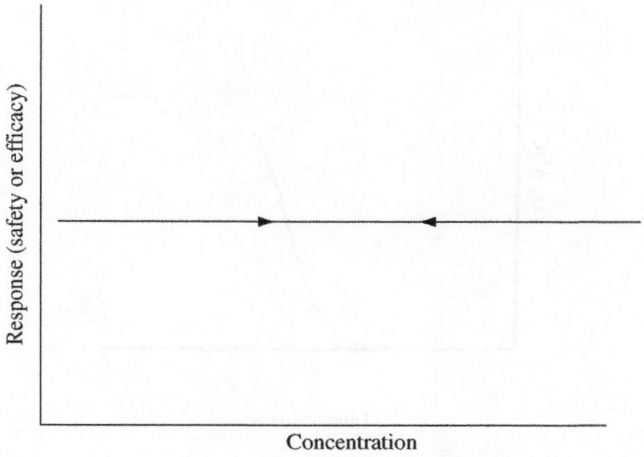

Figure 1.6 Relationship between response and pharmacokinetics after repeat doses.

This could be compared to an illustrative (hoped for) PK/PD relationship from after repeat dosing, given in Figure 1.6, where the PD response is constant relative to both time and the pharmacokinetics.

In terms of drug development, it is important to quantify any relationship between exposure and safety and/or efficacy throughout the development process. For example, the US Food and Drug Administration (FDA, 2003) stated that, for meetings between the regulators and developers at the end of the early stages of Phase II development (Phase IIa):

> The overall purpose of these meetings is to discuss the exposure response information during early drug development. The exposure response will be pertinent to both favorable (*sic*) and adverse effects.

1.6 DOSE PROPORTIONALITY

Probably one of the most important assumptions (or properties) in drug development is that of dose proportionality. Figure 1.7 gives an illustrative example of what the pharmacokinetics (in terms, here, of AUC) across a dose range may look like. The wish would be to concentrate future dose selections in clinical outcome studies on the linear part of the dose curve. This is because after a point in this example, increasing dose does not equate to increasing amount-of-drug concentration, and thus there is unlikely to be any benefit from these higher doses.

Dose proportionality would be assessed preliminarily in the first-into-man study before a later definitive study is performed. Having dose-proportional pharmacokinetics is important, as not only does this assumption drive dose selection in patient studies but it also effects

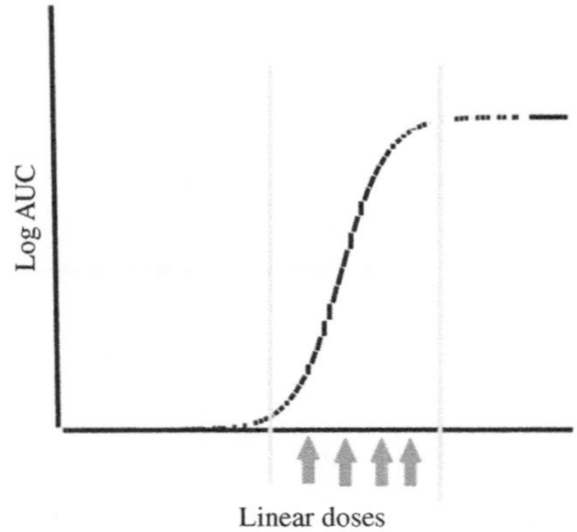

Figure 1.7 Anticipated relationship between pharmacokinetic AUC and dose.

decisions such as those of dose adjustments for special populations, and also underpins prediction of repeat-dose pharmacokinetics and interpolation in PK/PD modelling.

Without dose proportionality a compound could still be viable. However, there are consequent complications. Not only does it impact on the analyses described above but it can also complicate bioequivalence studies, for example, which may need to be undertaken with several doses.

Chapters 2, 8 and 10 give details on dose proportionality in the context of drug development, as well as how to design and analyse studies to make the assessment.

1.7 DOSE RESPONSE

The context of dose here is in terms of clinical response both for efficacy and for safety. The selection of dose is important; too low and the compound could be proceeding with a suboptimal level of efficacy; too high and unnecessary tolerability concerns may become an issue.

Figure 1.8 illustrates the points considered in dose response. This figure is a little naughty in that it has two response axes in the same graph, but it does summarize the considerations nicely. It illustrates a scenario where after a given dose there is no additional clinical benefit but the number of adverse responses is greatly increasing. This dose is referred to as the maximum effective dose (MED), and in adjudicating on harm, a decision on doses beyond this would tend to be against their selection.

Initially the safety cut off would have come from animal data and would be based on a fraction of the dose given to the most sensitive animal – often referred to as the no-observed-effect level (NOEL). After proceeding with drug development, however, this may relate to the maximum tolerated dose (MTD) given to man. This maximum dose could be different in different populations; for example the MTD in healthy volunteers could be considerably lower than that for patients, in certain indications.

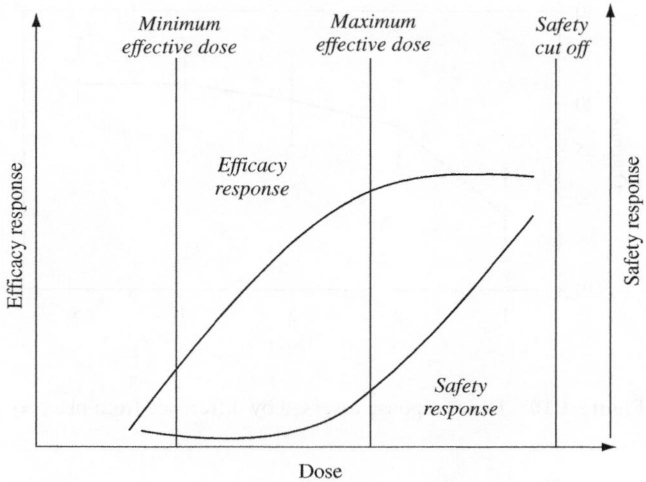

Figure 1.8 Anticipated relationship of dose response with safety and efficacy.

The dose range up to the safety cut off is referred to as the safety window – as highlighted in Figure 1.9. The wish is to have this window as wide as possible, as a compound could be misused or abused, or there may be unanticipated pharmacodynamic or pharmacokinetic interactions in the subsequent trial populations. Another consideration is absentmindedness, with patients forgetting they have taken their medication already and hence taking it twice. In double-dummy randomized controlled trials there

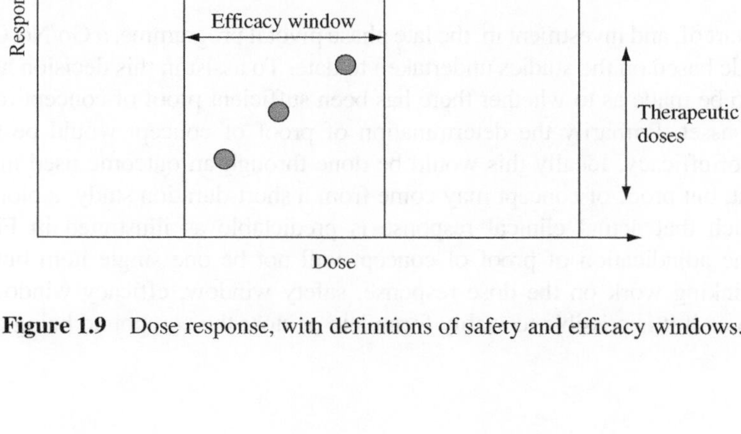

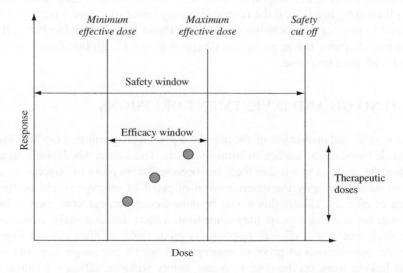

Figure 1.9 Dose response, with definitions of safety and efficacy windows.

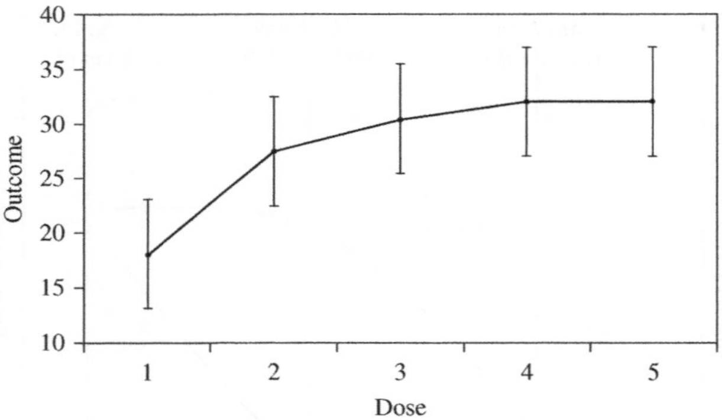

Figure 1.10 Dose response assessed by difference from placebo.

can be evidential support of absentmindedness from tablet count data. Hence, it is beneficial to have as big a safety window as possible.

In terms of clinical response to treatment as well as the maximum tolerated dose, the minimum effective and maximum effective dose need to be determined. The distance between the minimum effective and maximum effective dose is termed the efficacy window (see Figure 1.8 and Figure 1.9).

When designing trials to assess dose response it is optimal to select doses falling within this range, as illustrated by the three dots in Figure 1.9. Of course doses are not selected outside of this range on purpose, but often it is hard to judge what the efficacy window is. Figure 1.10 illustrates this point. Does the outcome plateau after dose 4, or is it randomly scattered about a true linear response? Dose selection is difficult and, in the case of the scenario given in Figure 1.10, if the response is truly linear (but dose 4 is carried forward) it could lead to smaller effects being observed in Phase III compared to Phase II.

Subsequent chapters, but in particular Chapters 6 and 12, go into detail on the issues associated with dose response.

1.8 GO/NO GO AND INVESTMENT DECISIONS

Before the start of, and investment in, the late phase pivotal programme, a Go/No-Go decision must be made based on the studies undertaken to date. To assist in this decision an adjudication needs to be made as to whether there has been sufficient proof of concept (or efficacy) for a given asset. Primarily the determination of proof of concept would be through an assessment of efficacy. Ideally this would be done through an outcome used in late-phase development, but proof of concept may come from a short-duration study, a biomarker or a surrogate such that actual clinical response is predictable as illustrated in Figure 1.11. However, the adjudication of proof of concept will not be one single item but would be a package linking work on the dose response, safety window, efficacy window and also aspects such as if it is possible to viably formulate or store the compound being developed.

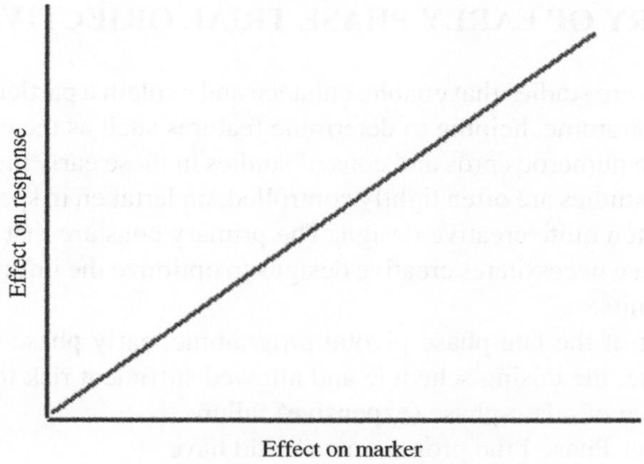

Figure 1.11 Linking later clinical responses with responses on a marker.

The definition of 'proof' in the context of drug development of course varies. 'Definitive' here means to provide convincing proof to a sceptic arbiter. Usually this would be a regulatory agency on behalf of society as a whole. Initially, however, the arbiter would be the sponsor of the clinical programme itself. As a consequence the level of proof required from early phase studies is to facilitate appropriate decisions such as Go/No Go and investment decisions.

Of course, just because the level of proof is for an internal arbiter does not mean that the rigour required is any less. However, the context may be in terms of risk discharged through the programme. The sponsor will wish to maximize risk discharged as early as possible in the programme, as a fast-fail decision for an individual compound could free resource and speed development for other compounds in the portfolio. These fast-fail decisions could be made (or facilitated) through assessing whether there has been proof of presence for a compound – determining if the drug gets to the site of action – or if there has been proof of mechanism – determining if the compound affects the *a-priori* hypothesized mechanism for efficacy. There is a logical hierarchy of different types of proof, as illustrated in Figure 1.12, such that with a proven mechanism for a compound, proof of concept may be achieved though proof of presence or through proof of mechanism.

Chapter 15 describes how Go/No-Go criteria may be formed.

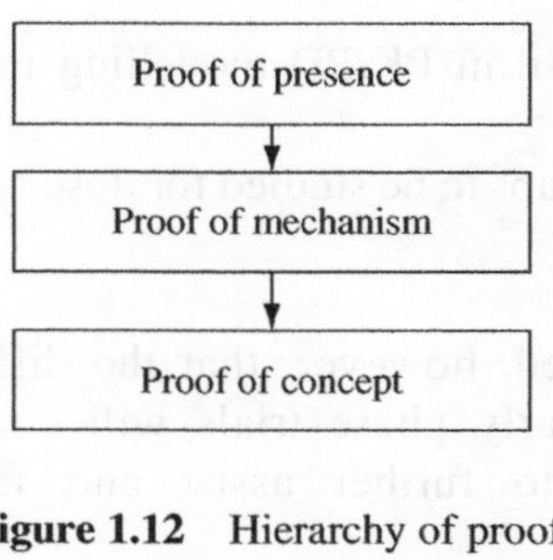

Figure 1.12 Hierarchy of proof.

1.9 SUMMARY OF EARLY PHASE TRIAL OBJECTIVES

Early phase studies are studies that enable, enhance and explain a particular compound for a development programme, helping to determine features such as the efficacy and safety windows. There are numerous pros and cons of studies in these early phases. The primary pros being that the studies are often tightly controlled, undertaken in specialist centres and allow the use of often quite creative design. The primary cons are that they have limited resource, which often necessitates creative designs to optimize the information we can get within the fixed limits.

Prior to the start of the late-phase pivotal programme, early phase trials should have determined the dose, the dosing schedule and allowed sufficient risk to be discharged to minimize the chance of a late-phase (expensive) failure.

In particular, after Phase I the programme should have

1. Quantified a range of safe (and potentially efficacious) doses – including the maximum tolerated dose (MTD).
2. Described pharmacokinetic exposure levels of each dose.
3. Facilitated the choice of dose and posology (dose titration, dose interval for later studies).
4. Described the pharmacodynamics at each dose (including biomarkers and surrogates).
5. Developed initial models for use in PK/PD modelling, including efficacy– and safety–exposure.

While at the end of Phase II the programme should have

1. Established the efficacy and safety windows in the target population, including
   (i) The minimum effective dose
   (ii) The maximum effective dose
   (iii) The maximum tolerated dose.
2. Identified the time interval needed to see efficacy or tolerability effects.
3. Provided the dose and schedule for dosing for Phase III, including
   (i) Response-guided titration steps
   (ii) Dosing intervals.
4. Developed a model for use in PK/PD modelling including efficacy– and safety–exposure.
5. Identified potential subgroups to be studied for dose adjustment in Phase III (e.g. age, gender).

It must again be highlighted, however, that the different phases of development at not mutually exclusive; early phase trials will continue whilst a compound is in late-phase development to further assist and facilitate in the compound's development.

2 Introduction to Pharmacokinetics

2.1 INTRODUCTION

An objective of many early phase studies is to describe the pharmacokinetics of a given compound. This usually is achieved by the derivation of a concentration–time profile for each individual given the compound. As with most forms of statistical comparison, however, a concentration–time profile is usually described through a series of summary parameters that we will introduce, such as area under the curve (AUC), maximum concentration (C_{max}), and the elimination rate and half-life. Once these summary parameters are determined for each individual, then inferences across all the subjects in the study may be drawn through appropriate analyses.

Pharmacokinetics is one of the areas where improving technologies of trials has had significant impact. It was only comparatively recently that, for many treatments, lower doses could not be fully quantified due to concentrations needing to be relatively high to be assessed. However, as the minimum level for quantification has fallen, the amount of possible pharmacokinetic analysis has thereby increased. This progress has enabled better characterization of the pharmacokinetics of different drugs, including lower doses.

In this chapter we describe how pharmacokinetic parameters are derived. As most statistical methodologies are developed by statisticians, they have statistically phrased outcomes that often require a clinical interpretation, such that the clinical interpretation has to be built around the statistics. A consequence is that what is straightforward to statisticians may not be so to others.

In contrast, much of the pharmacokinetics methodology has been developed by non-statisticians, often independently of analogous statistical areas. Hence pharmacokinetics often has a different nomenclature for 'standard' statistical terms. A consequence is that statistical methodologies have been specifically designed to fit around clinical terms to facilitate clinical interpretation.

Ease of interpretation is in the eye of the reader, however, as evidenced by the sea of differential equations that you often read when discussing pharmacokinetics; and because there is a different nomenclature it can be difficult to bridge the gap to analogous statistical texts. This chapter will try to keep things at a relatively simple

An Introduction to Statistics in Early Phase Trials Steven A. Julious, Say Beng Tan and David Machin

level with emphasis on straightforward pharmacokinetic derivation, and attempt to highlight nomenclatural differences. These descriptions will be made for pharmacokinetic parameters that are derived using both compartmental and noncompartmental approaches.

You do not have to be a mechanic to drive a car, and as such the objective of this chapter is not to describe how to 'do' pharmacokinetics *per se*, but to introduce some of the basic terms so that when reading protocols or published papers some of the most common terms can be understood.

2.2 BASICS OF PHARMACOKINETICS

The definition of pharmacokinetics is the effect of the body on the drug. Once a drug is introduced into the body, an individual's pharmacokinetic profile such as described in Figure 2.1 can be anticipated.

Fortunately for an individual, the full pharmacokinetic profile does not have to be analysed. Summary measures to describe a profile may be used instead. The two most common summaries are AUC (area under the curve) which measures the extent of exposure, and C_{max} (maximum concentration).

As mentioned earlier, pharmacokinetics-driven studies form the basis of much early drug development work. They are used to assess how much drug is in the body at a given dose (at a given time). As drug exposure is usually linked to both efficacy and safety, the pharmacokinetics for a given drug can in turn be used as a surrogate for efficacy and safety. As a consequence, through pharmacokinetics we can undertake activities such as assessing equivalence of two formulations – termed bioequivalence (discussed in Chapter 9) and facilitate the investigation of clinical subgroups such as the elderly, or possible interactions (discussed in Chapter 10) without the necessity to perform full clinical studies.

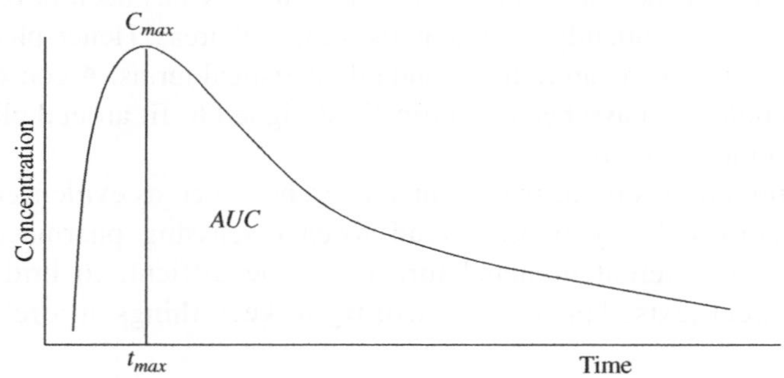

Figure 2.1 A pharmacokinetic profile.

2.3 DERIVATION OF PHARMACOKINETIC PARAMETERS

2.3.1 SINGLE DOSE

2.3.1.1 Compartmental Approach for Intravenous Dose: Single Compartment

In this section a brief description of the derivation of pharmacokinetic parameters will be given for the simple case of a dose being administered intravenously via a bolus (which allows for a quick delivery of the drug). A more detailed description of how these parameters are derived can be obtained from a standard pharmacokinetic text (Rowland and Tozer, 1995).

Figure 2.2 gives a simple illustration of what the pharmacokinetic profile for a single intravenous dose of a drug might look like. In turn, this concentration–time curve can be represented by the following equation

$$c(t) = Ae^{-\lambda t}, \tag{2.1}$$

where $c(t)$ is the concentration at time t, $A = c_0 = c(0)$ the concentration at $t = 0$, and λ the terminal rate constant. A in this context therefore is an Amount, and is a drug concentration (with appropriate units). In (2.1) A could be replaced by c_0; however, we will use A here to be consistent with other sections in the chapter.

It is evident from (2.1) that the assumption here is that the concentration in the body falls exponentially at a constant rate, λ. This terminal rate is the rate at which the drug is eliminated from the body. It can be calculated by deriving (2.1), through a nonlinear regression model of the data. Alternatively, a linear regression model of the semi-logarithmic data: log (concentration) against time, of the form given in Figure 2.3, can be used to fit a model to the log-transformed data. For the latter situation this is just a linear regression of the form $y = mt + c$, but on the semi-log scale, that is,

$$log_e(c) = log_e(A) - \lambda t. \tag{2.2}$$

Here λ, although the same as in (2.1), is interpreted now as the slope of the line in Figure 2.3. It should be noted that this approach assumes that the errors from the regression

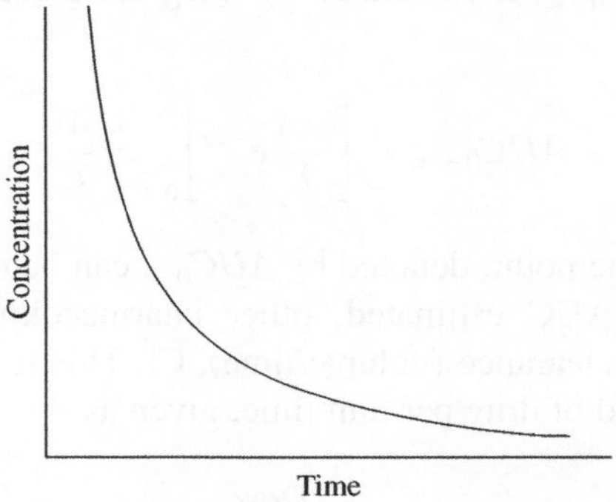

Figure 2.2 Pharmacokinetic concentration–time curve for an intravenous dose.

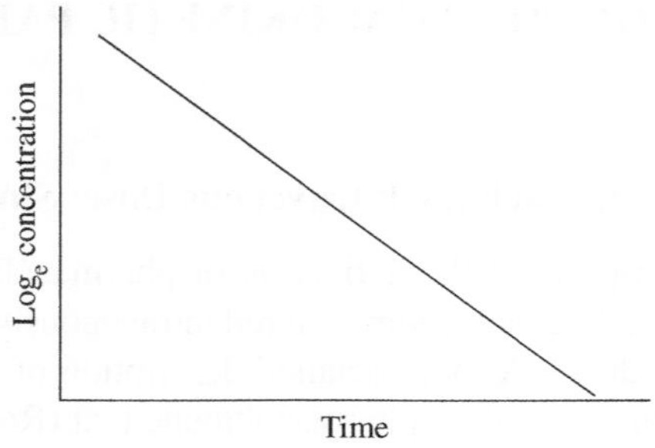

Figure 2.3 A semi-logarithmic pharmacokinetic concentration–time curve for an intravenous dose.

from (2.2) are Normally distributed on the $\log_e$ scale (i.e. they are log-Normally distributed), inferring that the results are conditional on an exponential error on the original scale.

Instead of the elimination rate constant, the elimination half-life ($t_{½}$) is usually more usefully used to summarize the time profile. This is the time taken for the drug concentration in the plasma to fall by one-half. It can be derived directly from (2.1), such that

$$c(t) = 2\ c(t + t_{½}),\ \text{which implies}\ \frac{A\,exp\,(-\lambda t)}{A\,exp\,(-\lambda(t + t_{½}))} = 2 \tag{2.3}$$

and hence

$$t_{½} = \frac{log_e(2)}{\lambda}. \tag{2.4}$$

This is a common result that crops up in other applications. For example it is often assumed in a survival analysis that the survival function can be expressed exponentially, and (2.4) can be used to calculate the median survival time of cancer patients receiving a particular treatment.

With the derivation of (2.1), AUCs can be estimated. An AUC is a measure of the total amount of drug in the body over a given period of time for a given dose. The usual measure of AUC, denoted by $AUC_{0-\infty}$, is calculated by integrating equation (2.1) from 0 to ∞. Thus, we have

$$AUC_{0-\infty} = \left[\frac{-A}{\lambda}e^{-\lambda t}\right]_0^{\infty} = \frac{A}{\lambda}. \tag{2.5}$$

An AUC to a given time point, denoted by AUC_{0-t}, can be calculated using the same methodology. With the AUC estimated, other pharmacokinetic parameters can be derived, such as the total clearance (volume/time), Cl. This is defined as the volume of plasma irreversibly cleared of drug per unit time, given as

$$Cl = \frac{Dose}{AUC_{0-\infty}}. \tag{2.6}$$

The apparent volume of distribution, defined as the hypothetical volume of plasma that would be required to dissolve the total amount of drug at the same concentration as that found in the blood, is

$$V = \frac{Cl}{\lambda}. \tag{2.7}$$

It is thus evident, from the above equations for $t_{1/2}$, V and Cl, that once $AUC_{0-\infty}$ and λ are estimated, then most other parameters can be also, as

$$t_{1/2} = \frac{log_e(2)V}{Cl}, \qquad AUC = \frac{Dose}{Cl} \quad \text{and} \quad AUC = \frac{Dose}{V\lambda}, \tag{2.8}$$

and

$$c(t) = \frac{Dose}{V}\,\mathrm{e}^{-\lambda t}. \tag{2.9}$$

A point to make here is that, though statistically the unknowns in the equation are the slope (λ) and the intercept term (A), if you have an estimate for the clearance (Cl) and the volume of distribution (V) for a given dose, you also you have an estimate of λ and A. This point is important as some software packages ask for initial estimates to begin iteration procedures to estimate (2.1), and require inputs in terms of Cl and V.

2.3.1.2 Compartmental Approach for Intravenous Dose: Two Compartments

A two-compartment pharmacokinetic profile could take the form of Figure 2.4, where there are two distribution phases to the pharmacokinetics. The two-compartment nature of Figure 2.4 becomes clearer if a semi-log plot of such a profile is used, as in Figure 2.5.

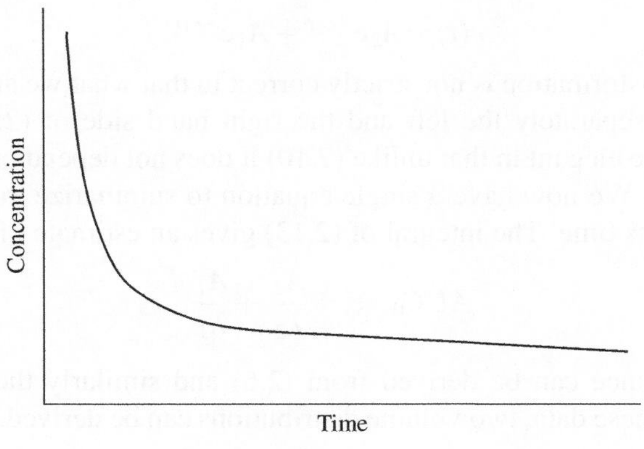

Figure 2.4 A two-compartment pharmacokinetic concentration–time curve for an intravenous dose.

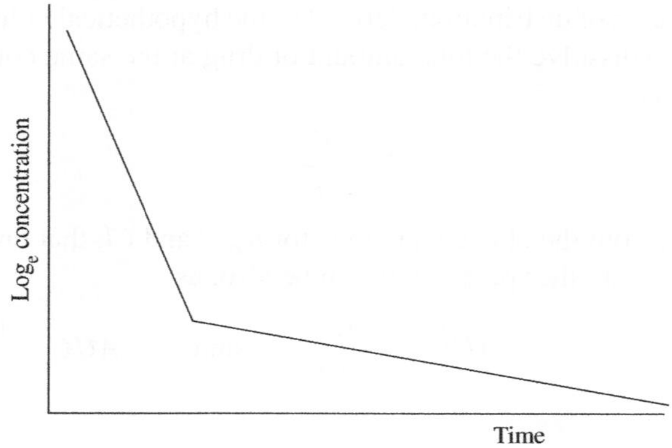

Figure 2.5 A two-compartment pharmacokinetic $\log_e$ concentration–time curve for an intravenous dose.

The data from Figure 2.5 can be summarized as a piece-wise regression model of the form

$$log_e(c) = log_e(B) - \mu t \qquad t \leq \delta \tag{2.10}$$

$$log_e(c) = log_e(A_2) - \lambda_2 t \qquad t \leq \delta \ .$$

It is rare to see the concentration–time relationship represented in a form such as (2.10). More usually the next step after (2.10) is to subtract the expression post-change-point from that pre-change-point; a process known as data stripping. This gives

$$\log_e c(t) = (\log_e B - \log_e A_2) - (\mu - \lambda_2)t + (\log_e A_2) - \lambda_2 t, \tag{2.11}$$

which can be rewritten, with $A_1 = (\log_e B - \log_e A_2)$ and $\lambda_1 = (\mu - \lambda_2)$, as

$$\log_e c(t) = log_e A_1 - \lambda_1 t + \log_e A_2 - \lambda_2 t. \tag{2.12}$$

Finally, back on the original scale

$$c(t) = A_2 e^{-\lambda_2 t} + A_1 e^{-\lambda_1 t}. \tag{2.13}$$

Note, this back-transformation is not strictly correct in that what we are in effect doing is back-transforming separately the left and the right hand side of (2.12). However, the result. (2.13) is quite elegant in that unlike (2.10) it does not depend on the change-point, δ, on the time axis. We now have a single equation to summarize the entire pharmacokinetic profile across time. The integral of (2.13) gives an estimate of $AUC_{0-\infty}$ as

$$AUC_{0-\infty} = \frac{A_2}{\lambda_2} + \frac{A_1}{\lambda_1}. \tag{2.14}$$

Likewise the clearance can be derived from (2.6) and similarly the half-life for each compartment. For these data, two volume distributions can be derived. The initial volume of distribution

$$V_1 = \frac{Dose}{A_1}, \tag{2.15}$$

and the distributional volume

$$V = \frac{Dose}{AUC_{0\text{-}\infty}\lambda_1}. \tag{2.16}$$

The latter is defined as the notional volume in which the drug must be distributed to observe the given drug concentration.

2.3.1.3 Compartmental Approach for Extravascular Dose: Single Compartment

In contrast to an intravenous dose profile, the single-dose extravascular pharmacokinetics would be anticipated to take the form described in Figure 2.6, which on the semi-log scale could be represented as Figure 2.7. For a single-compartment extravascular dose with first-order absorption the pharmacokinetic profile can be determined from

$$c(t) = -A_2 e^{-\lambda_2 t} + A_1 e^{-\lambda_1 t}, \tag{2.17}$$

where , (2.17) would be derived through nonlinear modelling or through data stripping as described for (2.10). In (2.17) the term $-A_2 e^{-\lambda_2 t}$ would equate to the absorption phase, while $A_1 e^{-\lambda_1 t}$ would equate to elimination.

Note that, often even when there are two compartments evident after intravenous dosing, following extravascular dosing only one compartment may be evident due to relatively slow absorption masking other compartments.

Here, λ_1 is defined as the elimination rate constant, that is, the slope of the log(concentration)–time curve during the terminal phase, and λ_2 is the absorption rate constant, defined as the slope of the semi-logarithmic curve during the absorption phase. The

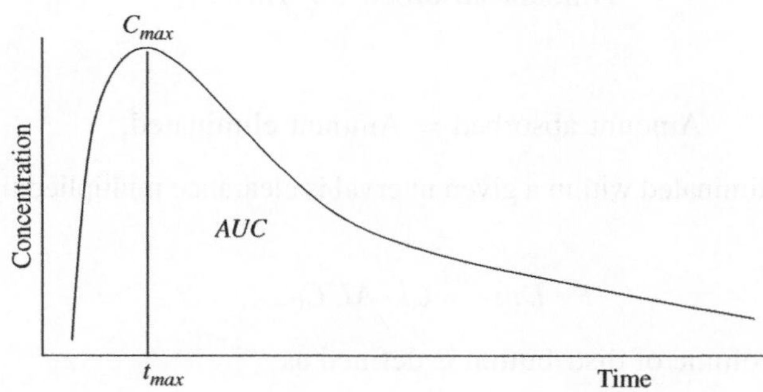

Figure 2.6 A one-compartment pharmacokinetic concentration–time curve for an extravascular dose.

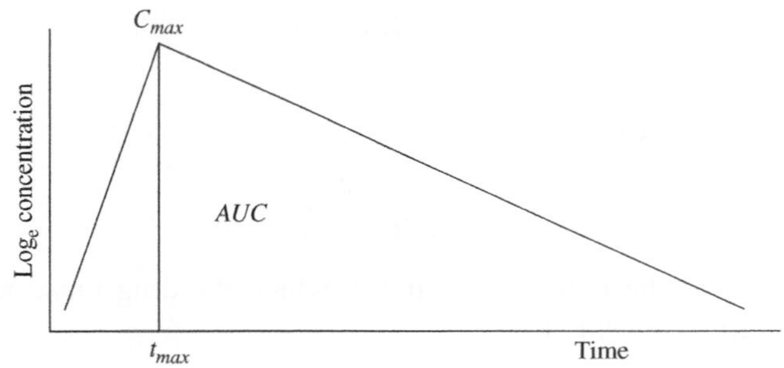

Figure 2.7 A one-compartment pharmacokinetic $\log_e$ concentration–time curve for an extravascular dose.

corresponding elimination and absorption half-lives can be derived from the rate constants

$$t_{1/2}^{\lambda_1} = \frac{log_e(2)}{\lambda_1} \text{ and } t_{1/2}^{\lambda_2} = \frac{log_e(2)}{\lambda_2}. \tag{2.18}$$

Similar to the parameter for intravenous dosing, the area under the curve until infinity can be calculated by integrating equation (2.17) between 0 and ∞

$$AUC_{0-\infty} = \left[\frac{A_2}{\lambda_2}e^{-\lambda_2 t} - \frac{A_1}{\lambda_1}e^{-\lambda_1 t}\right]_0^\infty = \frac{A_1}{\lambda_1} - \frac{A_2}{\lambda_2}. \tag{2.19}$$

Clearance is now defined a little differently as we need to know the bioavailability of the compound. Bioavailability will be discussed in Chapter 9, but here it is defined as the amount of drug that gets into the body relative to an intravenous dose. This relative comparison is abbreviated through the fraction, F, absorbed intact in the circulation. In the case of an extravascular dose, $F < 1$. Now for clearance we have

$$\text{Amount absorbed} = F \cdot Dose. \tag{2.20}$$

Then

$$\text{Amount absorbed} = \text{Amount eliminated}, \tag{2.21}$$

where the amount eliminated within a given interval is clearance multiplied by concentration over time. Thus

$$F \cdot Dose = Cl \cdot AUC_{0-\infty}. \tag{2.22}$$

Consequently the volume of distribution is defined as

$$F \cdot Dose = V \cdot AUC_{0-\infty} \cdot \lambda_1, \tag{2.23}$$

and hence we have

$$V = \frac{Cl}{\lambda_1}. \tag{2.24}$$

Note, however, it is usually Cl/F and V/F that are estimated in studies and are termed the apparent clearance and volume respectively.

In addition to the parameters, further empirical estimates can also be obtained for each subject: the maximum concentration observed is $C_{\max}$, and corresponding time value $t_{\max}$.

$C_{\max}$ for an extravascular dose is the point where the amount of drug absorbed into the body equals the amount eliminated, that is, $A_1 = A_2 = A$, and hence

$$c(t) = A\left(e^{-\lambda_1 t} - e^{-\lambda_2 t}\right). \tag{2.25}$$

Absorption still continues after $C_{\max}$, and it can be estimated from (2.25). It would be A in this equation; however, for an individual subject the actual observed $C_{\max}$ would be a point estimate and would depend on the estimation of $t_{\max}$. As such it is comparatively inaccurate and has higher statistical variability across subjects.

By integration of (2.25) we have

$$AUC_{0-\infty} = \frac{A(\lambda_2 - \lambda_1)}{\lambda_2 \lambda_1}, \tag{2.26}$$

and hence for clearance

$$Cl = \frac{F \cdot Dose}{AUC_{0-\infty}} = \frac{\lambda_1 \lambda_2 F \cdot Dose}{A(\lambda_2 - \lambda_1)} \tag{2.27}$$

and consequently

$$A = \frac{\lambda_1 \lambda_2 F \cdot Dose}{Cl(\lambda_2 - \lambda_1)} = \frac{\lambda_2 F \cdot Dose}{V(\lambda_2 - \lambda_1)}. \tag{2.28}$$

Further, from (2.28) and . (2.24) we can rewrite (2.25) as

$$c(t) = \frac{\lambda_2 F \cdot Dose}{V(\lambda_2 - \lambda_1)}\left(e^{-\lambda_1 t} - e^{-\lambda_2 t}\right). \tag{2.29}$$

This result is commonly seen in the literature. Hence from (2.29) it is evident that we can summarize a nonlinear model for a single-compartment extravascular model for a given dose in terms of the clearance (Cl), the distribution volume (V), the elimination rate (λ_1), absorption rate (λ_2) and F.

Note that as well as being derived empirically, $C_{\max}$ and $t_{\max}$ can be estimated from a compartmental model. From (2.29), if we differentiate with respect to t we obtain

$$\frac{\mathrm{d}c(t)}{\mathrm{d}t} = \frac{\lambda_2 F \cdot Dose}{V(\lambda_2 - \lambda_1)} \left(\lambda_2 \mathrm{e}^{-\lambda_2 t} - \lambda_1 \mathrm{e}^{-\lambda_1 t}\right), \tag{2.30}$$

which, if we set to zero, gives an estimate for $t_{\max}$ as

$$t_{max} = \frac{log_e \lambda_2 - log_e \lambda_1}{\lambda_2 - \lambda_1}. \tag{2.31}$$

Consequently, $C_{\max}$ can be estimated by taking the predicted concentration at this point:

$$C_{\max} = \frac{\lambda_2 F \cdot Dose}{V(\lambda_2 - \lambda_1)} \left(\mathrm{e}^{-\lambda_2 t_{max}} - \mathrm{e}^{-\lambda_1 t_{max}}\right) \tag{2.32}$$

From this it is apparent that instead of using Cl, V, F, λ_1 and λ_2, the parameters $C_{\max}$, $t_{\max}$, F, λ_1 and λ_2 could be used to the same effect.

This highlights two different approaches to modelling pharmacokinetic data. One approach is to estimate the terms in model (2.25) and from this derive parameters (volume of distribution, clearance, etc.). The other is the reverse process: to have outputs such as volume of distribution and clearance and from these obtain the model (2.25).

The point is not necessarily a trivial one, since numerical methods have to be used for fitting nonlinear models; for example, the Gauss–Newton algorithm. This requires initial estimates to begin the iterative procedure for estimation. For such an approach it is the values of the measure on the time axis that are the main influence on estimation. If just values of Cl, V, F, λ_1 and λ_2 are used for the initial iterations, then when converted to the form of (2.25) these may be nonsensical. Also, there is the issue of obtaining the best-fitting model for a given set of data. Figure 2.8 illustrates an issue when using the Gauss–Newton algorithm for an artificial problem analogous to (2.13) on the semi-log scale. This algorithm gets caught in local minima for δ, the change-point, when trying to estimate the best model; something that may not be anticipated when using Cl, V, F, λ_1 and λ_2 as initial estimates.

2.3.1.4 Noncompartmental Approach for Extravascular Dose with Single Compartment

The previous focus has been on compartmental-based derivation of pharmacokinetic parameters. We will now discuss noncompartmental derivation. Although this form of estimation of parameters is probably the most common, the form of estimation we have used previously with compartmental modelling is a requisite to understanding the noncompartmental derivation.

Suppose we have observed concentrations $C_1, C_2, C_3, \ldots, C_t$ assessed at different times $t_1, t_2, t_3, \ldots, t_t$. As for compartmental modelling, to estimate $AUC_{0-\infty}$ for these data we must integrate the data from 0 to ∞. This integration is performed in two stages. The first stage is to numerically integrate across the observed data. This can be accomplished using two approaches.

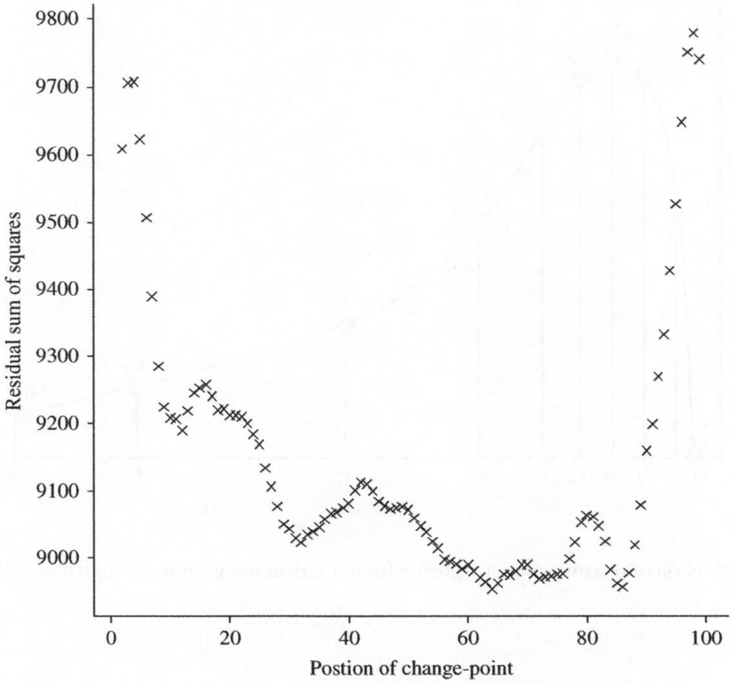

Figure 2.8 Local minima arising while estimating the change-point for a two-line model.

The first is the linear trapezoidal method. To do this you divide the data into sections corresponding to the observed data points as illustrated in Figure 2.9. For each section we work out the AUC. For the first section this would be the difference between the two time points, $t_0 - t_1$; multiplied by the average of the heights, $(C_0 + C_1)/2$, so that the corresponding area is

$$AUC_{0-1} = \frac{1}{2}(t_1 - t_0)(C_1 + C_0). \tag{2.33}$$

We actually wish to have AUC_{0-t}, and so we need to repeat (2.33) for all sections, and then add them together to obtain

$$AUC_{0-t} = \sum_{i=1}^{t} \frac{1}{2}(t_i - t_{i-1})(C_i + C_{i-1}). \tag{2.34}$$

The second approach is to use the log-linear trapezoidal method. As the name implies, this approach allows for the fact that pharmacokinetic data may take a log-linear form. Again we calculate the AUC for each section, but for each we need to work out the slope. For example, in Figure 2.10 the slope is taken as the ratio of the difference in heights divided by the difference in widths, or

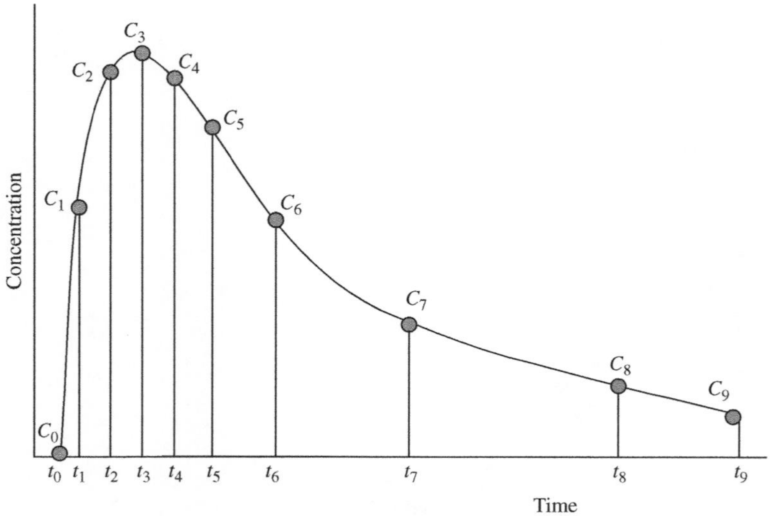

Figure 2.9 Division of pharmacokinetic profile for numerical integration through trapezoidal methods.

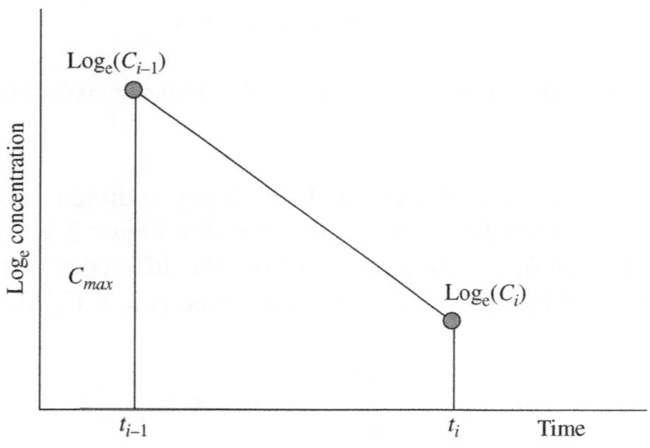

Figure 2.10 Numerical integration for a section of the log-linear trapezoidal method.

$$\lambda_i = \frac{log_e(C_i) - log_e(C_{i-1})}{(t_i - t_{i-1})} = \frac{log_e(C_i/C_{i-1})}{(t_i - t_{i-1})}. \tag{2.35}$$

We then calculate the area under the curve for each section by calculating $AUC_{t_i-\infty}$ and $AUC_{t_{i-1}-\infty}$ using an approach like (2.5) and then taking their difference, $AUC_{t_i-\infty} - AUC_{t_{i-1}-\infty}$. Here, $AUC_{t_i-\infty}$ is defined as

$$AUC_{t_i-\infty} = \left[C_i e^{-\lambda_i t}\right]_{t_i}^{\infty} = \frac{C_i}{\lambda_i} = C_i \cdot \frac{(t_i - t_{i-1})}{log_e(C_i/C_{i-1})}, \tag{2.36}$$

and AUC_{0-t} the sum of all the sections, formally defined as

$$AUC_{0-t} = \sum_{i=1}^{t} (t_i - t_{i-1}) \frac{(C_{i-1} - C_i)}{log_e(C_{i-1}/C_i)} \tag{2.38}$$

We have now described two approaches for estimating AUC_{0-t}, either of which could be used in practice. They are often used in combination: for example linear trapezoidal while concentrations are increasing and log-linear while they are decreasing.

We actually need to estimate $AUC_{0-\infty}$, which moves us to the second stage. To do this we first need to estimate $AUC_{t_{last}-\infty}$, which is done by first estimating the elimination rate λ. This is achieved through logging Figure 2.9 so that it appears like Figure 2.7 and then, ignoring all other possible phases or compartments, estimating the slope for the final elimination phase from the observed data. $AUC_{t_{last}-\infty}$ would then be estimated again as in (2.5) by

$$AUC_{t_{last}-\infty} = \left[\frac{-C_{last}}{\lambda} e^{-\lambda t}\right]_{t_{last}}^{\infty} = \frac{C_{last}}{\lambda}. \tag{2.39}$$

Note, the assumption here is that C_{last} is the minimum concentration, and this is used for the calculation. However, this need not be the case, and another observed concentration at a time prior to t_{last} can be utilized.

We can now calculate $AUC_{0-\infty}$ from

$$AUC_{0-\infty} = AUC_{0-t} + \frac{C_{last}}{\lambda}. \tag{2.40}$$

Other pharmacokinetic parameters such as clearance and volume of distribution can now be estimated as before, while C_{max} and t_{max} can be estimated empirically.

2.3.2 REPEAT DOSE

As well as single-dose pharmacokinetics, estimation of repeat-dose pharmacokinetics is also important, particularly when the pharmacokinetics has reached a steady state. Steady state is the point when there is no more accumulation in the pharmacokinetics, such that the amount of drug being carried forward from previous doses is the same as the amount being carried forward from the current point to future doses; that is, it is the point when input equals output.

A repeat-dose time interval for dosing is referred to using the Greek symbol τ. Recall from earlier in the chapter how the area under the curve to a given time point, *t*, can be calculated for single doses. Hence, similar to single dosing, $AUC_{0-\tau}$ is the AUC within a given dosing interval at steady state. What is interesting is the link between single- and repeat-dose pharmacokinetics.

Imagine repeat dosing where the doses were administered every 12 hours. The steady-state $AUC_{0-\tau}$ would hence be total amount of drug expected from a single dose (AUC_{0-12});

Table 2.1 Example of accumulation prediction from a single dose

Time	Dose 1	Dose 2	Dose 3	Dose 4	Dose 5	Dose 6	Dose 7	Dose 8	Dose 9	Dose 10	Total
0	24										24
6	12										12
12	6	24									30
18	3	12									15
24	1.5	6	24								31.5
30	0.75	3	12								15.75
36	0.375	1.5	6	24							31.875
42	0.1875	0.75	3	12							15.9375
48	0.0938	0.375	1.5	6	24						31.9688
54	0.0469	0.188	0.75	3	12						15.9844
60	0.0234	0.094	0.375	1.5	6	24					31.9922
66	0.0117	0.047	0.1875	0.75	3	12					15.9961
72	0.0059	0.023	0.0938	0.375	1.5	6	24				31.9981
78	0.0029	0.012	0.0469	0.1875	0.75	3	12				15.9990
84	0.0015	0.006	0.0234	0.0938	0.375	1.5	6	24			31.9995
90	0.0007	0.003	0.0117	0.0469	0.1875	0.75	3	12			15.9998
96	0.0004	0.001	0.0059	0.0234	0.0938	0.375	1.5	6	24		31.9999
102	0.0002	7E−04	0.0029	0.0117	0.0469	0.1875	0.75	3	12		15.9999
108	9E−05	4E−04	0.0015	0.0059	0.0234	0.0938	0.375	1.5	6	24	32.0000
114	5E−05	2E−04	0.0007	0.0029	0.0117	0.0469	0.188	0.75	3	12	16.0000
120	2E−05	9E−05	0.0004	0.0015	0.0059	0.0234	0.094	0.375	1.5	6	8.0000
126	1E−05	5E−05	0.0002	0.0007	0.0029	0.0117	0.047	0.1875	0.75	3	4.0000
132	6E−06	2E−05	9E−05	0.0004	0.0015	0.0059	0.023	0.0938	0.375	1.5	1.0000
138	3E−06	1E−05	5E−05	0.0002	0.0007	0.0029	0.012	0.0469	0.1875	0.75	1.0000

plus the amount of dose within the current interval from the previous dose ($AUC_{12\text{–}24}$); plus the amount from the dose before ($AUC_{24\text{–}36}$) and so on, such that

$$AUC_{0-\tau} = AUC_{0-12} + AUC_{12-24} + AUC_{24-36} + AUC_{36-48} + \ldots = AUC_{0-\infty}. \tag{2.41}$$

Therefore, $AUC_{0\text{–}\tau}$ at steady state is approximately equal to $AUC_{0\text{–}\infty}$ of a single dose. This reinforces the importance of $AUC_{0\text{–}\infty}$, for not only does it allow you to ascertain the total exposure to drug for a single dose, it also allows a prediction of $AUC_{0\text{–}T}$ independent of dosing schedule, under the assumption of dose proportionality. This assumption of dose proportionality is the key and is one of the crucial assumptions in clinical research. It is an assumption we will revisit throughout the book, with Chapters 6 and 10 detailing how it is assessed.

From a single dose, therefore, once $AUC_{0\text{–}\infty}$ has been estimated we can estimate the predicted accumulation ratio

$$R_p = \frac{AUC_{0-\infty}}{AUC_{0-t}}, \tag{2.42}$$

which we can use to multiply all the points in a single-dose pharmacokinetic profile, such as from Figure 2.2, Figure 2.4 or Figure 2.6, to estimate what the steady-state pharmacokinetic profile is anticipated to resemble. Also, for a given single-dose profile, repeat-dose accumulation can be predicted from the calculation illustrated in Table 2.1. You simply cut and paste the results from a single dose into adjacent columns to represent the additional exposure for subsequent doses. By adding these columns together the predicted pharmacokinetic profile across several accumulative doses is obtained.

Figure 2.11 gives an illustration of Table 2.1. From both of these it is clear that within five terminal half-lives steady state is anticipated to have been reached. The reason for this is that after five half-lives very little of the dose exposure more than five half-lives away would be anticipated to have been carried forward to the current dose.

So far we have only talked of predictions. Once a repeat-dose study has been conducted the observed accumulation ratio (R_o) can be estimated

$$R_o = \frac{AUC_{0-\tau}}{AUC_{0-t}}, \tag{2.43}$$

as well as the ratio

$$R_s = \frac{AUC_{0-\tau}}{AUC_{0-\infty}}, \tag{2.44}$$

which should equal 1 if assumptions hold.

Empirical C_{max} (and C_{min}) values can also be estimated at steady state, as well as values such as clearance

$$Cl = \frac{Dose}{AUC_{0-\tau}}. \tag{2.45}$$

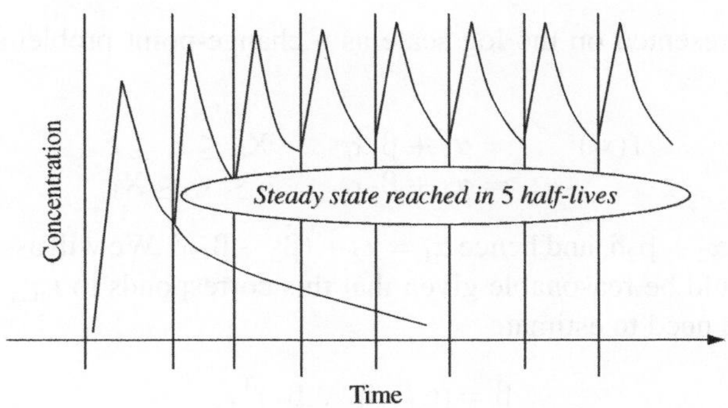

Figure 2.11 Example of accumulation to steady-state pharmacokinetics.

2.3.2.1 Extending Single-Dose Compartmental Approaches

We will not go into great detail on this other than to say that if compartmental models have been estimated then it is straightforward to use these to estimate parameters at steady state. Obviously $AUC_{0-\tau}$ is straightforward to estimate, but also for a single-compartment intravenous dose where *Dose/V* is an estimate of single-dose $C_{\max}$ (from (2.9)), steady-state $C_{\max,ss}$ is estimated by

$$C_{max,ss} = \frac{Dose}{V} \cdot R_p = \frac{Dose}{V} \cdot \frac{AUC_{0-\infty}}{AUC_{0-t}} = \frac{Dose}{V} \cdot \left(\frac{\frac{Dose}{V\lambda}}{\frac{Dose}{V\lambda}\left(1 - e^{-\lambda\tau}\right)} \right) = \frac{Dose}{V(1 - e^{-\lambda\tau})}, \tag{2.46}$$

where τ here is the dosing interval. Following on from this,

$$C_{min,ss} = \frac{Dose \cdot e^{-\lambda\tau}}{V(1 - e^{-\lambda\tau})}. \tag{2.47}$$

Similarly for single-compartment extravascular dose, $C_{\max,ss}$ and $C_{\min,ss}$ can be estimated from

$$C_{\max,ss} = \frac{\lambda_1 F \cdot Dose}{V(\lambda_1 - \lambda_2)(1 - e^{-\lambda_2\tau} + e^{-\lambda_2\tau})}, \tag{2.48}$$

$$C_{\min,ss} = \frac{\lambda_1 F \cdot Dose\left(e^{-\lambda_2\tau} - e^{-\lambda_1\tau}\right)}{V(\lambda_1 - \lambda_2)(1 - e^{-\lambda_2\tau} + e^{-\lambda_1\tau})}. \tag{2.49}$$

2.4 FURTHER ISSUES WITH PHARMACOKINETIC ANALYSIS

2.4.1 SIMPLE COMPARTMENTAL ANALYSIS MODEL

Consider (2.17) presented on the log scale as a change-point problem; then we have a model defined as

$$\begin{aligned} f(x_i) &= \alpha_1 + \beta_1 x_i \qquad && X_0 \le x_i \le \delta \\ &= \alpha_2 + \beta_2 x_i && \delta \le x_i \le X_1, \end{aligned} \tag{2.50}$$

where $\alpha_1 + \beta_1\delta = \alpha_2 + \beta_2\delta$, and hence $\alpha_1 = \alpha_2 + (\beta_2 - \beta_1)\delta$. We will assume here that δ is known, which would be reasonable given that this corresponds to $t_{\max}$ for extravascular data. We therefore need to estimate

$$\beta = (\alpha_2,\ \beta_1\ ,\ \beta_2)^{\mathrm{T}}. \tag{2.51}$$

To do this we need to construct a design (X) matrix of the form

$$X=\begin{pmatrix} 1 & x_1-\delta & \delta \\ 1 & x_2-\delta & \delta \\ \vdots & \vdots & \vdots \\ 1 & x_t-\delta & \delta \\ 1 & 0 & x_{t+1} \\ 1 & 0 & x_{t+2} \\ \vdots & \vdots & \vdots \\ 1 & 0 & \mathrm{x_T} \end{pmatrix} \tag{2.52}$$

which can in turn be solved for using normal equations, so that

$$\hat{\boldsymbol{\beta}}=(\mathbf{X}^T\mathbf{X})^{-1}\mathbf{X}^T\mathbf{Y}. \tag{2.53}$$

For the special case of $\delta=0$ we have the following result for the design matrix

$$X=\begin{pmatrix} 1 & x_1 & 0 \\ 1 & x_2 & 0 \\ \vdots & \vdots & \vdots \\ 1 & x_t & 0 \\ 1 & 0 & x_{t+1} \\ 1 & 0 & x_{t+2} \\ \vdots & \vdots & \vdots \\ 1 & 0 & x_T \end{pmatrix} \tag{2.54}$$

Now here is why we are introducing this theory. Obtain any dataset and take away the 'change-point' – which for extravascular pharmacokinetic data would be $\delta=t_{\max}$ – and we would then have a design matrix of the form (2.54), which forces $a_1=a_2$. The practical application of this is that we can use basic statistical procedures available in many software packages to derive the parameters in (2.50). Example SAS code and corresponding output are given in Figure 2.12.

With slight modification the previous model can be adapted for more than one subject and even for random intercepts and slopes as appropriate. Obviously, for more complicated models (e.g. more compartments) this model may not be suitable. However, the objective was to highlight how at the basic level what we have in compartmental modelling is a simple regression analysis.

If there was a simple linear relationship between time and concentrations (such as for (2.2)) then the model would be trivial, but even for more complicated nonlinear relationships the principles are the same. Many compartmental pharmacokinetic analyses at a basic level can be thought of in terms of regression analyses, even population approaches, which we discuss below.

(a)

```
DATA PK;
INPUT time conc lconc;
time1 = time-1.25;
A_time = time1*(time1 < 0);
B_time = time1*(time1 > 0);
DATALINES;
0.5     1.50  0.408
0.75    2.12  0.751
1       3.63  1.291
1.25    5.49  1.703
2       4.60  1.526
3       4.25  1.448
4       3.94  1.371
6       2.87  1.055
10      1.50  0.406
12      1.30  0.262
16      0.74  -0.303
24      0.28  -1.262
;
PROC glm DATA = PK;
MODEL lconc = A_time B_time /solution;
RUN;
QUIT;
```

(b)

Source	DF	Sum of Squares	Mean Square	F Value	Pr > F
Model	2	8.35788271	4.17894135	1190.58	<.0001
Error	9	0.03158996	0.00351000		
Corrected Total	11	8.38947267			

R-Square	Coeff Var	Root MSE	lconc Mean
0.996235	8.213292	0.059245	0.721333

Source	DF	Type I SS	Mean Square	F Value	Pr > F
A_time	1	0.00879282	0.00879282	2.51	0.1479
B_time	1	8.34908989	8.34908989	2378.66	<.0001

Source	DF	Type III SS	Mean Square	F Value	Pr > F
A_time	1	1.66392925	1.66392925	474.05	<.0001
B_time	1	8.34908989	8.34908989	2378.66	<.0001

Parameter	Estimate	Standard Error	t Value	Pr > |t|
Intercept	1.667918719	0.02716243	61.41	<.0001
A_time	1.711574946	0.07861072	21.77	<.0001
B_time	-0.131218839	0.00269048	-48.77	<.0001

Figure 2.12 Example SAS code and output for a single-compartment model. (a) SAS Code, (b) SAS output.

2.4.2 SUMMARIZING PHARMACOKINETIC DATA

We will not discuss in greater detail how to analyse pharmacokinetic data, but will briefly describe how to determine summary statistics for pharmacokinetic parameters. Thus far it has been demonstrated that most common pharmacokinetic parameters, with the exception of the empirical parameters C_{max} and t_{max}, are derived under the assumption of an exponential half-life. An implication of this is that these parameters should be summarized on the log scale. Previous work has also empirically shown that common noncompartmental (Lacey *et al.*, 1997) and compartmental (Mizuta and Tsubotani, 1985) pharmacokinetic variables are log-Normally distributed. In particular, for bioequivalence and other regulatory guidance documents, regulatory guidelines state that either a log-transformed analysis should be undertaken, or (implicitly) should be undertaken on C_{max} and AUC (FDA, 1998a, 1999a, 1999b, 2000, 2001, 2002a; CPMP, 1997, 1998a). The actual details of these studies will be discussed throughout the book.

There should be a distinction, however, between formal statistical analysis and a descriptive statistic to summarize the sample observed. For such a summary statistic a measure of central tendency is required. To get this you can either quote the median or calculate the geometric mean. To calculate the geometric mean you simply log the data and then calculate the mean on the transformed data, as you would a conventional mean. Then exponentiate this value back to the original scale. For log-Normal data this measure will be a measure of central tendency (and should be concurrent with the median).

A common mistake to make with pharmacokinetic data is to quote arithmetic means. However, due to the heavily skewed distributional form of pharmacokinetic data, this is not a measure of central tendency. Table 2.2 illustrates this point, highlighting how, for a particularly variable dataset, the arithmetic mean could have up to 70% of a population (not 50%) falling below it, depending on the size of the standard deviation on the log scale. An empirical illustration of the points raised is given in Table 2.3, which gives C_{max} data from a food-effect bioavailability study (Julious and Debarnot, 2000). For these data, 31 / 44 observations fall below the arithmetic means (16 / 22 fasted and 15 / 22 fed), equating to 70% of the observations,

Table 2.2 Proportion of the population anticipated to fall below the arithmetic mean when calculated from pharmacokinetic data which has a log-Normal form

SD of logs	Percentage below arithmetic mean
0.1	52.08
0.2	53.98
0.3	55.86
0.4	57.89
0.5	59.85
0.6	61.83
0.7	63.60
0.8	65.55
0.9	67.40
1.0	69.22

Table 2.3 Maximum observed plasma concentration C_{max} (ng ml^{-1}) from a food-effect bioavailability study

Subject	Fasted	Fed
01	5.808	5.930
02	3.618	5.810
03	2.398	2.040
04	0.333	0.632
05	20.024	14.889
06	2.465	4.632
07	2.436	4.274
08	4.879	5.083
09	9.290	10.277
10	3.602	10.165
12	0.768	1.414
13	4.913	4.851
14	6.302	11.646
15	1.844	1.459
16	26.559	18.080
17	1.757	2.222
18	9.491	6.071
19	5.276	5.498
20	1.040	1.648
22	13.885	9.512
23	2.158	1.171
24	22.610	17.176
N	22	22
Arith. mean	6.884	6.567
SD	7.400	5.222
Minimum	0.333	0.632
Median	4.249	5.291
Maximum	26.559	18.080
Geom. mean	4.055	4.578
CV (%)	15.6	12.0

whilst 19 / 44 of observations fall below the geometric mean (11/22 fasted and 8/22 fed), equating to 43% of the observations. The most striking feature of these data though is the direction of the treatment difference measured as arithmetic means and geometric means. For arithmetic means the fasted values are higher, 6.9 fasted compared to 6.6 fed, whilst for geometric means fasted values are lower, 4.1 fasted compared to 4.6. For both fasted and fed arms the geometric mean concurred most closely with the median. Therefore, depending on what scale you analysed the data on, you could conclude that subjects given the regimen fasted have both higher and lower bioavailability compared to subjects given the regimen fed.

The log-transformation is a special transformation as it gives values that are easy to understand (Keene, 1995). This is because, after logging the data for comparisons to estimate possible treatment differences, once these differences are back-transformed, values of the treatment difference are equivalent to a ratio of the geometric treatment means for a parallel group study, and a mean of the individual treatment ratios for a crossover study. Both of which are easily understood.

The log-transformation is also special because it has a measure of variability which can be interpreted easily on the original scale, through the relationship between the standard deviation (s) on the log scale and the coefficient of variation (CV) on the original scale. This link is due to following relationships for the log-Normal (Julious and Debarnot, 2000)

$$CV = \sqrt{e^{s^2} - 1}. \tag{2.55}$$

Hence, for small standard deviation s (< 0.30), the following result holds

$$CV \approx s. \tag{2.56}$$

The link to the CV highlights another advantage of logging, in that for pharmacokinetic data the standard deviation is proportional to the mean; this means that you must quote a separate standard deviation for every dose if on the arithmetic scale. However, by logging, the standard deviation is stabilized, enabling us to quote an overall figure across all doses.

2.4.3 POPULATION APPROACHES

Thus far in this chapter we have discussed the situation where we have the full profile for all subjects. This would usually be the case when a compound is in early development, but not necessarily in later development where sparse sampling may be conducted on a larger patient sample. Such an analysis is termed a population approach, which is defined as an assessment of the pharmacokinetics in a patient population receiving clinically relevant doses. The advantage of a population approach is that it may better reflect the true pharmacokinetics profile within a patient population.

There are other advantages to a population approach. For an analysis of summary measures (like AUC), the assumption is that all data are measured with the same precision. This is not necessarily true, such that with a population approach we may find that the elimination rate estimate will be estimated with different precision across subjects. This doesn't get factored in to a standard summary-measures AUC analysis, but a population analysis could account for this.

The question of interest would then be how to derive the main pharmacokinetic parameters, and finally how to summarize these parameters through appropriate geometric means and so on. We may have a few samples from several subjects, but when all these subjects are combined we will have sufficient information to estimate an entire profile as in Figure 2.13. We can therefore use this within- and between-subject information to make within- and between-subject inferences; that is, we could estimate the full profile for an individual subject even though we only have a few observations.

In a population approach, instead of undertaking a two-stage procedure of deriving the individual parameters and then summarizing these to make inferences, you do this in one multiple regression across all subjects. The analysis is a little complicated, as first an underlying model for the shape of the pharmacokinetic profile needs also to be entered. But on top of this, terms for age, gender, concomitant medical

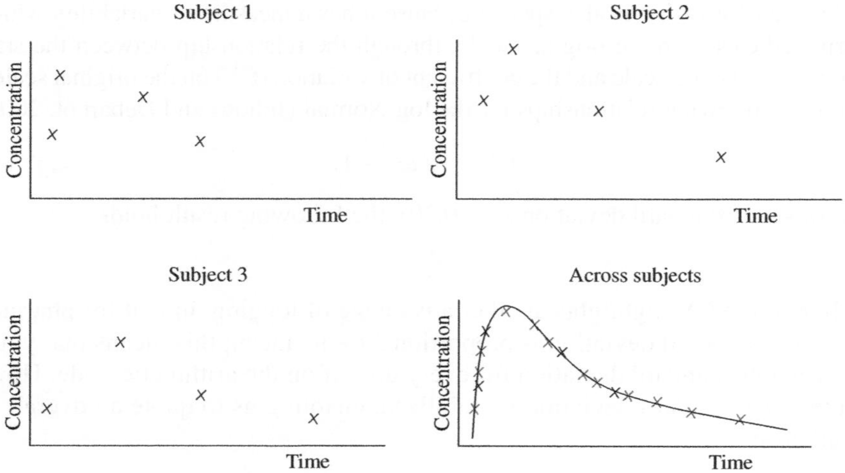

Figure 2.13 Sparse samples across subjects to obtain a full profile.

Table 2.4 Checklist for reviewing a pharmacokinetic analysis

Checklist	***Acceptable***
Was the objective of the study sufficiently described? Is it exploratory or confirmatory?	
Are statistical procedures adequately described and referenced?	
Were the statistical analyses appropriate?	
For any differences observed were the groups comparable at baseline? Were covariates adequately considered?	
Were there a large number of analyses? Multiple factors tested? Was Type I error controlled?	
Were both clinical and statistical significance considered? Are confidence intervals given for the main results? For example 'Significant difference between groups' may not be supported if confidence interval is enclosed within 0.80 and 1.25. How consistent are the findings with prospective studies (for example for drug interactions?	
Were any subgroup analyses conducted? May be one of the main reasons for the analysis? If so were they interpreted correctly?	

treatment and so on can also be entered, to assess whether they have a significant effect on the pharmacokinetics. If they do then a model can be used to predict the response.

In reality, things are a little more complicated for pharmacokinetic modelling, as aspects such as route of administration and whether single or repeat dosing would need to be considered, but the basic principles hold. However, this chapter is targeted at readers who will be reviewers of population analyses and not necessarily 'doers'. In which case the nuts and bolts are less important than the principles.

To this end we recommend the following checklist be used when reviewing population analyses. The CHMP (2006a) and FDA (1999c) also have guidelines on performing population analyses.

3 Sample Size Calculations for Clinical Trials

3.1 INTRODUTION

A sample size justification should be provided for all clinical studies. For early phase trials this justification could range from a formal powered sample size based on a hard clinical outcome to a situation where the main justification is that the sample size is based on feasibility. Even for the latter, sample size calculations can be provided, as we can determine the precision the trial would need to have in order to estimate the main effects, as well as what difference could be detected with a calculated level of power.

An issue with sample size calculations for early phase trials, however, is that, by definition, we often have very little information on which to base the sample size calculation. We will also discuss how this impacts on computations, with particular emphasis on assessing the sensitivity of the study to the trial design assumptions.

The chapter will concentrate on trials where the primary outcome is continuous and expected to take a Normal distribution form and on trials designed to assess superiority as well as precision-based studies. The calculations for bioequivalence-type studies will be discussed in Chapter 9, while some discussion on other primary outcomes will take place in Chapter 13.

3.2 GENERAL PRINCIPLES IN SAMPLE SIZE CALCULATIONS

3.2.1 SPECIFICATIONS OF RESPONSE, PRECISION OR MARGIN (RPM)

In subsequent sections we will discuss the details of sample size calculations, but one of the main drivers in the calculation of the sample size is an *a priori* specification of a response, precision or margin (RPM), or effect size of interest (discussed in Section 3.3); level of precision required (discussed Section 3.4) or margin of equivalence for the pharmacokinetics (discussed in Chapter 9).

In terms of superiority for early phase trials there may be few instances where we would wish to show a definitive level of proof on what may be a primary late-phase clinical outcome. Therefore there is less need for any observed differences to stand as definitive

---

An Introduction to Statistics in Early Phase Trials Steven A. Julious, Say Beng Tan and David Machin

evidence of effect. However, often we could be designing a study based on a surrogate (or biomarker) that would need to stand internal scrutiny as, depending on the evidence in the early phase trials, we proceed or not to further studies.

3.2.2 ESTIMATE OF POPULATION VARIANCE

Given that we have a specified RPM, we need to have a planning value of the population variance, σ^2. What makes things convenient with early phase trials is that we would usually expect to have all the data to assess variability in-house, and so there is no need to perform an extensive literature review (this is not meant to imply that there should be no literature review at all). The bad news, however, is that there may not be much data upon which to make the estimate of the population variance. As the population variance may be the only thing which we would need to anticipate for the sample size calculations it may be the one thing to which the sample size and consequently the study design is sensitive. It is recommended that this sensitivity is formally assessed at the design stage and we describe how to do this in Section 3.6.

3.2.3 TYPE I AND TYPE II ERROR

Basically, for trials designed to prove, at a given level of significance, whether there is or there is not a true difference between regimens, a level for the Type I and Type II errors needs to be set.

The Type I error is defined as the probability of rejecting the null hypothesis when it is true. We can reduce the risk of this error by demanding a more stringent level of 'statistical significance'. The level at which a result is declared significant is known as the Type I error rate, α. The significance level is usually set at the 'magic' 5%.

The Type I error is often referred to as a regulatory or society risk, as it is upon these that the cost of this error is incurred, as a new regimen (declared falsely superior) may enter the market with the result that patients are switched to a treatment that does not truly work. For early phase trials the risk is also the sponsor's risk, however, as a falsely significant result may lead to large, pivotal, and thereby expensive, but fruitless, late-phase studies being undertaken.

The Type II error is to reject the alternative hypothesis when it is true, and β is defined here as the anticipated probability of making this error when starting the study. A usual level for β is 0.1 to 0.2, with an acceptable Type II error typically being larger than a Type I error as the cost to society from this error is usually lower. The Type II error is often referred to as the sponsor's risk as it is upon the sponsor that the cost of this error falls. For early phase trials it could mean not progressing with a treatment which may actually work. There is a societal component also, as a patient may be deprived of a potentially beneficial treatment.

Often, instead of referring to the Type II error, reference is made to the power of a study. The power is the probability that we will detect a difference of a specified size, if there is one. That is, it is the probability of *not* making a Type II error, $1 - \beta$. The power, therefore, is probability of accepting the alternative hypothesis when it is true.

We said earlier that the Type II error is usually set between 0.1 and 0.2. However, often researchers talk in terms of power, and here moving from 0.90 to 0.80 does not seem such a great step to make, but in effect we are doubling the Type II error for a modest actual reduction (around 25%) in the sample size.

3.2.4 EVALUABLE SAMPLE SIZE

So far we have discussed the sample size in terms of the Type I error rate, α; Type II error rates, β; the population variance σ^2 and the specifications of response, precision or margin (RPM). As will be highlighted through this chapter, the sample size goes up for smaller α; goes up for smaller β (i.e. larger power); goes up for smaller RPM but goes down for smaller σ^2.

The sample size calculation, however, is only the first step in determining the required sample size, as what it estimates is the number of evaluable subjects required for the study. What is also required is the total sample size needed to ensure the evaluable number of subjects for analysis. For example, subjects may drop out prior to the first assessment session and so this may need to be accounted for in calculations. Thus, there may need to be a determination of the proportion of subjects that will comprise the analysis population. Particularly pertinent to early phase trials, there may be a need to determine the proportion of subjects that are expected to complete a multiperiod crossover trial. An assessment of these proportions could allow an estimate of the total sample size to enable a sufficient evaluable sample size at the end of the study.

3.3 SAMPLE SIZE CALCULATIONS FOR SUPERIORITY TRIALS

In a superiority trial the objective is to determine whether there is evidence of a statistically significant difference in the endpoint of interest between the regimens, with reference to the null hypothesis that the regimens are the same. The null (H_0) and alternative (H_1) hypotheses may take the form:

H_0: The two treatments are not different with respect to the mean response ($\mu_A = \mu_B$).
H_1: The two treatments are different with respect to the mean response ($\mu_A \neq \mu_B$).

In the definition of the null and alternative hypotheses, μ_A and μ_B refer to the mean response on regimens A and B respectively. For a superiority trial there are two chances of rejecting the null hypothesis and thus making a Type I error. The null hypothesis can be rejected if the trial data suggest $\mu_A > \mu_B$ or $\mu_A < \mu_B$ by a statistically significant amount. As there are two chances of rejecting the null hypothesis the statistical test is referred to as a two-tailed test, with each tail allocated an equal amount of the Type I error (2.5% each). The sum of these tails adds up to the overall Type I error rate of 5%. Thus, the null hypothesis can be rejected if the test of $\mu_A > \mu_B$ is statistically significant at the 2.5% level or the test of $\mu_A > \mu_B$ is statistically significant at the 2.5% level.

The purpose of the sample size calculation is hence to provide sufficient power to reject H_0 when in fact some alternative hypothesis is true.

3.3.1 PARALLEL-GROUP TRIALS

The sample size for regimen A in a parallel-group study can be estimated from

$$n_A = \frac{(r+1)(Z_{1-\alpha/2} + Z_{1-\beta})^2\sigma^2}{rd^2}, \tag{3.1}$$

and that for regimen B from $n_B = rn_A$, where r is the allocation ratio, σ^2 is the known population variance, d is treatment difference of interest, and $Z_{1-\alpha/2}$, $Z_{1-\beta}$ denote the respective percentage points of a standard Normal distribution for α and β. The total study size is $n = n_A + n_B$, which is minimized when $r = 1$.

The result (3.1) has a number of advantages, not least being that the computations are relatively simple and enable direct hand calculation to be performed easily. It has a disadvantage in that it is 'less precise', because it assumes that the variance is known, which will not be true in practice. Most sample size packages and texts do not use it but use instead the following formula (Julious, 2004a)

$$1-\beta = 1 - \text{Probt}\left(t_{1-\alpha/2,\, n_A(r+1)-2},\ n_A(r+1)-2,\ \sqrt{\frac{rn_A d^2}{(r+1)\sigma^2}}\right). \tag{3.2}$$

Here $\text{Probt}(t, \nu, \delta)$ is defined as the cumulative density function of a noncentral t-distribution with ν degrees of freedom and noncentrality parameter δ. Here, the nomenclature for Probt(•) is taken from the noncentral t function in the statistical package SAS. To estimate the sample size from (3.2) an iteration on n_A is required until a nominal level of power is reached. Table 3.1 gives sample sizes using (3.2) for various standardized differences ($\delta = d/\sigma$).

The hand calculations from (3.1) compared to (3.2) would be 1 or 2 subjects out (underestimating the sample size) with bigger differences expected for smaller studies. Such small discrepancies are not an issue for larger trials but could become an issue when sample sizes are small, as is common in early phase studies. For example:

- To detect a difference of 15 (= d) for a standard deviation of 100 (= σ) at the two-sided 5% level of significance with 90% power, (3.1) estimates the sample size to be 934 subjects per arm. From (3.2) the power for this sample size would be 89.993%, and the sample size should be 935 to obtain 90% power. The difference is thus trivial.
- To detect a difference of 35 for a standard deviation of 27.5 for the same significance level and power, (3.1) estimates the sample size to be 13 subjects per arm. From (3.2) the power for this sample size would be 87.5% and the sample size should be 15 to obtain 90% power. A small but potentially important difference in study size.

Table 3.1 Sample sizes for one group, n_A ($n_B = rn_A$) in a parallel-group study for various standardized differences $\delta = d/\sigma$ and allocation ratios, for 90% power and a two-sided Type I error of 5%.

	Allocation ratio (r)			
δ	1	2	3	4
0.05	8407	6306	5605	5255
0.10	2103	1577	1402	1314
0.15	935	702	624	585
0.20	527	395	351	329
0.25	338	253	225	211
0.30	235	176	157	147
0.35	173	130	115	108
0.40	133	100	89	83
0.45	105	79	70	66
0.50	86	64	57	53
0.55	71	53	47	44
0.60	60	45	40	37
0.65	51	38	34	32
0.70	44	33	30	28
0.75	39	29	26	24
0.80	34	26	23	21
0.85	31	23	20	19
0.90	27	21	18	17
0.95	25	19	17	15
1.00	23	17	15	14

To allow for the approximation, a correction factor of $Z^2_{1-\alpha/2}/4$ can be added to equation (3.1)

$$n_A = \frac{(r+1)\left(Z_{1-\beta} + Z_{1-\alpha/2}\right)^2 \sigma^2}{rd^2} + \frac{Z^2_{1-\alpha/2}}{4}.$$

This correction, for a two-sided 5% level of significance, is effectively the same as increasing n_A by 1 in (3.1), as $Z_{0.975} = 1.96$. For quick calculations the following formula, for 90% power and a two-sided 5% Type I error rate, can be used

$$n_A = \frac{10.5\sigma^2}{d^2}\frac{(r+1)}{r}, \tag{3.4}$$

or for $r = 1$

$$n_A = \frac{21\sigma^2}{d^2}. \tag{3.5}$$

The final result is particularly useful to remember for quick calculations.

3.3.2 CROSSOVER TRIALS

Details of crossover trials will be discussed in Chapters 3 and 4 along with the relative merits of such study designs. In this chapter we concentrate on sample size calculations.

For a crossover trial, the total sample size, n, can be estimated from

$$n = \frac{2\left(Z_{1-\beta} + Z_{1-\alpha/2}\right)^2 \sigma_w^2}{d^2}, \tag{3.6}$$

where $\sigma^2{}_w$ is the known within-subject population variance and d is the treatment difference of interest. The calculation has the same advantages and disadvantages as those for the parallel group calculation discussed earlier. A more precise result is

$$1 - \beta = 1 - \text{Probt}\left(t_{1-\alpha/2,n-2},\ n-2,\ \sqrt{\frac{nd^2}{2\sigma_w^2}}\right). \tag{3.7}$$

Again, you solve for n in the same manner as for a parallel-group study, through iteration. Compared to this, (3.6) underestimates the sample size a little. This calculation assumes a two-period crossover design but in Chapter 5 we visit sample size calculations for more than two periods. A correction factor of $Z^2_{1-\frac{\alpha}{2}}/2$ can be added to (3.6) to give

$$n = \frac{2(Z_{1-\alpha/2} + Z_{1-\beta})^2 \sigma_w^2}{d^2} + \frac{Z^2_{1-\alpha/2}}{2}. \tag{3.8}$$

When discussing crossover trials, the following result:

$$n = \frac{(Z_{1-\alpha/2} + Z_{1-\beta})^2 \sigma_d^2}{d^2}, \tag{3.9}$$

may also be seen instead of (3.6). This will be discussed in Chapter 4, but the main difference is that (3.9) has an estimate of the population variance of the difference, σ_d^2, as opposed to a within-subject variance, $2\sigma_w^2$, in (3.6). However, note that (3.9) is equivalent, as $\sigma_d^2 = 2\sigma_w^2$.

For quick calculations we can adapt (3.6) for the computation of sample sizes (estimated with 90% power and a two-sided 5% Type I error rate) to

$$n = \frac{21\sigma_w^2}{d^2}. \tag{3.10}$$

Table 3.2 gives sample sizes using (3.7) for various standardized differences ($\delta = d/\sigma_w$).

Table 3.2 Total sample size for two-period crossover study for various standardized differences $\delta = d/\sigma_w$.

δ	n
0.05	3076
0.10	771
0.15	344
0.20	195
0.25	126
0.30	88
0.35	66
0.40	51
0.45	41
0.50	34
0.55	28
0.60	24
0.65	21
0.70	19
0.75	17
0.80	15
0.85	14
0.90	13
0.95	12
1.00	11

3.4 SAMPLE SIZE CALCULATION BASED ON PRECISION

So far, methodologies have been described for sample size calculations where we wish to demonstrate statistically the presence of a given clinical effect. However, often in early clinical development what we are actually undertaking is a preliminary or pilot investigation with the objective of estimating any possible clinical effect, *d*, with a view to performing a later definitive study (Julious, 2004a; Julious and Patterson, 2004).

Early in drug development, it will often be the case that reliable estimates of between-subject and of within-subject variation for the endpoint of interest in the reference population are available, but the desired magnitude of the treatment difference of interest will be unknown. This may be the case, for example, when considering the impact of an experimental treatment on biomarkers or other measures not known to be directly indicative of clinical outcome, but potentially indicative of pharmacologic mechanism of action. In this situation, drug and biomarker development will be in such an early stage that no prespecified treatment difference could be declared *a priori* to be of interest. In such exploratory or 'learning' studies, we propose that the sample size be selected in order to provide a given level of precision, and not power in the traditional fashion for a (in truth unknown) desirable and prespecified difference of interest.

For precision-based studies, rather than testing a formal hypothesis, an estimation approach, through the provision of confidence intervals (CIs) for the effect size, *d*, is more appropriate. In this section the concentration will not be on assessing statistical significance but on estimation. If the sample size is based on estimation, then the protocol should clearly state this as the study objective and as the basis for the corresponding study.

3.4.1 PARALLEL-GROUP TRIALS

In a two-group study where the outcome measure is a continuous, Normally distributed variable, we can construct a confidence interval to describe a range of plausible values for the population difference in means of two groups, A and B

$$\gamma = \mu_A - \mu_B,$$

using the sample estimate

$$d = \bar{x}_A - \bar{x}_B.$$

A $100(1-\alpha)\%$ confidence interval for γ has the following half width

$$w = t_{1-\alpha/2,\upsilon}\sqrt{\mathrm{Var}(d)} \tag{3.11}$$

where $t_{\frac{\alpha}{2},\upsilon}$ is the appropriate two-sided t-statistic, on υ degrees of freedom, and Var(d) is the variance of the difference in means. Hence, a half width (w) of the confidence interval is a measure of precision for the trial. Thus, to enable the calculation of a sample size we need to specify w and Var(d). For Normally distributed data and using earlier notation,

$$\mathrm{Var}(d) = \frac{(r+1)\sigma^2}{rn_A} \tag{3.12}$$

Therefore, for a given half confidence interval width, w, the following property must be met to obtain the sample size per group for $r = 1$ (Julious, 2004a)

$$n_A \geq \frac{2\sigma^2 t^2{}_{1-\alpha/2,2n_A-2}}{w^2.} \tag{3.13}$$

To solve (3.13) you must iterate up to find the sample size, n_A, for which the property holds. Alternatively, the sample size, with a correction factor, can be derived approximately, directly from

$$n_A = \frac{2\sigma^2 Z^2_{1-\alpha/2}}{w^2} + \frac{Z^2_{1-\alpha/2}}{4}. \tag{3.14}$$

In practice, (3.14) can be used for initial values to start the calculations for (3.13).

Table 3.3 Sample sizes required per group at the two-sided 95% confidence level for various values of the standardized width ($\theta = w/\sigma$).

	Allocation ratios			
θ	1	2	3	4
0.05	3075	2306	2050	1922
0.10	770	578	513	481
0.15	343	257	229	214
0.20	194	145	129	121
0.25	125	94	83	78
0.30	87	65	58	54
0.35	64	48	43	40
0.40	50	37	33	31
0.45	40	30	26	25
0.50	32	24	22	20
0.55	27	20	18	17
0.60	23	17	15	14
0.65	20	15	13	12
0.70	17	13	12	11
0.75	15	12	10	10
0.80	14	10	9	9
0.85	12	9	8	8
0.90	11	8	7	7
0.95	10	8	7	6
1.00	9	7	6	6

Table 3.3 uses (3.13) and gives the sample size required for various values of the standardized width, defined as

$$\theta = \frac{w}{\sigma}, \tag{3.15}$$

and assuming two-sided 95% confidence intervals are to be constructed at the end of the trial.

3.4.2 CROSSOVER TRIALS

Following similar arguments as for parallel groups, for two-period crossover trials the required sample size could be estimated approximately from

$$n = \frac{2\sigma_{\mathrm{w}}^2 Z_{1-\alpha/2}^2}{w^2} + \frac{Z_{1-\alpha/2}^2}{2}. \tag{3.16}$$

However, using the more appropriate t-statistic, this becomes

$$n \geq \frac{2\sigma_{\mathrm{w}}^2 t_{1-\alpha/2,n-2}^2}{w^2}. \tag{3.17}$$

In this latter expression, n is obtained through iteration and σ_{w}^2 relates to the within-subject variance with degrees of freedom, $df = n - 2$. In Chapter 5 we discuss sample size calculations for more than two periods.

Table 3.4 gives the sample size required for various values of the standardized width, θ.

Table 3.4 Total sample size for a two-period crossover study for various standardized widths, θ, with 95% confidence intervals for the precision estimates ($\theta = w / \sigma_w$).

θ	n
0.05	3076
0.10	771
0.15	344
0.20	195
0.25	126
0.30	88
0.35	66
0.40	51
0.45	41
0.50	34
0.55	28
0.60	24
0.65	21
0.70	19
0.75	17
0.80	15
0.85	14
0.90	13
0.95	12
1.00	11

3.5 SAMPLE SIZE BASED ON FEASIBILITY

A similar situation occurs where the sample size is determined primarily by practical considerations, or feasibility, with the trial not being powered to detect any prespecified effect. Here, as you now have values for n, σ^2, β and α, from (3.2) the value of the difference (d) that can be detected for the given, fixed, sample size is calculated.

An alternative approach in such circumstances may be to give the precision for the fixed sample size in the study.

3.5.1 PARALLEL-GROUP TRIALS

For parallel groups of equal size, n, the $100(1-\alpha)\%$ confidence interval is

$$\bar{x}_A - \bar{x}_B \pm t_{1-\alpha/2,2(n-1)}\sqrt{\frac{2s^2}{n_A}}. \tag{3.18}$$

Where n_A is the sample size for group A and B (assuming $r = 1$). Hence, for prespecified n and s^2 (the sample estimate of the population variance), the anticipated precision can be estimated by

$$w = t_{1-\alpha/2,2(n-1)}\sqrt{\frac{2s^2}{n_A}}. \tag{3.19}$$

3.5.2 CROSSOVER TRIALS

Similarly, for a two-period crossover trial the confidence interval is defined as

$$\bar{x}_A - \bar{x}_B \pm t_{1-\alpha/2,n-2}\sqrt{\frac{2s_w^2}{n}}, \tag{3.20}$$

where n is the total sample size and s_w^2 the sample estimate of the within-subject variance.

Hence the anticipated precision for a given sample size n and s_w^2 is

$$w = t_{1-\alpha/2,n-2}\sqrt{\frac{2s_w^2}{n}}. \tag{3.21}$$

3.6 SENSITIVITY ANALYSIS

As previously mentioned, a study design may be very sensitive to factors such as the variance estimate used in calculations. With respect to sensitivity, ICH Topic E9 (ICH, 1998b) includes the following general comment, where the emphasis is that of the authors,

> The method by which the sample size is calculated should be given in the protocol, together with the estimates of any quantities used in the calculations (such as variances, mean values, response rates, event rates, difference to be detected)... It is important to investigate the ***sensitivity*** of the sample size estimate to a variety of deviations from these assumptions

The sensitivity of the trial design to the variance is relatively straightforward to investigate and can be done using the degrees of freedom around the variance estimate used in the calculations.

First of all, calculate the sample size conventionally using an appropriate variance estimate. Next, using the degrees of freedom for this variance and the chi-squared distribution, calculate the upper one-tailed 95th percentile for the variance using the following formula (Julious, 2004b)

$$s^2(95) < \frac{df}{\chi^2_{0.05,df}}s^2. \tag{3.22}$$

This upper, and plausibly high, estimate of the variance can then be used to investigate the loss in power from (3.2) or (3.7) as appropriate, or precision from (3.19) or (3.21) with the sample size estimated from the point estimate for the variance. This would give an assessment of the sensitivity of the study to deviations from the variability assumptions, by investigating changes in a study's power due to an extreme value that the variance could plausibly take.

The more degrees of freedom about the variance we have, the less sensitive calculations are to assumptions about the variance (Julious, 2004b). However, often when calculating a sample size, a great deal of information is thrown away. One approach that is commonly used when calculating sample sizes is to tabulate all the variances estimated from previously observed studies and then take the maximum of these variances. Another is to calculate a crude arithmetic mean across the studies to obtain an overall estimate. Both these approaches may be appropriate if the variances originate from studies of similar size. However, in many instances the studies are of diverse sample size with diverse estimates of the variance. The most extreme variance estimates are also often those from the smallest studies and thus by taking the maximum or by taking the arithmetic mean one may be giving undue weight to the studies with the poorest estimates of variance.

If there are several early phase studies with variance estimates available, each of which is in a similar patient population and also ostensibly the same for all relevant clinical factors that may affect outcome, then it is recommended that an overall estimate of the population variance is obtained from the following

$$s_p^2 = \frac{\sum_{i=1}^{k} df_i s_i^2}{\sum_{i=1}^{k} df_i}, \tag{3.23}$$

where k is the number of studies, s_i^2 is the variance estimate from the ith study, and df_i are the degrees of freedom about this variance. The pooled variance estimate, s_{p}^2, is the minimum variance unbiased estimate of the population variance, and is estimated with the following degrees of freedom

$$df_{\mathrm{p}} = \sum_{s=1}^{n} df_i. \tag{3.24}$$

This estimate of the variance has two obvious advantages. The first is that appropriate weight is given to the variances with the smallest and largest degrees of freedom. The second advantage is that the overall estimate has degrees of freedom assigned to it which can be used in sensitivity calculations. Thus, by appropriately combining the variance estimates one is both maximizing the degrees of freedom about the overall estimate and minimizing the sensitivity of the study to this estimate.

It is worth noting again here the point about the pooled studies being ostensibly similar. If they are not then the 'increased' precision in the variance estimates may be spurious.

Table 3.5 Possible response with confidence intervals for the precision expected in the trial.

Response	Lower 90% CI	Upper 90% CI
0.90	0.76	1.06
0.95	0.81	1.12
1.00	0.85	1.18
1.05	0.89	1.24
1.10	0.93	1.30

3.6.1 WORKED EXAMPLE: PRECISION SAMPLE SIZE CALCULATIONS

We are planning a two-period crossover study to compare the bioavailability of two formulations. The sample size is fixed at 24 and we are anticipating 20 subjects to complete. You have an estimate of the within-subject variance on the $\log_e$ scale of $s_w = 0.09$.

What we wish to estimate is the anticipated precision of the estimates assuming 90% confidence intervals are to be calculated.

Note: the calculations will be performed on the log scale. To transform back to the original scale we exponentiate our results and deduct from 1, that is, $1 - \exp(-w)$.

With 20 subjects (and 18 degrees of freedom), $t_{0.95,18} = 1.734$; hence on the $\log_e$ scale the precision would be $\sqrt{2} \times 1.734 \times 0.3/\sqrt{20} = 0.165$. Back on the original scale the precision would be $1 - \exp(-0.165) = 0.152$.

It is usually worth presenting the precision in terms of 'Given different observed results what would the confidence interval look like?' For different possible responses in the trial Table 3.5 can be constructed.

The results in Table 3.5 are only 'hypothetical' results. The table would be applied by saying 'Suppose we observed a ratio of 1.00 in the trial, then the confidence intervals would infer that a plausible range of values would be 0.85 to 1.18.' The same would hold for the other values in the table.

Suppose, however, the variance was estimated with just 10 degrees of freedom. If we take the 95th percentile as a high plausible value, the precision for the study if such an extreme variance was observed would be calculated as follows:

The chi-squared value for 10 degrees of freedom would be 31.41 and hence, from (3.22), a high plausible value for the variance would be $0.09 \times 10 / 3.94 = 0.228$.

From this the precision would be 0.262 on the log scale or 0.231 on the original scale.

3.7 MINIMUM SAMPLE SIZE REQUIRED

As we have stated, when designing an early phase clinical trial an appropriate justification for the sample size should be provided in the protocol. This justification could be based on formal power calculations or on other considerations such as the precision of the estimates of interest. However, there are a number of settings when designing an initial pilot investigation where there is no prior information upon which to base the sample size.

For example, in very early Phase I we could be designing a bioavailability study for a new chemical entity, while for a later phase the study could be with a novel endpoint or in a previously unstudied group of patients (for the compound).

Any recommendation in such a situation would be a 'finger-in-the-air' number; however, for situations where the intention is that later, more definitive, studies may be carried out, Julious (2005a) gave three reasons for recommending a sample size of 12 per group. These were based on: feasibility; gains in the precision about the mean and variance; and regulatory considerations, which will now be highlighted.

3.7.1 REASON 1: FEASIBILITY

The first argument is somewhat *ad hoc* and is not in the context of future trials, but in the design of a parallel-group trial a sample size of 12 per group is a good round number with nice properties. It is divisible by 2, 3, 4 and 6, and so facilitates the setting of a variety of block sizes. Thus one could have block sizes of 2, 3, 4, 6, 8 or 12 if you had 2 groups and a total sample size of 24.

For multiperiod crossover studies, discussed in Chapter 4, which are common with early Phase I investigations, a total sample size of 12 gives 2-, 3-, 4- and 6-, or even 12-period crossover trials with balanced Williams squares designs. For a 5-period crossover trial you need a sample size that is divisible by 10 and so feasibility considerations may then reduce the sample size to 10.

3.7.2 REASON 2: PRECISION ABOUT THE MEAN AND VARIANCE

3.7.2.1 Precision about the Mean

Obviously, the greater the sample size the smaller the standard error and as a consequence the greater the precision about the mean difference – as assessed by its confidence interval. A two-sided confidence interval for a parallel-group trial is defined as (3.18). The situation we are considering here is to assess, with a finite sample size, what gain in precision do we have for every unit increase in the sample size per group. This could be calculated using the right hand side of (3.18) and the following

$$\text{Gain} = \frac{t_{1-\alpha/2,\,2n-2}\sqrt{2}s}{\sqrt{n}} - \frac{t_{1-\alpha/2,\,2(n+1)-2}\sqrt{2}s}{\sqrt{n+1}}. \tag{3.25}$$

From (3.25) Figure 3.1 can be derived. This was estimated assuming a unit variance ($s^2=1$) and that a two-sided 95% confidence interval would be used in the planned trial.

The point associated with '4' on the x-axis gives the gain in precision of an increase in sample size of 1 over 3. The point associated with '5', the gain over 4, and so on. Therefore, from Figure 3.1 it seems that for small sample sizes there is a marked gain for each increase of 1 in the sample size per group but that the gains are less pronounced by the point where the sample size has reached 12.

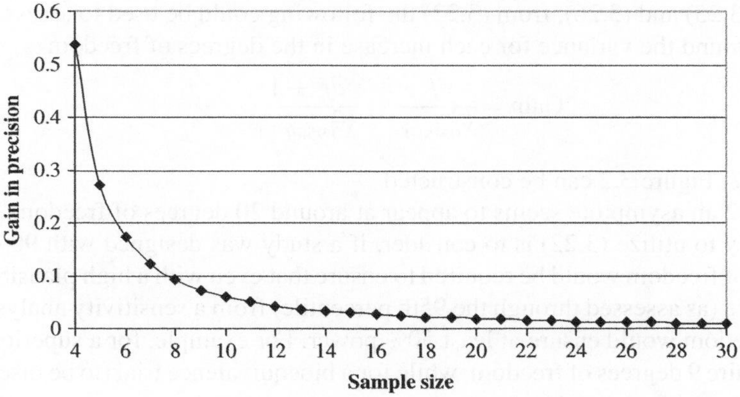

Figure 3.1 Gain in precision for each increase of one in the sample size per arm for a parallel-group trial.

Note, in Figure 3.1 (and in the subsequent Figure 3.2) the left hand axis, although calculated using a unit variance, could be considered as a multiple of the estimated standard deviation.

Equivalent to (3.25), the following can be used for crossover trials to estimate the gain in precision for each increase in the total sample size of one

$$\text{Gain} = \frac{t_{1-\alpha/2,\,n-2}\sqrt{2}s_w}{\sqrt{n}} - \frac{t_{1-\alpha/2,\,(n+1)-2}\sqrt{2}s_w}{\sqrt{n+1}}, \tag{3.26}$$

where s_w^2 is the within-subject estimate of the variance. The degrees of freedom associated with the t-statistic here are given assuming the trial is a two-period crossover study analysed using an analysis of variance with period fitted in the model. Similar to parallel-group trials, after a sample size of 12 the gains in precision become less pronounced.

3.7.2.2 Precision about the Variance

As well as quantifying an estimate of the possible effect in a pilot study, it is also important to provide an estimate of the variance as this may be used in a formal sample size calculation in a subsequent study. One way of assessing the precision of the variance would be to determine the sensitivity of the future, formally powered study to the estimate of the (now assumed unknown) variance, as discussed earlier in the chapter.

What is therefore required from a pilot study is a sample size sufficiently large to have appropriate degrees of freedom for s^2 in a sensitivity analysis in the future study. As a reminder, the process in the formal sample size calculation in the future study would be to obtain an estimate of the variance (s^2) from your pilot study and calculate the sample size from this variance. With this sample size we would then determine what would be the sensitivity of the study to the assumptions about the variance. The sensitivity could be assessed as a loss in power, to a high plausible value fors^2 taken from (3.22).

Similar to (3.25) and (3.26), from (3.22) the following could be used to assess the gain in precision around the variance for each increase in the degrees of freedom

$$\text{Gain} = \frac{df}{\chi^2_{0.95,df}} - \frac{df+1}{\chi^2_{0.95,df+1}}, \tag{3.27}$$

and from (3.27) Figure 3.2 can be constructed.

In Figure 3.2 an asymptote seems to appear at around 20 degrees of freedom.

Another way to utilize (3.22) is to consider, if a study was designed with 90% power what degrees of freedom would be required to ensure that even with a high plausible value for the variance (as assessed through the 95th percentile) from a sensitivity analysis, what degrees of freedom would ensure at least 50% power. For example, for a superiority trial we would require 9 degrees of freedom, while for a bioequivalence trial (to be discussed in Chapter 9) we would require 16.

3.7.3 REASON 3: REGULATORY CONSIDERATIONS

For general guidance for a sample size calculation, ICH Topic E9 (ICH, 1998b) simply states:

> The number of subjects in a clinical trial should always be large enough to provide a reliable answer to the questions addressed. This number is usually determined by the primary objective of the trial. If the sample size is determined on some other basis, then this should be made clear and justified.

Hence if a study is a pilot with the sample size based on feasibility it should be expressly stated as such in the protocol. If based on feasibility you may wish to calculate the precision for the confidence interval(s) around the primary endpoint(s) and include this as part of the justification for the sample size.

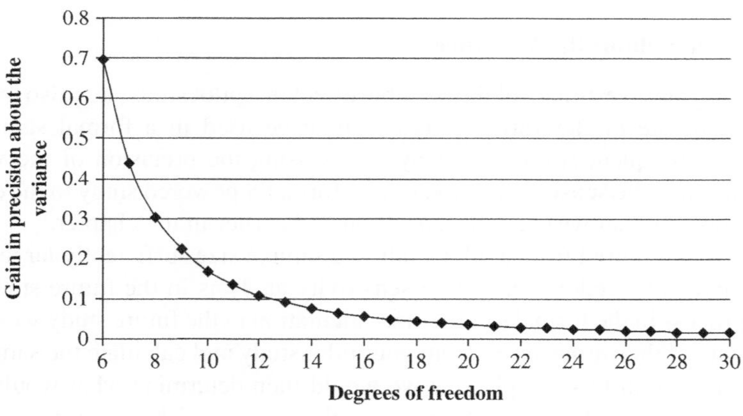

Figure 3.2 Gain in precision for each increase of one in the degrees of freedom.

For pilot bioavailability (BA) and food investigations there is some regulatory justification for choosing a sample size of 12 – justification that could be extended to other types of Phase I studies. For food-effect studies, FDA Guidance (2002a) states:

> A minimum of 12 subjects should complete the food-effect BA and fed BE (bio-equivalence) studies.

Hence, you should over-recruit to ensure you have 12 subjects for the assessment of food-effect studies. Similarly, for assessing BA and BE, FDA Guidance (2001) states:

> A minimum number of 12 evaluable subjects should be included in any BE study.

However, the most interesting justification comes in general-considerations guidelines on BA/BE from the FDA (2003b).

> If the sponsor chooses, a pilot study in a small number of subjects can be carried out before proceeding with a full BE study. The study can be used to validate analytical methodology, assess variability, optimize sample collection time intervals, and provide other information. A pilot study that documents BE can be appropriate, provided its design and execution are suitable and a sufficient number of subjects (e.g., 12) have completed the study.

4 Crossover Trial Basics

4.1 INTRODUCTION

In previous chapters we have described some generic basics for early phase trials, and here we continue this theme by introducing crossover trials. This trial design is used commonly in early development and is applied from the first-time-in-man studies through to the later stages of Phase II. In Chapter 5 we will describe in detail multiperiod crossover trials, but in this chapter we concentrate on two-period designs to introduce the basic concepts. To put crossover trials into context we will first discuss parallel-group studies.

4.2 PARALLEL-GROUP TRIALS

A *parallel-group trial* is one in which there are at least two arms to be investigated and subjects are to be randomized to each of these arms. Note that in this context 'arm' is a generic term to describe the groupings in trials. Subjects may be assigned to two or more different arms, where these arms could be (in the context of this book) different treatments.

When randomizing subjects to the different arms in the trial, an important consideration is to maintain balance for the interventions to which subjects are being randomized. This is particularly important in small studies where by chance there can easily be a particularly large imbalance in the number of subjects on the respective arms. One tool to ensure that groups are balanced is to introduce 'blocks' into the randomization. Basically, a block is a device to help ensure balance in the randomization – balance being important as it leads to more efficient estimates. It is best to illustrate this with a simple worked example.

Consider the case of two groups. We wish to randomly allocate individuals to either group A or group B. In this example we could toss a coin and record either heads (H) or tails (T), so that we can then use the order to allocate individuals to groups (i.e. if heads then group A, if tails then group B). If we set the block size to be four we need to ensure that after every four tosses there are two heads and two tails. For example:

Block 1: T T (H H)
Block 2: T T (H H)
Block 3: T H T (H)
Block 4: T H H (T).

An Introduction to Statistics in Early Phase Trials Steven A. Julious, Say Beng Tan and David Machin

The terms in brackets in the above sequences are not the result of coin tossing but we are forced to enter these to ensure balance. For example, in Block 1 the first 2 tosses were tails. We thus made the next 2 heads so that after '4 tosses' we had a balance. Notice that after '16 tosses' by blocking we have 8 heads and 8 tails.

Another important consideration is stratification. Stratification is similar to blocking but here, as well as ensuring balance after a requisite block size, we also ensure balance by strata. These strata are usually clinically important subgroups such as gender or age group. Again it is best to illustrate by example. Suppose we are repeating the same coin tossing to create a randomization list. For this randomization we wish to ensure balance for a two-level stratification factor. Operationally this would be the same as completing the coin-tossing exercise twice: once within each stratum.

Stratum 1

Block 1: T T (H H)
Block 2: T T (H H)

Stratum 2

Block 1: T H T (H)
Block 2: T H H (T)

Now after '16 tosses' we have balance both in terms of heads and tails and also for heads and tails by stratum.

4.3 CROSSOVER TRIALS

The distinction between *parallel-group designs* and *crossover designs* is that, in parallel-group designs, subjects are assigned at random to receive only one treatment, and as a result of the randomization the groups are essentially the same in all respects other than the investigation made. However, with a crossover trial all subjects receive all the investigations but it is the order in which subjects receive the investigations that is randomized. A crossover trial therefore is one in which subjects are allocated to sequences of treatment with the object of studying differences between individual treatments (or subsequences of treatment). The big assumption with crossover trials is that prior to starting each investigational period all subjects return to their baseline condition and that the order in which subjects have the investigations does not affect their response to the them.

4.3.1 TWO-PERIOD AB/BA DESIGN

In the simplest case, for a two-arm investigation (comparing A with B, say) subjects will be randomized to receive either A in Period 1 followed by B in Period 2 (sequence AB) or to the reverse: B followed by A (BA). AB and BA are called sequences and represent the order in which subjects receive the investigations. In practice, subjects are randomly assigned to either the sequence AB or the sequence BA, and to ensure balance, blocking can still be used.

Block size in the context of crossover trials is used to maintain balance for sequences across a certain number of subjects. For example, for a block size of four in the coin-tossing example discussed earlier, instead of A and B being assigned to H and T, the sequences AB and BA are assigned. Thus

Block 1: BA BA (AB AB)
Block 2: BA BA (AB AB)
Block 3: BA AB BA (AB)
Block 4: BA AB AB (BA).

There are a number of approaches to analysis of crossover trial data and we will now describe each and make comparisons between them.

4.3.1.1 Paired t-tests

A paired t-test, as the name implies, is a test that is appropriate for data which is paired in some form, such before–after a treatment, or two different treatments on the same subject. The main assumptions are that we expect the differences to be distributed at random about a true treatment effect and for the treatment differences to be from a Normal population.

To undertake a paired t-test we would follow the following steps:

- Place the n observed individual effects on the two treatments in two columns – one for A and one for B, ignoring the sequences from which they come.
- For each subject a treatment difference is calculated and consequently a mean of these differences, $\overline{d}$ (which estimates the difference in the treatment means, $\mu_A - \mu_B$).
- We then obtain an estimate of the population standard deviation of the differences, s_d $\left(\text{where } s_d = \sqrt{\frac{1}{n-1}\sum_{i=1}^{n}\left(d_i - \overline{d}\right)^2}\right)$.

The test statistic is thus

$$\frac{\overline{d}\sqrt{n}}{s_d}, \tag{4.1}$$

which is compared to the t-distribution on $n-1$ degrees of freedom; the t-distribution being an approximation to the Normal distribution which is used for small sample sizes.

4.3.1.2 Worked Example 4.1

The data and SAS code for analysing a crossover trial through a paired t-test is given in Figure 4.1a. This analysis ignores the order in which the treatments are administered to subjects. The corresponding output for this analysis is given in Figure 4.1b, and the calculated P-value = 0.2907.

If this calculation was undertaken by hand we would have $\overline{d} = 3.59$ and $s_d = 11.20$. From (4.1) we would therefore have a test statistic of $\frac{\overline{d}\sqrt{n}}{s_d} = \frac{3.59\sqrt{12}}{11.20} = 1.11$.

From t-values from Table 16.4 in the appendix, using the line corresponding to 11 degrees of freedom, we therefore have a P-value of $0.25 < P < 0.30$ or $P < 0.30$, which is consistent with the more accurate result from SAS.

(a) Data and SAS code.

```
TITLE 'Paired t-test';
DATA trialdat;
INPUT ID A B d;
DATALINES;
1.00    116.35  120.97  4.62
2.00    125.87  127.26  1.39
3.00    102.16  89.49   -12.67
4.00    125.24  146.58  21.34
5.00    127.20  129.03  1.83
6.00    151.41  147.69  3.72
7.00    123.29  110.4   -12.85
8.00    107.14  122.27  15.13
9.00    141.03  151.86  10.83
10.00   130.21  126.41  -3.80
11.00   152.75  155.09  2.34
12.00   129.78  148.41  18.63
;
PROC ttest DATA = trialdat;VAR d;
RUN;
```

(b) SAS output.

Paired t-test

The TTEST Procedure

Statistics

Variable	N	Lower CL Mean	Mean	Upper CL Mean	Lower CL Std Dev	Std Dev	Upper CL Std Dev	Std Err
d	12	-3.528	3.5892	10.706	7.9348	11.201	19.018	3.2335

T-Tests

Variable	DF	t Value	Pr > |t|
d	11	1.11	0.2907

P-value of 0.2907

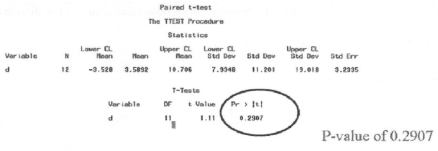

Figure 4.1 Example data, SAS code and output for paired t-test.

4.3.1.3 Period-Adjusted t-tests

In contrast to the paired t-test just described, a period-adjusted test takes account of the order in which the treatments are given to each subject (Senn, 2002). Hence, for each treatment sequence (AB or BA) calculate either a mean difference, $\bar{d}_{AB}$ (estimating $\mu_A - \mu_B$) or $\bar{d}_{BA}$ (estimating $\mu_B - \mu_A$).

A variance for each sequence is then calculated. However, assuming that there is equal allocation to each sequence, $n_{AB} = n_{BA} = n/2$, and the within-sequence variances, $s^2_{d_{AB}} = s^2_{d_{BA}} = s^2_d$, are the same (i.e. the standard deviations of the difference from each sequence equal each other), then the mean difference of interest, $(\bar{d}_{AB} - \bar{d}_{BA})/2$, has variance $s^2_d(1/n_{AB} + 1/n_{AB})/4 = s^2_d/n$, which is used here for the test statistics.

The test statistic for testing the difference between treatments is

$$\frac{(\bar{d}_{AB} - \bar{d}_{BA})/2}{s_d/\sqrt{n}}, \tag{4.2}$$

which is compared to the t-distribution on $n - 2$ degrees of freedom. Note that we lose a degree of freedom when compared to (4.1), from $(n - 1)$ to $(n - 2)$, as we are adjusting for any period effect.

If there is truly no period effect, then,

$$\frac{(\bar{d}_{AB} - \bar{d}_{BA})/2}{s_d/\sqrt{n}} \approx \frac{((\mu_A - \mu_B) - (\mu_B - \mu_A))/2}{s_d/\sqrt{n}} \approx \frac{\bar{d}\sqrt{n}}{s_d}. \tag{4.3}$$

In which case, we would have an equivalent test to a paired t-test of (4.1), but with one fewer degrees of freedom.

4.3.1.4 Worked Example 4.2

The SAS code for analysing the trial through a period-adjusted t-test is given in Figure 4.2a for the same data as in Worked Example 4.1.

Note here that what we have is the difference between treatments for each subject, with 'sequence' being a between-group term. The data are hence analysed through a parallel-group test, here a two-group t-test, with sequence entered as the class variable.

Example output for the analysis is given in Figure 4.2b. As highlighted in the figure, the estimate of the mean in the output is twice as large as it should be. This is because the procedure only takes a *difference* of the mean differences and not the *average* of the mean differences as in (0.1). It does not matter for the test statistic, however, as it estimates the standard error as $2s_d/\sqrt{n}$ for the test statistic as opposed to $s_d/\sqrt{n}$. This means the standard errors are also twice as big, which cancels out the doubling of the estimate of the mean difference.

(a) Data and SAS code.

```
TITLE 'Period-Adjusted t-test';
DATA trialdat;
INPUT ID d Sequence;
DATALINES;
1.00      4.62     1
2.00      1.39     1
3.00      12.67    2
4.00      -21.34   2
5.00      1.83     1
6.00      3.72     2
7.00      12.85    2
8.00      15.13    1
9.00      10.83    1
10.00     3.80     2
11.00     0.34     1
12.00     -18.63   2
;
PROC ttest DATA = trialdat;CLASS sequence;VAR d;
RUN;
```

(b) SAS output.

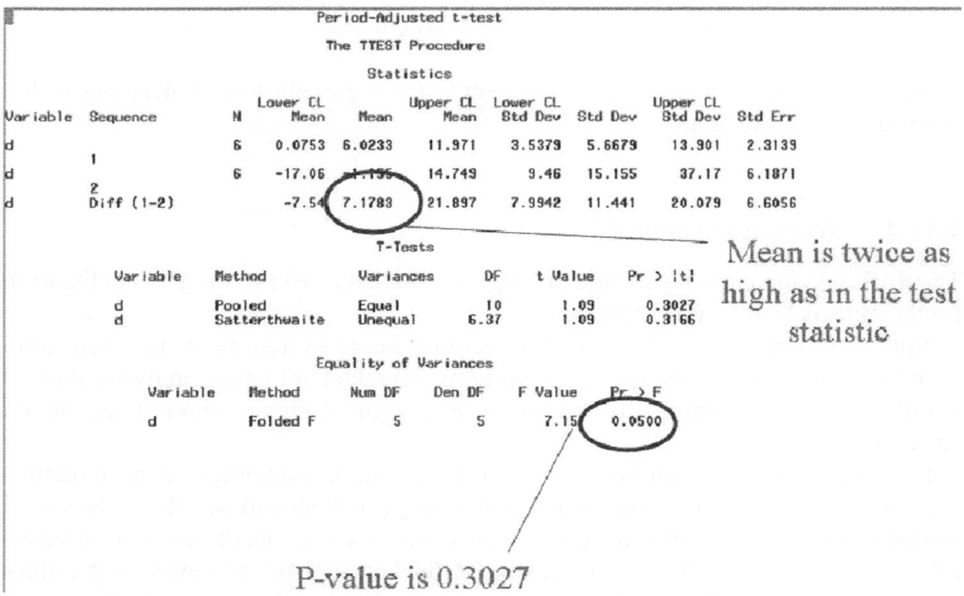

Period-Adjusted t-test

The TTEST Procedure

Statistics

Variable	Sequence	N	Lower CL Mean	Mean	Upper CL Mean	Lower CL Std Dev	Std Dev	Upper CL Std Dev	Std Err
d	1	6	0.0753	6.0233	11.971	3.5379	5.6679	13.901	2.3139
d	2	6	-17.06	-1.155	14.749	9.46	15.155	37.17	6.1871
d	Diff (1-2)		-7.54	7.1783	21.897	7.9942	11.441	20.079	6.6056

T-Tests

Variable	Method	Variances	DF	t Value	Pr > |t|
d	Pooled	Equal	10	1.09	0.3027
d	Satterthwaite	Unequal	6.37	1.09	0.3166

Equality of Variances

Variable	Method	Num DF	Den DF	F Value	Pr > F
d	Folded F	5	5	7.15	0.0500

Figure 4.2 Example data, SAS code and analysis output for period-adjusted t-test.

Here the test statistic gives a P-value of 0.3027.

Note, the fact that the mean differences are twice as high needs to be accounted for when quoting any mean effects and corresponding confidence intervals.

If we were to do this calculation by hand: $\overline{d}_{\mathrm{AB}} = 6.02$ and $\overline{d}_{\mathrm{BA}} = -1.16$, and a standard deviation of the difference, $s_{\mathrm{d}} = 11.44$. Hence, from (4.2) we have

$$\frac{(\overline{d}_{\mathrm{AB}} - \overline{d}_{\mathrm{BA}})/2}{s_{\mathrm{d}}/\sqrt{\mathrm{n}}} = \frac{(6.02 - (-1.16))/2}{11.44/\sqrt{12}} = 1.09.$$

With t-values from Table 16.4 in the appendix, using the line corresponding to 11 degrees of freedom, we therefore have a P-value of $0.30 < P < 0.40$ or $P < 0.40$, which is consistent with the more accurate result from SAS.

4.3.1.5 Nonparametric Tests

We will not go into great detail, but the nonparametric equivalent to the paired t-test is the Wilcoxon signed rank test. While, like the period-adjusted t-test, to undertake a nonparametric analysis you would perform a Mann–Whitney test (or Wilcoxon rank sum) on the sequence differences. For a period-adjusted analysis, a confidence interval would also be calculated on the sequence differences.

4.3.1.6 Analysis of Variance (ANOVA)

To analyse the data through an analysis of variance (ANOVA) the question needs to be reconsidered a little. Suppose we have two groups of observations: $x_{11}, x_{12}, \ldots, x_{1n}$ in group 1 and $x_{21}, x_{22}, \ldots, x_{2n}$, each measured on n subjects in two periods such that each subject receives both treatments, where it is the mean difference that is of interest: $\overline{x}_1 - \overline{x}_2$. To undertake this analysis we would need to

- Fit a linear model using a procedure such as PROC MIXED or PROC GLM in SAS, entering the terms for subject, period and treatment (and other factors such as predose measures if appropriate).
- Then use contrasts to estimate the difference in means.

The test statistic will be constructed using the within-subject standard deviation (s_{w}) from the residual line of the ANOVA

$$t = \frac{\overline{x}_1 - \overline{x}_2}{(\sqrt{2}s_{\mathrm{w}})/\sqrt{\mathrm{n}}}. \tag{4.4}$$

Under the null hypothesis, t is distributed as Student's t, with $n-2$ degrees of freedom.

4.3.1.7 Worked Example 4.3

For the same trial data as discussed in Worked Example 4.1 and Worked Example 4.2, the structure of the data to be analysed through an ANOVA is given in Figure 4.3. The corresponding output shows that the inference from this analysis is exactly the same as that for the period-adjusted t-test (highlighted in the figure). Hence, the ANOVA approach adjusting for period is the same as the period-adjusted matched t-test.

The second analysis undertaken is given in Figure 4.4 and does not have period in the model. This approach gives the same result as that for a paired t-test.

The final analysis in Figure 4.5 is one which may be commonly seen and has an additional term for sequence in which subject is nested. Here inference has not changed, compared to the model with period in it, as sequence is a between-subject term and all information is within subject.

4.3.1.8 Summary of Analysis Approaches

We have highlighted how apparently different approaches to analysis give the same inference with respect to the P-value. For example, when comparing the ANOVA approach with the paired t-test approach when period is not fitted into the model, the estimated mean difference was 3.59 in the worked example for both approaches (see Figure 4.2 and Figure 4.3).

With respect to the variances there is a twofold difference, with the variance from the paired t-test of 125.46 ($= s_d^2$) being twice as big as that from an analysis of variance (without period), which was 62.73 ($= s_w^2$). However, we have $s_d^2 = 2s_w^2$, and from inspection of (4.1) and (4.2) we can see how the inference is the same.

From this point forth in the book the concentration will be on the analysis-of-variance approach. For comparison to other texts, however, the reader needs to aware of whether the text is referring to a t-test or analysis of variance.

Additional analyses for crossover trials will be discussed in Chapter 9 in the context of bioequivalence trials.

4.3.2 UTILITY OF CROSSOVER TRIALS

4.3.2.1 What is Good about Crossover Trials

To discuss the utility of crossover trials we must first remind ourselves of how a sample size is calculated. For a two-period crossover trial, the total sample size, n, can be estimated from

$$n = \frac{2\left(Z_{1-\beta} + Z_{1-\alpha/2}\right)^2 \sigma_w^2}{d^2}, \tag{4.5}$$

(a) Data and SAS code.

```
TITLE 'ANOVA Analysis';
DATA trialdat;
INPUT subject outcome period trt sequence;
DATALINES;
1.00     116.35   1   1   1
1.00     120.97   2   2   1
2.00     125.87   1   1   1
2.00     127.26   2   2   1
3.00      89.49   1   2   2
3.00     102.16   2   1   2
4.00     146.58   1   2   2
4.00     125.24   2   1   2
5.00     127.20   1   1   1
5.00     129.03   2   2   1
6.00     147.69   1   2   2
6.00     151.41   2   1   2
7.00     110.44   1   2   2
7.00     123.29   2   1   2
8.00     107.14   1   1   1
8.00     122.27   2   2   1
9.00     141.03   1   1   1
9.00     151.86   2   2   1
10.00    126.41   1   2   2
10.00    130.21   2   1   2
11.00    152.75   1   1   1
11.00    155.09   2   2   1
12.00    148.41   1   2   2
12.00    129.78   2   1   2
;
PROC mixed DATA = trialdat;CLASS subject period trt;
MODEL outcome = subject trt period;
ESTIMATE 'B-A' trt -1 1;
RUN;
QUIT;
```

(b) SAS output.

```
                    ANOVA Analysis
                  The Mixed Procedure
                    Fit Statistics
         BIC (smaller is better)          84.4

              Type 3 Tests of Fixed Effects

                      Num     Den
      Effect           DF      DF    F Value    Pr > F

      subject          11      10       8.50    0.0010
      trt               1      10       1.18    0.3027
      period            1      10       0.54    0.4781

                        Estimates

                         Standard
Label     Estimate        Error      DF    t Value    Pr > |t|

B-A         3.5892       3.3028      10       1.09      0.3027
```

P-value same as period-adjusted t-test

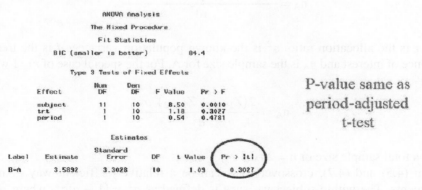

Figure 4.3 Example data, SAS code and output for an analysis of variance with period in the model.

(a) SAS code.

```
PROC mixed data = trialdat;
CLASS subject trt;
MODEL outcome = subject trt;
ESTIMATE 'B-A' trt -1 1;
RUN;
QUIT;
```

(b) SAS output.

ANOVA Analysis

The Mixed Procedure

Type 3 Tests of Fixed Effects

Effect	Num DF	Den DF	F Value	Pr > F
subject	11	11	8.87	0.0005
trt	1	11	1.23	0.2907

Estimates

Label	Estimate	Standard Error	DF	t Value	Pr > |t|
B-A	3.5892	3.2335	11	1.11	0.2907

P-value same as paired t-test

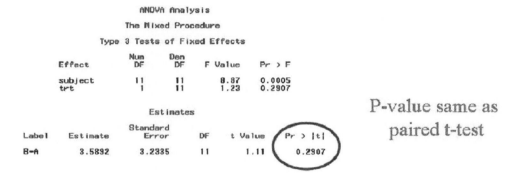

Figure 4.4 Example SAS code and output for an analysis of variance without period in the model.

where σ_w^2 is the known within-subject population variance and d is the treatment difference of interest. This compares to a parallel-group trial where the sample size for treatment group A is estimated from

$$n_A = \frac{(r+1)\left(Z_{1-\beta} + Z_{1-\alpha/2}\right)^2 \sigma^2}{rd^2}, \tag{4.6}$$

where r is the allocation ratio, σ^2 is the known population variance, d is the treatment difference of interest and n_A is the sample size for A. For the special case of $r = 1$ we have

$$n_A = \frac{2\left(Z_{1-\beta} + Z_{1-\alpha/2}\right)^2 \sigma^2}{d^2}, \tag{4.7}$$

giving a total sample size of $n = 2n_A$.

From (4.5) and (4.7), crossover trials can be a relatively efficient way of making assessments. The within-subject variance is defined as $\sigma_w^2 = (1-\rho)\sigma^2$, where ρ is the correlation between the two measures and σ^2 is the variance from a parallel-group study.

(a) SAS code.

```
PROC mixed DATA = trialdat;
CLASS subject sequence trt period;
MODEL outcome = subject(sequence) sequence trt period;
ESTIMATE 'B-A' trt -1 1;
RUN;
QUIT;
```

(b) SAS output.

```
                    ANOVA Analysis

                The Mixed Procedure

            Type 3 Tests of Fixed Effects

                     Num     Den
Effect                DF      DF    F Value    Pr > F

subject(sequence)     10      10       9.22    0.0008
sequence               1      10       1.33    0.2756
trt                    1      10       1.18    0.3027
period                 1      10       0.54    0.4781

                      Estimates

                     Standard
Label    Estimate       Error    DF    t Value    Pr > |t|

B-A        3.5892      3.3028    10       1.09      0.3027
```

Figure 4.5 Example SAS code and output for an analysis of variance with period and the term for sequence in the model.

Hence, $\sigma_w^2 = \sigma^2$ only for $\rho = 0$, so a crossover study would require, at worst, half the number of subjects compared to a parallel-group study.

As well as being relatively efficient, all the information for assessments is within subject, so no between-subject variability exists that could 'cloud' assessments. Hence, making assessments of both regimens in each subject is informative, as each subject acts as their own control and this permits a better determination of efficacy (and safety).

4.3.2.2 What is Bad about Crossover Trials

Here, when talking about what is bad with crossover trials we are mainly considering the context of studies designed with the objective to assess efficacy. For pharmacokinetics-driven studies there are generally fewer issues.

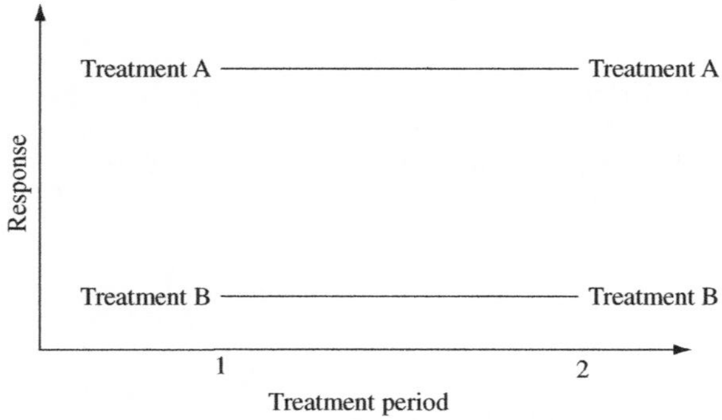

Figure 4.6 Idealized results from a crossover: no period effect.

Figure 4.6 gives an illustration of the crossover-trial results we would like to see in an ideal world. Here the responses for Treatment A, and likewise for B, are identical no matter whether assessed in Period 1 or Period 2.

Figure 4.7 gives a rather extreme example of the presence of a period effect. Here the individual treatment effects of A and B are both different in different periods. However, what is important is that the difference between treatments, A – B, remains constant over time.

Table 4.1 gives an example of how a period effect in a crossover trial may appear. The effects for A are indicated by the mean from Period 1: 2.40, and that for Period 2: 7.19. Clearly A does better in Period 2. Similarly for B, the Period 1 and 2 means are 4.53 and 8.50 and B also does better in Period 2. A period-adjusted estimate of the mean difference between A and B is $(-6.10 + 2.44)/2 = -1.72$. Here the mean difference, which ignores the ordering of treatments, gives the same result.

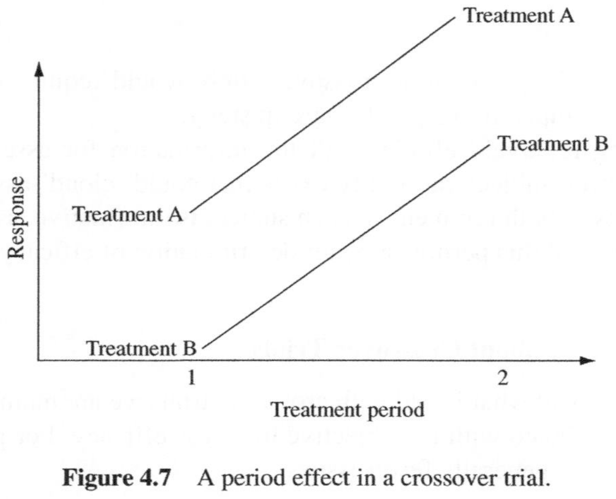

Figure 4.7 A period effect in a crossover trial.

Table 4.1 Example of a crossover trial with a period effect

Sequence AB				Sequence BA			
ID	A	B	A − B	ID	B	A	B − A
1	1.95	7.18	−5.23	3	6.29	5.51	0.78
2	4.58	8.17	−3.59	4	2.76	8.96	−6.20
5	0.16	10.80	−10.64	7	6.96	5.96	1.00
6	0.37	7.56	−7.18	8	4.96	6.58	−1.62
9	4.43	7.72	−3.28	10	5.24	9.67	−4.43
11	3.20	8.08	−4.89	12	2.27	5.91	−3.63
14	2.65	8.06	−5.42	13	6.04	7.54	−1.50
16	0.19	7.76	−7.57	15	4.28	5.95	−1.68
18	4.54	11.20	−6.61	17	2.65	9.36	−6.71
19	1.90	8.53	−6.63	20	3.82	6.43	−2.61
$\bar{x}_{AB}$	2.40	8.50	−6.10	$\bar{x}_{BA}$	4.53	7.19	−2.66

In reality data such as those described in Figure 4.6 and 4.7 would seldom be observed. Figure 4.8 gives a more common example of the form the data may take. Here there is a slight narrowing of the effect, although this could be down to chance variation alone.

Figure 4.9 gives an example of the type of result that we do not wish to see. Here the effect of treatment does not seem to be independent of period. It could be that there is a treatment-by-period interaction or maybe there could be carryover effects from previous periods.

The big question is, how do you separate out a treatment effect? If there is a carryover effect, then effects we observe for each treatment in the current period are dependent on the treatment of the previous period. Usually if we a have variable upon which an effect is dependent then we would fit this as a covariate in a statistical model. So here

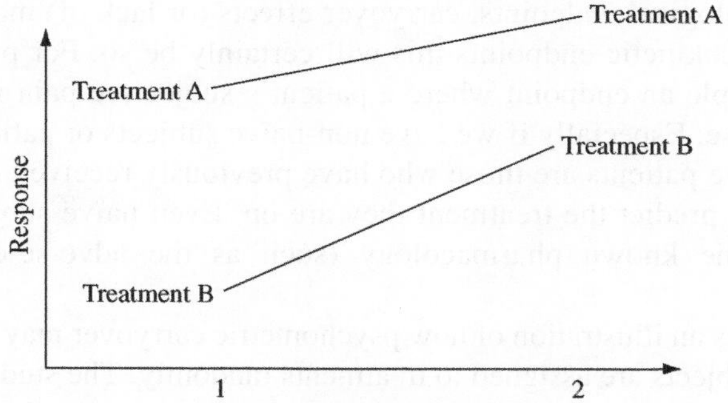

Figure 4.8 Illustration of what may be expected in a crossover trial.

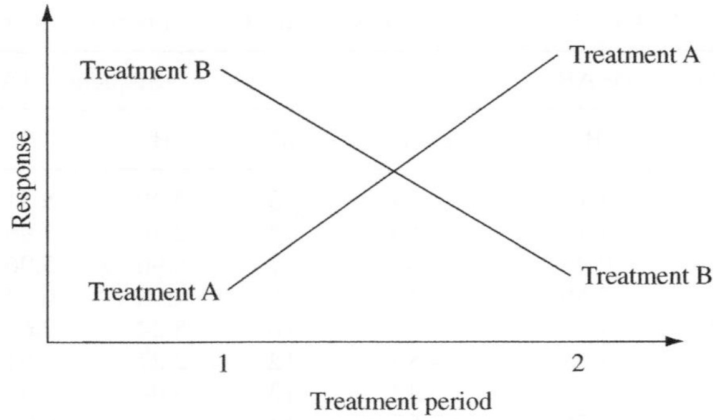

Figure 4.9 Illustration of a possible carryover effect in a clinical trial.

the desired solution would be to fit the previous period's treatment as a covariate. However, with an AB/BA crossover trial, A is always preceded by B and B is always preceded by A. Hence, the second-period treatment is totally confounded with what is received in the first period.

Note the assumption is not that there is *no* carryover effect, but rather that there is *equal* carryover effect with both treatments.

There is no real solution to the problem illustrated in Figure 4.9, except by modifying the basic design. Thus, *a priori* you could repeat the final period's treatment such that the sequences are now ABB and BAA. This design will be discussed in Chapter 9 on bioequivalence, as it brings the added advantage of reducing the number of subjects required by 25%.

Note, however, for a double-blind study, we would need to add additional sequences: BAB, ABA, BBA and AAB. Otherwise with just ABB and BAA, it would be known that the third period has the same treatment allocated as the second.

Probably though, the only solution if we anticipate a response such as in Figure 4.9 is not to do crossover studies?

For hard physiological endpoints, carryover effects (or lack of) may be predictable, while for pharmacokinetic endpoints this will certainly be so. For psychometric endpoints – for example an endpoint where a patient's subjective pain is recorded – this may not be the case. Especially if we have non-naïve subjects or patients enrolled into the trial. Non-naïve patients are those who have previously received the treatment and so may be able to predict the treatment they are on. Even naïve subjects may predict treatment from the known pharmacology (such as the adverse-event profile) of the drug.

Figure 4.10 gives an illustration of how psychometric carryover may manifest itself. In the first period, subjects are assigned to treatments randomly. The study is ostensibly set up as a double-blind trial. However, non-naïve patients are enrolled and, due to the pharmacology of the drug, they have a good chance of guessing the treatment. In the second period they swap treatments. Suppose Treatment A is placebo, then in the second

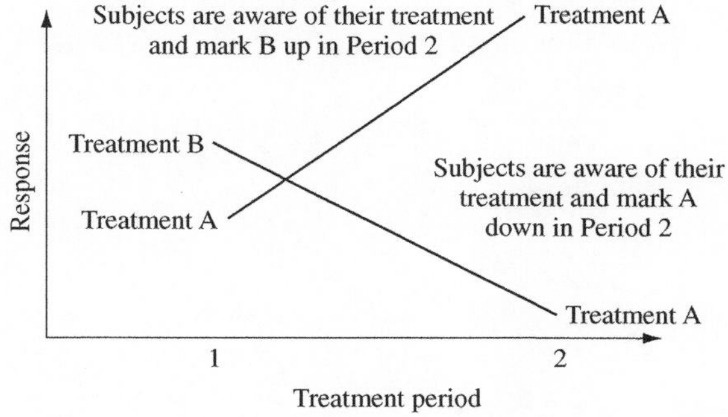

Figure 4.10 Psychometric carryover in a clinical trial.

period a subject may guess that they 'must be on a better treatment' and so mark the active arm, Treatment B, up in this period. While with the converse they mark Treatment A down as they know it must be worse.

Of course one 'solution' to this problem would be to perform a statistical test for any possible carryover and then, depending on this, decide upon the appropriate analysis to conduct. There is only one thing wrong with this approach, and that is that it is complete and utter nonsense. You should never conduct a second statistical test dependent upon the results of a preceding test. When designing a trial you should always design it to ensure that there is either no, or equal, carryover and then analyse the study under the assumption that there is no carryover.

Given what we have discussed, especially with respect to psychometric carryover, there may be instances, however, of a trial being proposed and designed where the assumptions with respect to carryover are questionable. What do we do then?

We could be dogmatic in approach and say that in such instances you should always conduct a parallel-group trial. But in truth the pragmatic consideration is to ask, who is the study trying to convince? For internal decisions or as a pre-pilot, would such a study be appropriate? Is a definitive pilot study to follow? As discussed in Chapter 3, the Type I error for early phase trials is a concern for the sponsor, as this error could necessitate the (unnecessary) initiation of other expensive activities. As such, a crossover trial in such circumstances could be a relatively efficient way to assess proof of concept, especially if once completed the plan is to proceed to a parallel-group trial. However, a determination of the risks to be taken would need to be made.

Conversely if the wish is to convince external agencies, then such issues could rule out a crossover trial and necessitate a parallel-group trial at this early stage.

5 Multi-period Crossover Trials

5.1 INTRODUCTION

Early phase trials commonly have multiple arms, often in a small number of subjects on whom a number of investigations are made, such as in an assessment of bioavailability for different formulations or a comparison of dose proportionality across several doses or, in the context of a proof of concept study, a comparison of several doses against negative and positive controls.

In Chapter 4 we discussed the basic two-period design. In this chapter we move on to more general multiperiod crossover studies, which by definition are trials where subjects receive a multiple number of regimens. For example with four regimens, A, B, C and D, all subjects will receive all regimens or at least a selection of them.

Like two-period crossover trials where subjects are randomized to the sequences AB or BA, it is the same for multiperiod crossovers. For example, for three arms with three treatments, subjects will be randomized to one of six sequences: ABC, BCA, CAB, BAC, ACB or CBA.

Multiperiod crossover trials are in fact analogous to many agricultural studies, where for subjects read blocks and for periods read plots. Indeed there is an irony in designing early phase clinical trials in that the first source to which some may turn is one on agricultural statistics. As a consequence, much of the nomenclature for multiperiod crossovers comes from agricultural work, such as Latin square designs and balanced incomplete blocks designs to which we will refer later in the chapter.

This chapter therefore will extend the earlier discussion to multiperiod crossovers and will look at designs pertinent to trials with many periods, such as Williams squares, and balanced incomplete blocks.

Note, multiperiod replicate designs will be discussed in Chapter 9 under bioequivalence.

5.2 ALL INVESTIGATIONS ARE MADE ON ALL SUBJECTS

Early phase trials can be complicated as they are often undertaken in a small number of subjects on whom a number of investigations are made, such as:

- A comparison of different therapies, or different doses of the same therapy, within a subject.
- An assessment of bioavailability across several formulations.
- A determination of dose proportionality.

An Introduction to Statistics in Early Phase Trials Steven A. Julious, Say Beng Tan and David Machin

It is quite commonplace, therefore, for 4 or more investigations to be made on the same subject. If 4 investigations are made, that would result in 24 different sequences for assigning subjects to these 4 investigations. This is all very well, but what if we have only 12 subjects in the trial?

Actually, for multiperiod investigations we do not necessarily need to use all possible sequences but can form special sequences, called Williams squares.

For example, in order to investigate an even number of interventions we can build a Williams square from the following general sequence:

$$0,\ 1,\ t,\ 2,\ t-1,\ 3,\ t-2, \ldots$$

Here t is the number of interventions to be compared minus 1.

Thus if we were to conduct 4 investigations then $t = 3$ and our sequences would include only the integers 0, 1, 2, 3. The first row is derived from the result above. We then form the second by adding 1 to each term in the first row, but where the number is 3 the new number becomes 0 (we are adding in base 3). The calculation is simpler than the explanation.

Sequence				
1	0	1	3	2
2	1	2	0	3
3	2	3	1	0
4	3	0	2	1

This is known as a Latin square: each investigation (0, 1, 2 or 3) appears in every row and column. The columns here could reflect the successive periods when, for example, investigations on different interventions are held.

A Williams square is a special form of Latin square such that, as well as being balanced for rows and columns, each investigation is preceded by each other investigation at least once; for example 1 is preceded by 0, 2, and 3. Here we are saying that as well as the order of investigations being important, the effect of the preceding investigations is too. Hence we ensure balance for the immediately preceding investigation. This is known as first-order balance.

First-order balance is important; as highlighted in Chapter 4, for an AB/BA crossover, what we are investigating in the second period is confounded with the first period's investigation, which can cause issues. There are fewer issues therefore if we have first-order balance.

If we were conducting a trial where we are to undertake 4 different investigations on 12 subjects, we would randomize the 4 sequences above so that each sequence appears 3 times.

For an odd number of investigations we need to build two Latin squares with starting sequences:

$$0,\ 1,\ t,\ 2,\ t-1,\ 3,\ t-2, \ldots$$

and

$$\ldots, t-2, 3, t-1, 2, t, 1, 0.$$

With 5 investigational drugs, $t = 4$ and we would therefore have

0	1	4	2	3
1	2	0	3	4
2	3	1	4	0
3	4	2	0	1
4	0	3	1	2

and

3	2	4	1	0
4	3	0	2	1
0	4	1	3	2
1	0	2	4	3
2	1	3	0	4

What is apparent from these 10 sequences is that one set of sequences is effectively the mirror of the other. For an odd number of treatments we need to have a number of sequences double the number of treatments to ensure that we have first-order balance. Note how in the first 5 sequences above (on the left), 3 is preceded only by 0 and 2. It is only in the second 5 sequences (on the right) that 3 is preceded by 1 and 4 to ensure first-order balance.

5.2.1 HOW TO ANALYSE

To analyse data where all subjects receive all treatments is relatively straightforward and an analysis such as described in the steps below could be applied:

- Fit a linear model using a procedure such as PROC GLM in SAS.
- Enter the terms for subject, period and treatment (also other factors such as predose measures if appropriate).
- Use contrasts (pairwise comparisons) to estimate the difference in means.
- The test statistic will be constructed using the within-subject standard deviation (s_w) from the residual line of the analysis of variance (ANOVA),

$$t = \frac{\bar{x}_1 - \bar{x}_2}{(\sqrt{2}s_w)/\sqrt{n}}. \tag{5.1}$$

- Under the null hypothesis, t is distributed as Student's t, with degrees of freedom taken from the residual line: $df = n(p - 1) - 2(p - 1)$, where p is the number of periods.

Note that the degrees of freedom may also be expressed as $df = n(p - 1) - p - t + 2$, but here we have $p = t$ and hence $df = n(p - 1) - 2(p - 1)$.

5.2.2 SAMPLE SIZE CALCULATIONS

5.2.2.1 Superiority Trials

To calculate the sample size for a superiority trial, the result for two-period crossover trials from Chapter 3 would need to be adapted to account for the extra degrees of freedom we have with respect to the estimated variance. Thus Equation (3.7) is replaced by

$$1-\beta = 1 - \text{Probt}\left(t_{1-\alpha/2,n-2},\ n(p-1)-2(p-1),\ \sqrt{\frac{nd^2}{2\sigma_{\mathrm{w}}^2}}\right). \tag{5.2}$$

Note, however, that most packages and texts provide calculations assuming a two-periodcrossover. For multiperiod crossover studies, using (3.6), repeated as (5.3) below, which is based on the large-sample Normal approximation, may provide an estimate of sample size quite close to (5.2).

$$n = \frac{2(Z_{1-\beta}+Z_{1-\alpha/2})^2\sigma_{\mathrm{w}}^2}{d^2}. \tag{5.3}$$

This is because using the result from a two-period crossover will understate how many degrees of freedom we have for the t-statistic and consequently overestimate the required sample size.

5.2.2.2 Precision-Based Trials

For precision-based trials the following result could be used, which again accounts for the degrees of freedom from the multiperiod model

$$n \geq \frac{2\sigma_{\mathrm{w}}^2 t_{1-\alpha/2,n(p-2)-2(p-1)}^2}{w^2}, \tag{5.4}$$

where w is the width of the $100(1-\alpha)\%$ confidence interval.

As for superiority trials, most texts and packages assume that the trial being planned is a two-period crossover, and a Normal approximation result

$$n = \frac{2\sigma_{\mathrm{w}}^2 Z_{1-\alpha/2}^2}{w^2}. \tag{5.5}$$

may give a close estimate of the sample size stipulated by (5.4).

For a trial based primarily on feasibility, as multiperiod trials often are, determining the precision for a given sample size, n, may be more appropriate.In this case, the anticipated width of the resulting confidence interval is given by

$$w = t_{1-\alpha/2, n(p-2)-2(p-1)} \sqrt{2s_{\mathrm{w}}^2/n}. \tag{5.6}$$

5.3 NOT ALL INVESTIGATIONS ARE MADE ON ALL SUBJECTS

Often in early clinical investigations there are logistical, practical and safety considerations to be taken into account. For example, we may wish to investigate four different formulations but there may be practical reasons why we can only schedule three dosing periods, or there may be safety reasons restricting how many times you can dose an individual subject, or even time pressures meaning there is only a finite time window in which the study can be undertaken. We can still construct Latin squares, but need to construct a special type of these known as a balanced incomplete block design (BIBD). Again we will illustrate by example.

5.3.1 EVEN NUMBER OF TREATMENTS

If we could have three sessions for each subject, but we have four investigations, then taking the sequences derived previously and removing the first column, and then repeating but now deleting the final column, gives

0	1	3	2
1	2	0	3
2	3	1	0
3	0	2	1

0	1	3	2
1	2	0	3
2	3	1	0
3	0	2	1

Then combining these gives the following eight sequences:

1	3	2
2	0	3
3	1	0
0	2	1
0	1	3
1	2	0
2	3	1
3	0	2

Hence we have balance for columns as well as first-order balance within these eight sequences. This approach works so long as the number of periods in the BIBD is greater than half the number of treatments, thus it will work for:

- Four periods with six treatments;
- Five periods with nine treatments, and so on.

To generalize, therefore, you remove the first column(s) from the Williams square and then match by also taking away the last.

5.3.1.1 Worked Example 5.1

A trial is being designed which has six treatments, but for timing reasons there will only be four periods. We wish therefore to derive the treatment sequences for the study, to account for the study limitations.

To derive the starting sequences we build a six-period Williams square. We then delete the first two and last two columns as in the shaded areas below.

0	1	5	2	4	3
1	2	0	3	5	4
2	3	1	4	0	5
3	4	2	5	1	0
4	5	3	0	2	1
5	0	4	1	3	2

0	1	5	2	4	3
1	2	0	3	5	4
2	3	1	4	0	5
3	4	2	5	1	0
4	5	3	0	2	1
5	0	4	1	3	2

The eight treatment sequences would thus be:

5	2	4	3
0	3	5	4
1	4	0	5
2	5	1	0
3	0	2	1
4	1	3	2
0	1	5	2
1	2	0	3
2	3	1	4
3	4	2	5
4	5	3	0
5	0	4	1

As a quick check it is usually beneficial to confirm that each treatment is indeed preceded by each other treatment in the eight sequences by having a little table as below and checking manually. For example, for the first row check that 0 is preceded by 1, 2, 3, 4 and 5, and so on.

	0	1	2	3	4	5
0		x	x	x	x	x
1	x		x	x	x	x
2	x	x		x	x	x
3	x	x	x		x	x
4	x	x	x	x		x
5	x	x	x	x	x	

5.3.2 ODD NUMBER OF TREATMENTS

For an odd number of sequences we use a similar procedure. Using our previous example of having five investigations, and assuming that we can only do three sessions, then we could delete the first two columns of the first five sequences and the last two columns of the next, to leave the unshaded blocks below, which are then stacked one above the other.

3	2	4	1	0
4	3	0	2	1
0	4	1	3	2
1	0	2	4	3
2	1	3	0	4

0	1	4	2	3
1	2	0	3	4
2	3	1	4	0
3	4	2	0	1
4	0	3	1	2

5.3.3 HOW TO ANALYSE

A fixed-effects approach such as from PROC GLM in SAS will only use within-subject information for comparisons, and so a random-effects approach may be appropriate, such as from PROC MIXED in SAS. This is because from this analysis we could extract within- and between-subject information. In reality, little information comes from between-subject comparison in relation to within for BIBD, but a random-effects approach could be considered to be preferable. Any formal comparisons would come from contrasts such as from (5.1).

5.3.4 SAMPLE SIZE

The results (5.2) to (5.5) could be used to estimate the sample size, except that for the results that use t-statistics, the degrees of freedom for the t-statistics should be replaced by $df = n(p-1) - 2(p-1) - (t-p)$. For a trial based primarily on feasibility, (5.6) could be used.

The sample size now, however, is the sample size for each paired contrast. There needs to be an inflation of the sample size, to ensure the appropriate number of subjects for the contrast. For example, for the BIBD example in Section 5.3.1, each treatment only appears with another treatment, for example 1 with 0, or 2 with 3, in half the sequences. Hence, the total sample would need to be doubled to ensure the appropriate number of subjects for each paired contrast.

5.4 NOT ALL INVESTIGATIONS ARE MADE ON ALL SUBJECTS BUT EVERYONE RECEIVES PLACEBO

A common situation when designing an early phase trial is where, for the reasons described earlier, not all subjects can receive all treatments, but a BIBD may be restricted by a requirement that all subjects receive placebo.

The reason for this could be because the primary objective is to compare each regimen in turn to placebo, and a BIBD may not be the most efficient design in this circumstance. Also, there may be a need to give all subjects placebo to enable a better assessment of tolerability.

There is no generic solution as for complete Williams squares and BIBD designs within a small number of sequences. However, for common designs, Williams squares can be constructed as we will now describe.

5.4.1 NUMBER OF PERIODS ONE LESS THAN THE NUMBER OF TREATMENTS

5.4.1.1 Even Number of Treatments in Odd Number of Periods

If the number of periods is just one less than the number of treatments, then the building of a Williams square is relatively straightforward.

For an even number of treatments into an odd number of periods, for example, six treatments in five periods, build the sequences as in Section 5.2, but in the left-hand-block leading diagonal, replace each member of the diagonal: 4, 4, 1, 3, 3 by placebo (P). Likewise for the descending diagonal, 3, 3, 1, 4, 4 of the right-hand block (Block 2), to obtain

0	1	4	2	P
1	2	0	P	4
2	3	P	4	0
3	P	2	0	1
P	0	3	1	2

P	1	4	2	3
1	P	0	3	4
2	3	P	4	0
3	4	2	P	1
4	0	3	1	P

These two blocks almost form a Williams square (which may be sufficient for most trials), but to complete the square we must also add the following two blocks (Blocks 3 and 4).

3	2	4	1	P
4	3	0	P	1
0	4	P	3	2
1	P	2	4	3
P	1	3	0	4

P	2	4	1	0
4	P	0	2	1
0	4	P	3	2
1	0	2	P	3
2	1	3	0	P

Hence we have first-order balance within 20 treatment sequences.

5.4.1.2 Odd Number of Treatments in Even Number of Periods

For an odd number of treatments in an even number of periods you can build the sequences as for four treatments (0, 1, 2 and 3) in four periods, as described in Section 5.2, then in the four successive 4 × 4 blocks, replace 0 by P in the first, 1 by P in the second, 2 by P in the third, and 3 by P in the last, to obtain

P	1	3	2
1	2	P	3
2	3	1	P
3	P	2	1

0	P	3	2
P	2	0	3
2	3	P	0
3	0	2	P

0	1	P	2
1	2	0	P
2	P	1	0
P	0	2	1

0	1	3	P
1	P	0	3
P	3	1	0
3	0	P	1

An alternative approach would be to take the same 4 × 4 block considered above, but replace the first column entries by P, as follows:

P	1	3	2
P	2	0	3
P	3	1	0
P	0	2	1

Then add a placebo arm and build four Williams squares (which would give the same result). The advantage of this approach is that it could be applied also to four treatments in three periods, for example, building Williams squares from starting sequences (P, 1, 0), (P, 1, 2) and (P, 0, 2).

5.4.2 NUMBER OF PERIODS TWO OR MORE LESS THAN THE NUMBER OF TREATMENTS

The Williams squares approach can also be applied for instances where the treatments outnumber the periods by more than one, provided that the number of periods is greater than half the number of treatments; that is, $t - p > 1$ provided $p > t / 2$. It is best to illustrate by example, using one approach.

For this approach we are using an example of six treatments in four periods where one of the treatments is placebo, which all subjects must receive. Take five sequences from a BIBD for five periods; delete the first two columns.

0	1	4	2	3
1	2	0	3	4
2	3	1	4	0
3	4	2	0	1
4	0	3	1	2

Then add a single column of placebo and use this square for the start sequences:

P	4	2	3
P	0	3	4
P	1	4	0
P	2	0	1
P	3	1	2

From these five sequences build five different Williams squares. The same process could be undertaken for an odd number of treatments in an odd number of periods (where treatments outnumber periods by more than two).

This approach is not the only solution and other approaches could be applied to the same effect.

5.4.2.1 Worked Example 5.2

We wish to design a study with six treatments in four periods where everyone must received placebo. There are a number of ways to derive the treatment sequences, but one approach is to start with the initial five combinations of treatments:

Sequence				
I	P	4	2	3
II	P	0	3	4
III	P	1	4	0
IV	P	2	0	1
V	P	3	1	2

We know from Section 5.2 that the following is a Williams square for four treatments:

0	1	3	2
1	2	0	3
2	3	1	0
3	0	2	1

Hence, for Sequence I of

P 4 2 3,

As 2 and 3 already appear, we replace 0 and 1 with P and 4 in the Williams square to obtain

P	4	3	2
4	2	P	3
2	3	4	P
3	P	2	4

For Sequence II, replace 1 and 2 with P and 4:

0	P	3	4
P	4	0	3
4	3	P	0
3	0	4	P

For Sequence III,

0	1	4	P
1	P	0	4
P	4	1	0
4	0	P	1

For Sequence IV,

0	1	P	2
1	2	0	P
2	P	1	0
P	0	2	1

and V,

P	1	3	2
1	2	P	3
2	3	1	P
3	P	2	1

A quick check of the 20 sequences confirms that there is first-order balance:

	0	1	2	3	4	P
0		x	x	x	x	x
1	x		x	x	x	x
2	x	x		x	x	x
3	x	x	x		x	x
4	x	x	x	x		x
P	x	x	x	x	x	

5.4.3 SAMPLE SIZE AND STATISTICAL ANALYSIS

With respect to the statistical analysis all information is now within subject, and so either a fixed- or random-effects approach can be used.

The sample size calculations are relatively straightforward. To calculate sample size we can use the results (5.2) to (5.5). For a trial based primarily on feasibility, the resulting confidence interval given by (5.6) could be used. All sample-size calculations would need account for the residual degrees of freedom as before. Also, the sample size calculation would actually be the number of subjects required for each contrast and so this would need to be inflated to account for the number of contrasts concerned, to give the total sample size.

5.5 NOT ALL INVESTIGATIONS ARE MADE ON ALL SUBJECTS BUT EVERYONE RECEIVES PLACEBO AND ACTIVE CONTROL

There is no generic solution to this problem, but on a case-by-case basis one can derive the sequences. For example, suppose there are five treatments in four periods where everyone must receive A and P. A Williams square can be formed from the following sequences APBC, APBD, and APCD.

5.5.1 WORKED EXAMPLE 5.3

Suppose we are designing a six-period crossover study with six treatments. The Williams square of sequences for subjects to be randomized to would therefore be

0	1	5	2	4	3
1	2	0	3	5	4
2	3	1	4	0	5
3	4	2	5	1	0
4	5	3	0	2	1
5	0	4	1	3	2

Suppose further that, due to practical limitations, the study is to be a BIBD in four periods. We then build the treatment sequences by deleting the appropriate columns as below to form the unshaded blocks.

0	1	5	2	4	3
1	2	0	3	5	4
2	3	1	4	0	5
3	4	2	5	1	0
4	5	3	0	2	1
5	0	4	1	3	2

0	1	5	2	4	3
1	2	0	3	5	4
2	3	1	4	0	5
3	4	2	5	1	0
4	5	3	0	2	1
5	0	4	1	3	2

To form:

5	2	4	0
0	3	5	1
1	4	0	2
2	5	1	3
3	0	2	4
4	1	3	5

0	1	5	2
1	2	0	3
2	3	1	4
3	4	2	5
4	5	3	0
5	0	4	1

To complicate matters further, suppose one of the five treatments was a placebo. The wish is still to have the trials in four periods, but the restriction is to be added that all subjects must receive placebo.

The initial sequences are:

P	1	2	3
P	2	3	4
P	3	4	5
P	4	5	1
P	5	1	2

The simplest thing to do in this example would be to build a four-period Williams square:

0	1	3	2
1	2	0	3
2	3	1	0
3	0	2	1

From this the following sequences can be derived:

P	1	3	2
1	2	P	3
2	3	1	P
3	P	2	1

P	4	3	2
4	2	P	3
2	3	4	P
3	P	2	4

P	4	3	5
4	5	P	3
5	3	4	P
3	P	5	4

P	1	4	5
1	5	P	4
5	4	1	P
4	P	5	1

P	1	5	2
1	2	P	5
2	5	1	P
5	P	2	1

A further consideration is that the sample size is to be fixed at 24 subjects, with only 20 subjects expected to complete the trial. With a within-subject standard deviation of 7.5 we wish to calculate the precision (as discussed in Chapter 3) for 95% confidence intervals for estimates of regimen compared to placebo for:

1. The complete Williams square (take 0 to be placebo).
2. The balanced incomplete block design (take 0 to be placebo).
3. The balanced incomplete block design where everyone receives placebo.

1. For the first design we anticipate having the following division of the degrees of freedom for an ANOVA:

Source	Degrees of freedom
Subject	19
Period	5
Treatment	5
Residual	90
Total	119

Hence, we expect to have 90 degrees of freedom about the within-subject variance. The precision for the first design is $\sqrt{2} \times 7.5 \times t_{0.975,90}/\sqrt{(20)} = 4.71$.

An example table, described in Chapter 3, to illustrate this precision for the protocol could be:

Precision	Difference	Lower 95% CI	Upper 95% CI
4.71	−10	−14.71	−5.29
4.71	−5	−9.71	−0.29
4.71	0	−4.71	4.71
4.71	5	0.29	9.71
4.71	10	5.29	14.71

2. Note, here for the precision estimates we take our sample size, n, to be the least number of times 0 appears with a regimen (e.g. regimen 3). For this precision calculation we will only use within-subject information.

   For the second design the degrees of freedom for the ANOVA will be

Source	Degrees of freedom
Subject	19
Period	3
Treatment	5
Residual	42
Total	79

With 24 subjects, 0 would appear eight times with regimen 3. In 20 subjects it could reduce to six.

The precision for the second design is $\sqrt{2} \times 7.5 \times t_{0.975,40} /\sqrt{6} = 8.70$.

3. For the third design we have

Source	Degrees of freedom
Subject	19
Period	3
Treatment	5
Residual	42
Total	79

In 20 subjects, placebo appearing with each other regimen 12 times. Hence, the precision for the third design is $\sqrt{2} \times 7.5 \times t_{0.975,40} /\sqrt{(12)} = 6.15$.

6 First Time into Man

6.1 INTRODUCTION

In previous chapters we have described the basic derivation of pharmacokinetics as well as the basic concepts around crossover trials. Here we will start to describe the different types of specific early phase trials by introducing first-time-into-man studies.

The first human clinical trials of any new chemical entity, referred to as first-time-into-man (FTIM) studies, are conducted with the primary objective to assess the safety and tolerability of a range of doses to use throughout drug development.

The safety and tolerability is assessed with increasing doses and relative to the preset safety cut offs. The safety cut off is based on the no-observed-adverse-event levels (NOAELs) observed preclinically. As a rule of thumb, the NOAEL is taken from the highest tolerated dose in the most sensitive animal species divided by 100 to give an indication of the starting dose in humans. The top dose is a 5th to a 10th of the NOAEL dose given to the most sensitive animal. The FDA (2002b) has guidelines on the topic, and it will be discussed again in Section 6.3.

FTIM studies also usually have the objective of characterizing, across a range of doses, a preliminary assessment of the pharmacokinetic profile, for example to determine where the C_{max} is, or when blood samples should be taken in order to obtain a profile. With the pharmacokinetics profile, an early assessment of dose proportionality across the range of doses can be made. For some new chemical entities there may also be an interest in assessing pharmacodynamics and its links to the pharmacokinetics. Statistically, FTIM studies are a compromise between learning and confirming. For example, the timing of blood samples for pharmacokinetic profiles is honed during the first initial doses. A consequence is that the pharmacokinetic parameters for these initial doses (e.g. C_{max} and AUC) may be estimated with less statistical precision than for subsequent doses.

As an aside, referring to the first study as FTIM is not a sexist nomenclature (first time into human or FTIH may also be used) but highlights operationally the nature of drug development. Except for a few notable exceptions, for example hormone therapies, compounds usually go first time into the male. This is because the minimum body of work to get a compound into men does not require reproductive toxicity data. Without reproductive toxicity results a compound can still be investigated in males provided they abstain from procreation for several months, by which time completely new sperm will have been produced. On the other hand, women are born with all their eggs, and produce no more, so that if they are given a compound which subsequently is found to have reproductive toxicity issues they must abstain from having children for life. In fact there is some evolutionary order to drug development, as a compound is

An Introduction to Statistics in Early Phase Trials Steven A. Julious, Say Beng Tan and David Machin

tested first on rats and if found to be safe in rats is then given to men. If found to be safe in men it is given to women, hence rats are the toxicity species for men and men are the toxicity species for women.

In FTIM studies the pharmacokinetics are often used as a surrogate, and the safety cut off definitions may well be given in terms of total exposures, for example AUC. Figure 6.1 gives an illustration of how a dose response may look for different scenarios. It is only in scenario (a) that a full planned profile may be investigated, as for the other two scenarios escalation would stop before reaching the end of the planned doses. The intended top dose would also be reviewed throughout the study, and the other planned doses and dose increments may be changed.

As previously mentioned, FTIM studies are usually performed in healthy (male) volunteers with the dose escalated on a log scale. As healthy volunteers are unable to derive any clinical benefit from any new chemical entity being investigated, a primary concern is therefore to ensure the safety of the volunteers. As well as drug exposure there

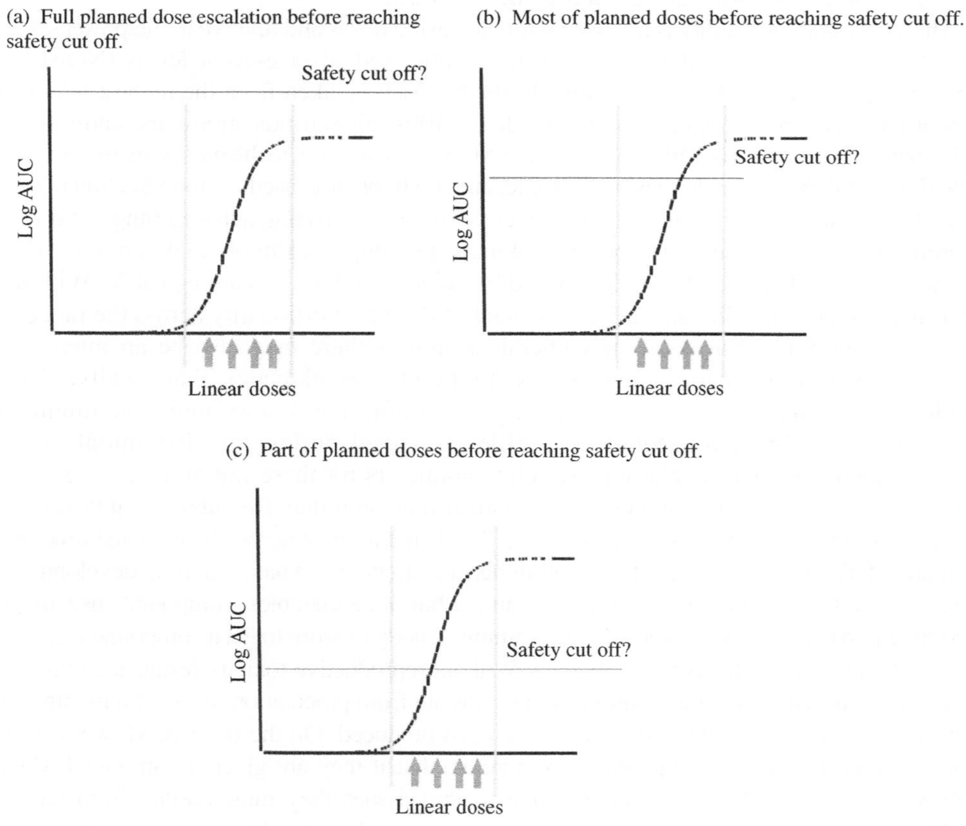

Figure 6.1 Schematic of exposure against dose.

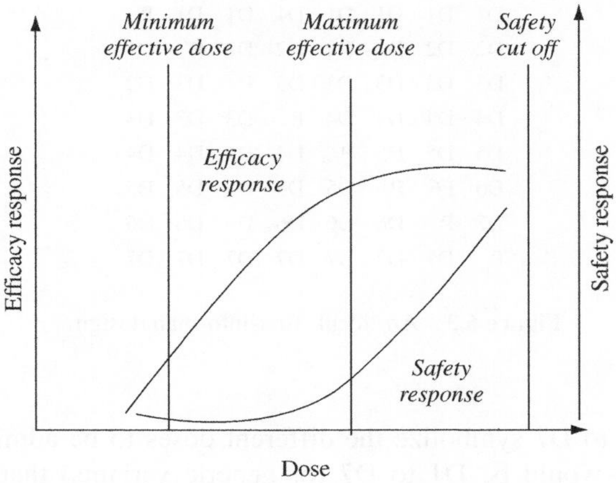

Figure 6.2 Schematic of dose response.

will be continuous safety monitoring, and dose escalation is stopped as soon as maximum tolerability is reached.

It is in both societies' and the sponsor's interest to identify the maximum tolerated dose (MTD), and to push the dose as high as possible in order to identify the safety window for a given compound. There are a number of reasons for this. For example, there may be potential for drug abuse with a given compound, or more simply patients may absentmindedly take prescribed medication twice (forgetting they have already taken it). It is therefore optimal to establish good general safety cover and to have as wide a safety window as possible. Figure 6.2 gives a schematic representation of the dose response curve for a given compound and how a safety cut off fits in context with efficacious doses.

6.2 STANDARD HEALTHY VOLUNTEER DESIGNS

In terms of statistical design, FTIM studies are a special form of the multiperiod crossover studies discussed in Chapter 5, in that subjects receive several single doses plus placebo across several periods, with the response to each dose evaluated prior to subsequent higher doses being administered.

Ideally a study design for a FTIM study would look like Figure 6.3. Here each column represents a different subject while each row represents a different period. Subjects are not randomized completely to each dose but simply either the planned dose for this session or placebo.

There are ethical and logistical issues with such designs – for example limitations as to the total amount of blood that can be taken – though the principles of this design are generic to all FTIM designs.

D1	D1	D1	D1	D1	D1	D1	P
D2	D2	D2	D2	D2	D2	P	D1
D3	D3	D3	D3	D3	P	D2	D2
D4	D4	D4	D4	P	D3	D3	D3
D5	D5	D5	P	D4	D4	D4	D4
D6	F6	P	D5	D5	D5	D5	D5
D7	P	D6	D6	D6	D6	D6	D6
P	D7	D7	D7	D7	D7	D7	D7

Figure 6.3 An 'ideal' first-into-man design.

Here D1 through to D7 symbolize the different doses to be administered across the different periods. It would be D1 to D7 (or generic variants) that would be used in randomization systems and databases initially. A protocol may say what D1 to D7 are planned but, in reality, these planned doses will more than likely change once the study starts.

We have the situation that dose is confounded with period, which may be a concern if the number of subjective adverse events increases across periods independent of treatment – this may be evidenced by adverse events on placebo increasing over successive periods.

An additional issue is that such FTIM designs cannot be truly blind – to be blind requires that it should not be possible to predict treatment allocation – but as dose is confounded with placebo this is not the case. However, here as safety concerns override purist design concerns, this is an issue that needs to be worked around.

Given the limitations of first-time-into-man designs, we will only describe some of the most common designs.

6.2.1 PLACEBO INTERRUPTING DESIGN

An example design for a first-time-into-man study is a placebo-controlled, dose-rising, four-period crossover study in a number of cohorts, as illustrated in Figure 6.4. Note that, depending on the objectives of the study, we may require three or five periods, but these designs would be similar in form to Figure 6.4. Here different subjects are represented in columns and each period is in a row. We have a sample size of 4 here for illustration, but the sample size could also be 6, 8 or 12 depending on the study. Typically the design would be of 2 or 3 subjects per treatment sequence with the sequences randomly assigned to subjects. The sample size, however, is usually based on feasibility considerations.

As Figure 6.4 illustrates, subjects are given the investigative treatments in cohorts, with each subject receiving several different doses in ascending order. For example in the first cohort each volunteer receives three escalating doses and a placebo which interrupts the escalation.

Cohort 1				Cohort 3			
P	D1	D1	D1	P	D7	D7	D7
D1	P	D2	D2	D7	P	D8	D8
D2	D2	P	D3	D8	D8	P	D9
D3	D3	D3	P	D9	D9	D9	P
Cohort 2				**Cohort 4**			
P	D4	D4	D4	P	D10	D10	D10
D4	P	D5	D5	D10	P	D11	D11
D5	D5	P	D6	D11	D11	P	D12
D6	D6	D6	P	D12	D12	D12	P

Figure 6.4 Placebo-interrupting first-time-into-man design.

As with the previous design, doses throughout the escalation can be amended in the light of the ongoing trial data, such that the actual doses administered, which may take the form of Figure 6.5, may bear little resemblance to the planned doses. The principle of the planned doses would remain, however, with the plan to start at 'homeopathic' doses and escalate up to the maximum tolerated dose (MTD).

The designs of Figure 6.4 and Figure 6.5 are quite conservative in terms of the dose escalation. Subjects are only dosed in a very limited range with all subjects receiving all doses assigned to a given cohort, plus placebo. As with the design of Figure 6.3, dose is once more confounded with period as well as cohort. This could be an issue if there is a cohort effect for a response, but as safety considerations are the main drivers for the study design such issues are unavoidable.

6.2.1.1 Summarizing the Data

Here we will begin by describing some basic graphs and statistics to summarize such studies, while in Section 6.4 we will more formally describe how to analyse FTIM studies.

Cohort 1				Cohort 3			
P	0.25	0.25	0.25	P	16	16	16
0.25	P	0.5	0.5	16	P	32	32
0.5	0.5	P	1	32	32	P	64
1	1	1	P	64	64	64	P
Cohort 2				**Cohort 4**			
P	2	2	2	P	125	125	125
2	P	4	4	125	P	250	250
4	4	P	8	250	250	P	500
8	8	8	P	500	500	500	P

Figure 6.5 A placebo-interrupting first-time-into-man design.

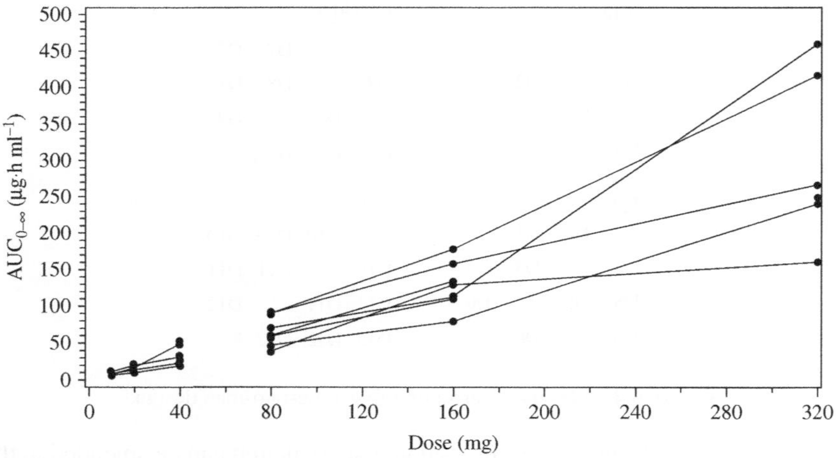

Figure 6.6 AUC against dose.

Figure 6.6 plots the raw AUC against dose for each individual subject. In this example, there are two cohorts of six patients, the subjects in the first cohort receive doses 10, 20 and 40 mg and those in the second 80, 160 and 320 mg. We can see that, by plotting on the arithmetic scale, the top dose cohort visually dominates the graph and hence too much emphasis is given to these.

Note also how on the arithmetic scale the variance seems to increase with dose and consequently, as discussed in Chapter 2, on this scale a measure of variability would need to be quoted for each dose.

The intercept for this graph should be at 0 if the data are dose proportional and so the figure is worth producing for this eye-ball inspection.

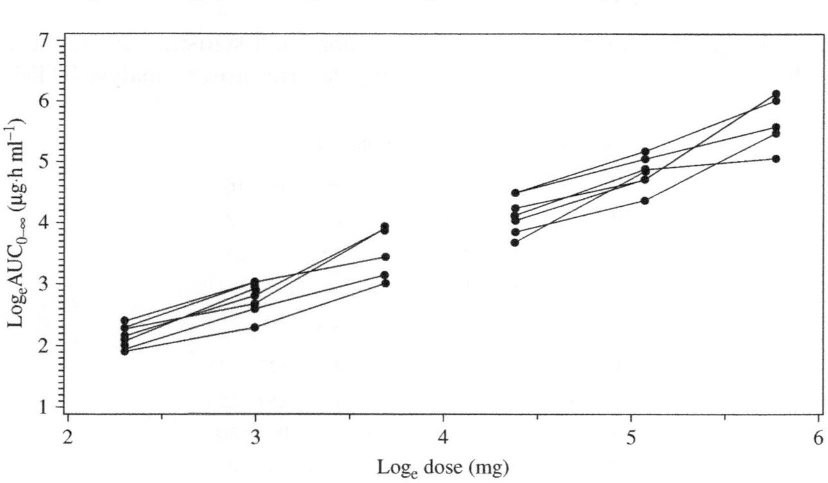

Figure 6.7 log$_e$ AUC against log$_e$ dose.

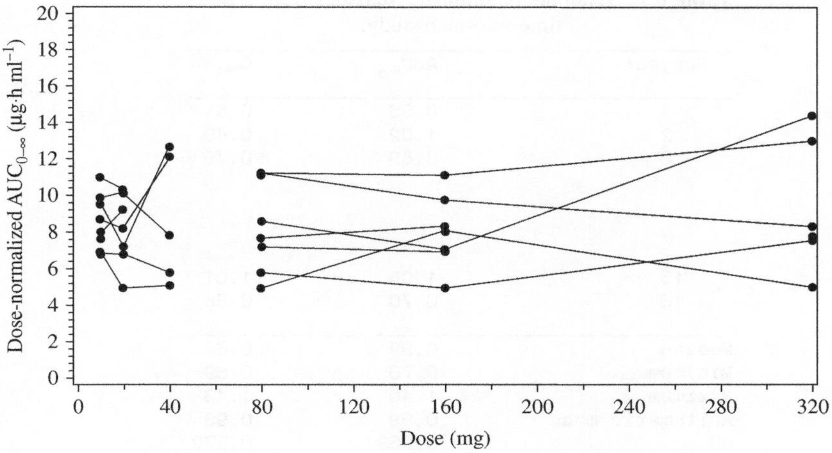

Figure 6.8 Dose-normalized AUC against dose.

A more useful approach is to plot both AUC and dose on the log scale as in Figure 6.7. Note how the variance is now stabilized – hence a single variability estimate can be given across all doses – and also how more equal emphasis is now placed on all the doses across the two cohorts. What is now more apparent is how the doses are confounded with the dosing cohorts (Cohort 1 – low doses, Cohort 2 – high doses).

If the data are dose proportional then the slope in this plot should be unity.

Figure 6.8 gives a plot of the dose-normalized AUC against dose. Dose-normalizing is done by dividing AUC by the dose given, and in this instance, further multiplied by 10. Here again the top doses are given too much emphasis, as was the case in Figure 6.6.

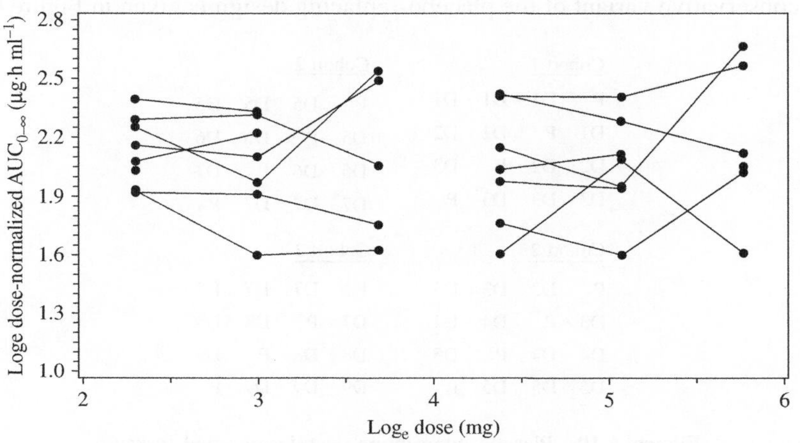

Figure 6.9 Dose-normalized $\log_e$ AUC against $\log_e$ dose.

Table 6.1 Example of summary statistics from a first-time-into-man study.

Subject	$AUC_{0-\infty}$	C_{max}
1	0.93	0.81
2	1.02	0.89
3	0.89	0.79
.		
.		
.		
15	1.05	1.01
16	0.70	0.68
Median	0.99	0.88
Minimum	0.70	0.69
Maximum	1.40	1.43
Arithmetic mean	0.99	0.93
SD	0.239	0.273

After dose normalizing, the slope should be zero. Note how here too the variability is stabilized. This is because variability multiplicatively rises with dose and so by dividing by dose, it is stabilized.

In the context of Figures 6.6 to 6.9, descriptive statistics could be obtained from the individual slopes for each subject in the study. For example, for each subject, individual regression analyses of log(AUC) against log(dose) could be computed and the slopes of these individual regressions used as the summary measure. We can then undertake descriptive statistics on these slopes, as in Table 6.1.

6.2.2 PLACEBO-INTERRUPTING DESIGN: LAST DOSE CARRIED FORWARD

A more conservative variant of the placebo-replacing design is given in Figure 6.10.

Cohort 1

P	D1	D1	D1
D1	P	D2	D2
D2	D2	P	D3
D3	D3	D3	P

Cohort 2

P	D5	D5	D5
D5	P	D6	D6
D6	D6	P	D7
D7	D7	D7	P

Cohort 2

P	D3	D3	D3
D3	P	D4	D4
D4	D4	P	D5
D5	D5	D5	P

Cohort 2

P	D7	D7	D7
D7	P	D8	D8
D8	D8	P	D9
D9	D9	D9	P

Figure 6.10 Placebo-interrupting last-dose-carried-forward first-time-into-man design.

Here, each dosing cohort is started with a dose known to be tolerable via evidence from a previous cohort, prior to escalating to new doses. In the same amount of time, it investigates 9 doses compared to 12 (Figure 6.4); but this conservativeness is probably the feature that may make the design preferable for certain investigative treatments.

6.2.3 PLACEBO-REPLACING DESIGN

Here, as the title of the design suggests, instead of interrupting a dose – such that a subject will receive all doses – in this design placebo actually replaces a dose, as summarized in Figure 6.11. For example, a subject who received placebo rather than D1 in period one then receives D2 in the second period without actually receiving D1. Hence, we would be relying on the safety and tolerability data of other subjects to escalate each individual subject if they previously had placebo. As compared to Figure 6.4, this design investigates 15 doses in the same timeframe and in the same number of subjects.

6.2.4 INTERLOCKING-COHORT PLACEBO-INTERRUPTING DESIGN

For most FTIM studies the aim would be to have two dosing sessions per week. However, there may be instances where the half-life of the compound (usually pharmacokinetic, but could also be pharmacodynamic) prevents having two dosing sessions, and in some cases even one each successive week would not be possible.

Interlocking the dosing cohorts could be a solution in this difficulty. Here, subjects in a second cohort are dosed during the washout phase of the first cohort as illustrated in

Cohort 1				Cohort 3			
P	D1	D1	D1	P	D9	D9	D9
D2	P	D2	D2	D10	P	D10	D10
D3	D3	P	D3	D11	D11	P	D11
D4	D4	D4	P	D12	D12	D12	P

Cohort 2				Cohort 4			
P	D5	D5	D5	P	D13	D13	D13
D6	P	D6	D6	D14	P	D14	D14
D7	D7	P	D7	D15	D15	P	D15
D8	D8	D8	P	D16	D16	D16	P

Figure 6.11 Placebo-replacing first-time-into-man design.

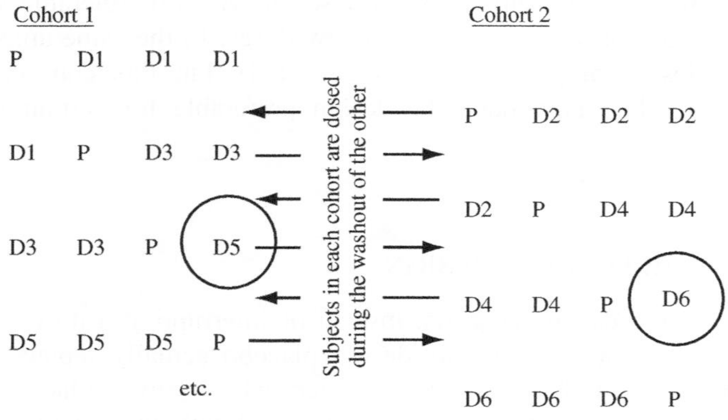

Figure 6.12 An interlocking-cohort study for a first-time-into-man design.

Figure 6.12. This has doubling dose increments across subjects and quadruple increments within subjects.

Such a design could have a major impact on the length of a study, potentially halving duration. For example if the design in Figure 6.4 was dosed once a week it would take 16 weeks, compared to 8 weeks if the cohorts were interlocked. This could lead to substantial saving especially as first FTIM studies are on the critical path.

One issue with the design, as highlighted in Figure 6.12, could be that very few subjects at different stages in a trial may be used before a dosing increment is made. Here we have just one subject receiving D5 before another subject receives D6. This may be less of an issue for studies with larger sample sizes.

An advantage of an interlocking design is that all subjects receive a greater range of doses, such that although dose cohorts are still confounded with dose they are not confounded with dose range. Thus, in Figure 6.12 Cohort 1 has doses ranging from D1 to D5 while Cohort 2 has doses ranging from D2 to D6. An example of the outcome from an interlocking first-time-into-man design is given in Figure 6.13.

6.2.5 INTERLOCKING-COHORT PLACEBO-REPLACING DESIGN

The design of Figure 6.14 is a variant of the interlocking design but with 'placebo replacing' rather than 'interrupting'. This design has an additional advantage, in that as well as going through the doses more rapidly it also has a greater number of subjects on each dose. Here, for the sample size of four, we always have three subjects on a dose prior to an escalation.

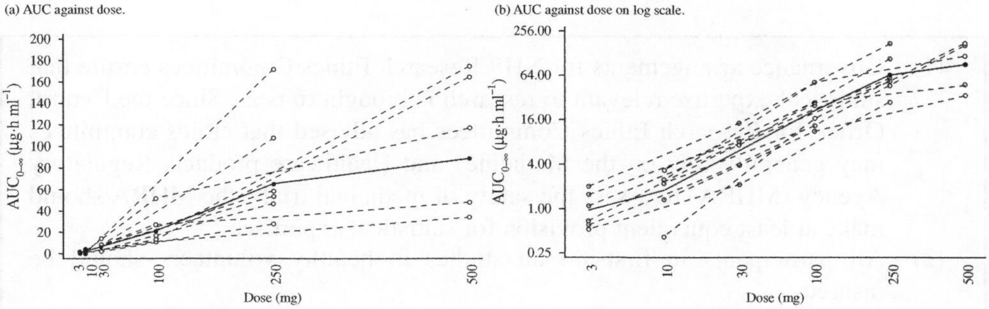

Figure 6.13 Results of a placebo-replacing first-time-into-man design.

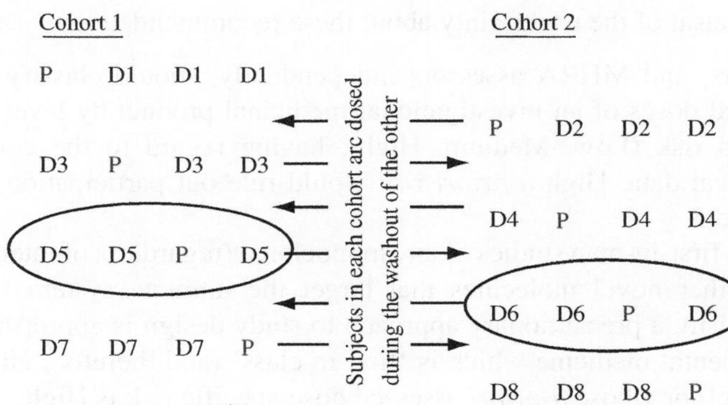

Figure 6.14 Placebo-replacing first-time-into-man design.

6.3 FIRST-TIME-INTO-MAN STUDIES IN LIGHT OF TGN1412

In light of the TeGenero trial of TGN1412 undertaken by Parexel at their Northwick Park Hospital trials unit, where subjects in a FTIM study suffered severe adverse reactions, the working party of Senn *et al.* (2007) issued a report on FTIM studies and made 21 recommendations as to the design and analysis. These recommendations are summarized below.

(1) Governance arrangements for NHS Research Ethics Committees ensure that statistical expertise relevant to research is brought to bear. Since the Central Office for Research Ethics Committees has advised that ethics committees may generally rely on the Medicines and Healthcare products Regulatory Agency (MHRA) to assess the safety of medicinal trials, the MHRA should make at least equivalent provision for statistical expertise.

(2) All participants in first-in-man studies in healthy volunteers should be insured.

(3) Studies wherein even the remote possibility of such complications as cytokine storm has been foreseen should be carried out only in hospitals with full facilities for giving tertiary care.

(4) Before proceeding to a first-in-man study, there should be:

- Quantitative justification of the starting dose – based on suitable preclinical studies and relevant calculations.
- *A priori* assessment of the risk level for the recommended study dose(s).
- Appraisal of the uncertainty about these recommendations.

(5) Sponsors, and MHRA assessors independently, should classify the finally proposed doses of an investigational medicinal product by level of *a-priori* assessed risk (Low, Medium, High), having regard to the confidence in preclinical data. High *a-priori* risk would rule out participation by healthy volunteers.

(6) Besides first-in-man studies of any monoclonal (regardless of intended target) or of other novel molecules that target the immune system via a novel mechanism, a precautionary approach to study design is appropriate for any experimental medicine which is 'first in class' (and therefore High *a-priori* risk level) or whose *a-priori* assessed dose-specific risk is High.

(7) Assessment described in 3 above should be available in a separate document – to be provided to research ethics committee, study participants, and insurers.

(8) Crude interspecies scaling may be inadequate for establishing the initial dose of 'biological' treatments in man. *In-vitro* studies using human cells will be necessary to establish the avidity of the ligands for their targets and assist in dose calculation.

(9) Unless arguments have been provided that the risk is so low that simultaneous treatments are acceptable, in order to allow early evidence of toxicity to halt the trial without risk to subsequent subjects, a proper, or sufficient, inter-administration interval needs to be proposed and observed.

(10) First-in-man study protocols should provide:

- Justification of the proper interval between administration to successive subjects.
- Justification of the dose steps the trial will use.

- Operational definition of 'safety' if investigating safety and tolerability.
- Delay between receiving biomarker or other laboratory results which determine 'safety' and having obtained the relevant biological sample.
- Prior estimates of the expected number (or rate) of adverse reactions by dose, especially those serious enough to raise questions about 'safety'.

(11) Appropriate sample sizes for first-in-man studies can be better justified statistically – rather than by mere custom and practice – when 'safety' has been given an operational definition.

(12) First-in-man study protocols should discuss their chosen design and its limitations together with the implications for analysis. For example, if an unequal allocation between treatment and placebo per dose step is chosen, this affects the ability of the data-safety monitors to assess tolerability most efficiently before proceeding to a further dose-escalation step.

(13) First-in-man study protocols should describe their intended analysis in sufficient detail to allow protocol reviewers (and the independent research ethics committee) to determine if the objectives, design and proposed analyses are compatible.

(14) The design of first-in-man trials and the analysis of the data should reflect realistic models of the pharmacokinetic data.

(15) The plan for blood sampling, and analysis and observation of vital signs should be based on information from preclinical studies.

(16) For first-in-man studies, the standard of informed consent to be observed is 'open protocol, hidden allocation' – that is, all aspects of the trial design shall be shared with subjects to be recruited.

(17) Public debate and research are needed about the maximum acceptable level of risk for first-in-man studies in healthy volunteers and about whether there should be risk-adjusted remuneration of healthy volunteers.

(18) Competent drug regulatory authorities should provide a mechanism for the pharmaceutical industry to collect and share data on serious adverse reactions in first-in-man studies – to improve *a-priori* risk assessment.

(19) Statistical reporting of preclinical studies should be improved to be comparable to the requirements by the International Conference on Harmonization for the reporting of clinical trials: see ICH E9.

(20) Greater use should be made of numerical, as opposed to verbal, descriptions of risk and statistical variation in the submissions made to, and accepted by, competent drug regulatory authorities.

(21) Mock applications to Competent Authorities convey expected standards. They should be revised to: (a) be in conformity with the preceding recommendations on the statistical reporting of preclinical studies, (b) require always that a proper interadministration interval between successive subjects is both specified and justified, (c) specify the waiting time for laboratory-based results which pertain to 'safety'.

Julious (2007) wrote a commentary on the report and, in addition to the recommendations above, made four additional suggestions:

- Volunteers should be paid according to risk.
- The group that decides on the dosing decisions should have a charter similar to that for data monitoring committees and should have core representation to make decisions including a physician and a statistician.
- For new areas where there could be a potential concern as to the reliability of the animal models, consideration should be given to having external representation on the group monitoring doses, maybe in the form of an independent chair.
- Consideration should be given to dose escalation decisions for subjects not being based on dose but on individual observed pharmacokinetic exposures, with the decision as to the next dose being made for each individual depending on their individual exposures.

The recommendations from the Royal Statistical Society themselves are not contentious and the document has been widely well received and had considerable impact. As a consequence, changes in the conduct of such trials have been initiated especially for new investigative treatments that target a new clinical pharmacology.

For certain compounds, however, it may not be appropriate to use healthy volunteers in the first-into-man study. When considering whether to use healthy volunteers or patients the CHMP (2007a) make the following general points:

> The choice of the study population, i.e. healthy subjects or patients, including special populations, should be fully justified by the sponsor on a case-by-case basis. Several factors should be considered, such as:
>
> (a) the risks inherent in the type of medicinal product – it is important that those risks (and uncertainty about them) be quantified and justified;
> (b) its molecular target;
> (c) immediate and potential long-term toxicity;
> (d) the lack of a relevant animal model;
> (e) the relative presence of the target in healthy subjects or in patients, e.g. cancer patients;
> (f) the possible higher variability in patients;
> (g) the ability of healthy volunteers to tolerate any potential side effects;
> (h) the potential pharmacogenomic difference between the targeted patient group and healthy subjects;
> (i) the patients' ability to benefit from other products or interventions; and
> (j) the predicted therapeutic window of the IMP [investigative medicinal product].

In addition for the starting dose, the CHMP (2007a), as well as discussing NOAEL, highlight the need to consider the dose which has the minimal anticipated biological effect:

> In general, the No Observed Adverse Effect Level (NOAEL) determined in nonclinical safety studies performed in the most sensitive and relevant animal species, adjusted with allometric factors or on the basis of pharmacokinetics gives the most important information. The relevant

dose is then reduced/adjusted by appropriate safety factors according to the particular aspects of the molecule and the design of the clinical trials. For investigational medicinal products for which factors influencing risk have been identified, an additional approach to dose calculation should be taken. Information about pharmacodynamics can give further guidance for dose selection. The 'Minimal Anticipated Biological Effect Level' (MABEL) approach is recommended. The MABEL is the anticipated dose level leading to a minimal biological effect level in humans. When using this approach, potential differences of sensitivity for the mode of action of the investigational medicinal product between humans and animals, need to be taken into consideration e.g. derived from *in-vitro* studies. A safety factor may be applied for the calculation of the first dose in human from MABEL as discussed below.

The calculation of MABEL should utilize all *in-vitro* and *in-vivo* information available from pharmacokinetic/pharmacodynamic (PK/PD) data.

6.3.1 IMPACT ON STUDY DESIGN

The study designs described so far in this chapter have been generic, to convey some of the main types used in first-time-into-man studies. However, consideration should be given to adjust these designs for compounds with a new pharmacology. A joint report by the Association of the British Pharmaceutical Industry (ABPI) and BioIndustry Association (BIA) made the following points for first-time-into-man studies (ABPI/BIA, 2006):

> Two or more subjects should only be dosed on the same day if there is no reason to expect significant adverse effects with delayed onset. If such effects are expected then subsequent subjects should only be dosed after the expected time period for the effects has expired. . . . In general subsequent subjects should be dosed in cohorts of no more than 3 or 4 and sometimes less. The absence of adverse effects in the first subject provides reassurance that adverse effects are not universal but adverse effects could still be quite common so increasing the numbers exposed at each dose level should be relatively gradual.
>
> It is recommended that at least three or four subjects receive a given dose level prior to any subjects receiving a higher dose.

We will now show how the general study designs can be applied to the situation where a drug is to target a new pharmacology.

6.3.1.1 Placebo-Interrupting Design

Previously we have used some basic dosing panels to describe how a design may be applied. We now go into a little more detail regarding the rows and columns as in Table 6.2, which gives just one cohort of eight subjects of a sequential cohort design where subjects and dosing sessions are labelled.

To minimize risk therefore, for any new dose only one subject can be given the new dose on a given day prior to the remainder of the subjects in the dosing cohort, as illustrated in Table 6.3. For example, for D1 (which is the first dose given) in Session 1 on Day 1, one

Table 6.2 Placebo-interrupting design for the first cohort.

	Dosing session			
Subject	1	2	3	4
1	P	D1	D2	D3
2	P	D1	D2	D3
3	D1	P	D2	D3
4	D1	P	D2	D3
5	D1	D2	P	D3
6	D1	D2	P	D3
7	D1	D2	D3	P
8	D1	D2	D3	P

subject receives this dose (and one receives placebo). On the next day in this session, five other subjects receive D1 (and one receives placebo). Session 2 and Session 3 are similar to Session 1 but for a new dose. In the final session, 4, because this uses a dose already given, all subjects can be dosed at the same time.

It is important to highlight that, although staggering administration of doses between two days within the same period won't have any major impact on randomization, it does need to be considered when randomizing subjects.

Generally we would randomize subjects to a certain sequence as if the design was not staggered. FTIM studies are generally single blind, and we can hence determine to which treatment sequence each subject has been randomized. For example, in Table 6.3 the sequences currently allocated to Subjects 2 and 3 may actually be assigned to Subject 1 and 7 (say), and so these subjects will come in for the first day's dosing. Hence we would know, for example, that on the first day of Period 1, Subject 1 has taken placebo (say) and Subject 7 has taken D1.

For double-blind studies, the statistician would randomize subjects as if the design was not staggered. Then someone involved in the study who is not blind (e.g. the pharmacist) would identify the subjects assigned to the appropriate sequence for each session.

Table 6.3 Placebo-interrupting design with staggered dosing for the first cohort.

	Dosing session						
	1		2		3		4
	Day		Day		Day		
Subject	1	2	1	2	1	2	
1		P		D1		D2	D3
2	P			D1		D2	D3
3	D1			P		D2	D3
4		D1	P			D2	D3
5		D1	D2			P	D3
6		D1		D2	P		D3
7		D1		D2	D3		P
8		D1		D2		D3	P

Table 6.4 Placebo-replacing design for the first cohort.

	Dosing session			
Subject	1	2	3	4
1	P	D2	D3	D4
2	P	D2	D3	D4
3	D1	P	D3	D4
4	D1	P	D3	D4
5	D1	D2	P	D4
6	D1	D2	P	D4
7	D1	D2	D3	P
8	D1	D2	D3	P

6.3.1.2 Placebo-Replacing Design

A placebo-replacing design is highlighted in Table 6.4, while Table 6.5 gives the same design but with staggered dosing. Note here how each dosing session, including the final one, has staggered dosing, as with each session subjects are given a new dose.

6.3.1.3 Interlocking-Cohort Placebo-Interrupting Design

An illustration of how a staggered dosing plan would work for an interlocking-cohort design (for example see Table 6.6) is given in Table 6.7.

6.3.1.4 Interlocking-Cohort Placebo-Replacing Design

An illustration of how a staggered dosing plan would work for an interlocking-cohort placebo-replacing design (for example, Table 6.8) is given in Table 6.9.

Table 6.5 Placebo-replacing design for the first cohort, with staggered dosing.

	Dosing session							
	1		2		3		4	
	Day		Day		Day		Day	
Subject	1	2	1	2	1	2	1	2
1		P		D2		D3	D4	
2	P			D2		D3		D4
3	D1			P		D3		D4
4		D1	P			D3		D4
5		D1	D2			P		D4
6		D1		D2	P			D4
7		D1		D2	D3		P	
8		D1		D2		D3		P

Table 6.6 Placebo-interrupting interlocking-cohort design for the first cohort.

		Dosing session			
Cohort	Subject	1	2	3	4
1	1	P	D1	D3	D5
	2	P	D1	D3	D5
	3	D1	P	D3	D5
	4	D1	P	D3	D5
	5	D1	D3	P	D5
	6	D1	D3	P	D5
	7	D1	D3	D5	P
	8	D1	D3	D5	P
2	9	P	D2	D4	D6
	10	P	D2	D4	D6
	11	D2	P	D4	D6
	12	D2	P	D4	D6
	13	D2	D4	P	D6
	14	D2	D4	P	D6
	15	D2	D4	D6	P
	16	D2	D4	D6	P

Table 6.7 Placebo-interrupting interlocking-cohort design for the first cohort, with staggered dosing.

		Dosing session						
		1		2		3		4
		Day		Day		Day		
Cohort	Subject	1	2	1	2	1	2	
1	1		P		D1		D3	D5
	2	P			D1		D3	D5
	3	D1			P		D3	D5
	4		D1	P			D3	D5
	5		D1	D3			P	D5
	6		D1		D3	P		D5
	7		D1		D3	D5		P
	8		D1		D3		D5	P
2	9		P		D2		D4	D6
	10	P			D2		D4	D6
	11	D2			P		D4	D6
	12		D2	P			D4	D6
	13		D2	D4			P	D6
	14		D2		D4	P		D6
	15		D2		D4	D6		P
	16		D2		D4		D6	P

Table 6.8 Placebo-replacing interlocking design for the first cohort.

		Dosing session			
Cohort	Subject	1	2	3	4
1	1	P	D3	D5	D7
	2	P	D3	D5	D7
	3	D1	P	D5	D7
	4	D1	P	D5	D7
	5	D1	D3	P	D7
	6	D1	D3	P	D7
	7	D1	D3	D5	P
	8	D1	D3	D5	P
2	9	P	D4	D6	D8
	10	P	D4	D6	D8
	11	D2	P	D6	D8
	12	D2	P	D6	D8
	13	D2	D4	P	D8
	14	D2	D4	P	D8
	15	D2	D4	D6	P
	16	D2	D4	D6	P

Table 6.9 Placebo-replacing interlocking design for the first cohort, with staggered dosing.

		Dosing session						
		1		2		3		4
		Day		Day		Day		Day
Cohort	Subject	1	2	1	2	1	2	1
1	1		P		D3		D5	D7
	2	P			D3		D5	
	3	D1			P		D5	
	4		D1	P			D5	
	5		D1	D3			P	
	6		D1		D3	P		
	7		D1		D3	D5		
	8		D1		D3		D5	P
2	9		P		D4		D6	D8
	10	P			D4		D6	
	11	D2			P		D6	
	12		D2	P			D6	
	13		D2	D4			P	
	14		D2		D4	P		
	15		D2		D4	D6		
	16		D2		D4		D6	P

6.4 ANALYSIS OF FIRST-TIME-INTO-MAN STUDIES

Although FTIM studies are mainly exploratory in nature, pharmacokinetic data from a wide range of doses is derived which could be analysed to give a preliminary assessment of the dose proportionality of the pharmacokinetics. Here we describe how to make such an early assessment, while Chapter 10 will discuss more definitive assessments.

6.4.1 ANALYSIS 1: ANALYSIS OF VARIANCE

The first approach is an ANOVA where the dose-normalized and logged dose-dependent pharmacokinetic parameters (such as AUC, C_{max}) for each dose are compared in a pair-wise manner with the reference dose. As the data are dose normalized (and hence dose independent), the ratio for each comparison should be unity.

SAS code from the analysis is given in Figure 6.15. Subject tends to have to be declared as a random term as in the contrasts there is a mixture of intra- (within cohort) and inter- (across cohort) comparisons.

There is an issue with this approach in that FTIM studies may have very little data with respect to the sample sizes and number of subjects per dose. Also the pharmacokinetic profile will often be poorly defined – particularly for early doses – as these are learning studies.

It should be noted also that often $AUC_{0-\infty}$ for the first dose(s) is not well characterized. The reference dose would hence be the first with a well characterized $AUC_{0-\infty}$.

Due to the small sample sizes a more appropriate approach could be the power method for assessment of dose proportionality.

6.4.2 ANALYSIS 2: POWER METHOD

The power method for AUC (or C_{max}) is described by

$$AUC = a(Dose)^b. \qquad (6.1)$$

```
PROC mixed noitprint order = internal DATA = pk;
 CLASS subject dose;
 MODEL lnauc = dose /p;
 RANDOM subject;
  ESTIMATE 'd1-d2'  TMT  1 0 0 0 -1 0 / cl alpha = 0.1 e;
  ESTIMATE 'd1-d3'  TMT  0 1 0 0 -1 0 / cl alpha = 0.1 e;
  ESTIMATE 'd1-d4'  TMT  0 0 1 0 -1 0 / cl alpha = 0.1 e;
  ESTIMATE 'd1-d5'  TMT  0 0 0 1 -1 0 / cl alpha = 0.1 e;
  ESTIMATE 'd1-d6'  TMT  0 0 0 0 -1 1 / cl alpha = 0.1 e;
RUN;
```

Figure 6.15 Example SAS code for the analysis of variance method.

(With the power method, instead of fitting dose as a class term in the ANOVA model, log dose is fitted as a linear term, as suggested by Gough *et al.* (1995)). Thus

$$log(AUC) = log(a) + b \cdot log(Dose). \tag{6.2}$$

Hence, for dose-dependent variables we should have $b = 1$, while for dose-independent variables we should have $b = 0$.

The power model is so called because the slopes can be back-transformed and represented in terms of a power. Supposing we were logging to base 2; we would have

$$log_2(AUC) = b \cdot log_2(Dose). \tag{6.3}$$

Hence, the power 2^b from the model would give you the ratio of AUCs per doubling of dose.

However, for dose-dependent pharmacokinetic measures a better transformation would be

$$2^{b-1}. \tag{6.4}$$

This is the ratio of dose-normalized AUCs per doubling of dose. This should equal unity if the data are dose proportional.

6.4.2.1 Worked Example 6.1

The following analysis is that of an indicative first-time-into-man study. The SAS code used for the analysis is given in Figure 6.16.

Note how here we use SAS ODS to output the data. The model has random slope and intercept. Note too the variance–covariance matrix is output. This will be used in additional analyses described in Section 6.4.3.

The model contrasts, given in Figure 6.17, are back-transformed to derive the ratio of dose-normalized AUC per doubling of dose. The point estimate and its corresponding confidence interval can be used for inference.

For the worked example, the slope and its 90% confidence interval are

$$b = 1.0061, \text{ CI } (0.9348 \textit{ to } 1.0775). \tag{6.5}$$

Hence, the ratio for dose-normalized AUCs per dose doubling and associated 90% CI are

$$2^{(1.0061-1)} = 1.004, \text{ CI } (0.956 \textit{ to } 1.055). \tag{6.6}$$

Can we declare the data to be dose proportional?

There are no clear guidelines on the assessment of dose proportionality. The Health Canada Expert Advisory Committee on Bioavailability and Bioequivalence (2003) states:

> ... evidence is provided to show that the dose-normalized concentrations deviate (increase or decrease) by less than 25% [sic] over the labeled dose range for the proposed indication.

```
***********************************************************;
**** Doing the Power Model with Random Slope and Intercept     ***;
***********************************************************;
ODS output solutionF = beta;
ODS output covb = covar;
ODS output estimates = est;
PROC mixed data = pkdata1 noitprint order=internal;
  CLASS subject1;
  MODEL lauc = ldose /s ddfm = satterth covb;
  RANDOM intercept ldose /subject = subject1;
  ESTIMATE 'ldose' ldose 1 /cl alpha = 0.1;
  RUN;

********************************************************;
***Dose-Normalized Back-Transformed Slope            ****;
********************************************************;
 DATA est1;
 SET est;
 r = 2**(Estimate-1);
 lowerr = 2**(lower-1);
 upperr = 2**(upper-1);
 RUN;

TITLE 'Output from Power Model';
PROC print;VAR b lowerb upperb; RUN;
```

Solution for Fixed Effects

Effect	Estimate	Standard Error	DF	t Value	Pr > |t|
Intercept	-0.2300	0.1556	21.6	-1.48	0.1538
ldose	1.0061	0.04175	24.8	24.10	<.0001

Covariance Matrix for Fixed Effects

Row	Effect	Col1	Col2
1	Intercept	0.02422	-0.00603
2	ldose	-0.00603	0.001743

Figure 6.16 Example SAS Code and output of $\log_e$ AUC against $\log_e$ dose from a first-time-into-man study.

Hence, assuming this implies that the limits 0.80 to 1.25 are to be used, and suppose the dose range is a fourfold one, then the point estimate and CI are

$$4^{(1.0061-1)} = 1.008, \text{ CI } (0.914 \text{ to } 1.113). \tag{6.7}$$

Output from Power Model
The Mixed Procedure

Type 3 Tests of Fixed Effects

Effect	Num DF	Den DF	F Value	Pr > F
ldose	1	24.8	580.70	<.0001

Estimates

Label	Estimate	Standard Error	DF	t Value	Pr > |t|	Alpha	Lower	Upper
ldose	1.0061	0.04175	24.8	24.10	<.0001	0.1	0.9348	1.0775

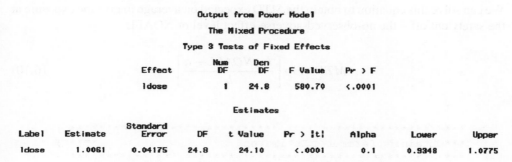

Figure 6.17 Example contrasts from a first-time-into-man analysis.

Consequently this could be considered as sufficient evidence for a claim of dose proportionality.

6.4.3 ADDITIONAL ANALYSES

We have the model

$$AUC = exp[a + b\,log(Dose)], \tag{6.8}$$

which in our example earlier was estimated by

$$AUC = exp[-0.231 + 1.0061 \cdot log(Dose)]. \tag{6.9}$$

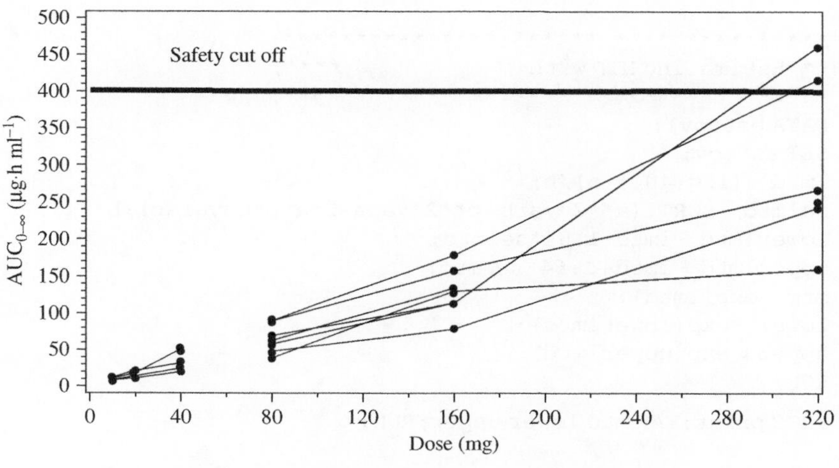

Figure 6.18 First-time-in-man study with safety cut off.

We can solve this equation to obtain the MTD expected on average to give the exposure at the safety cut off – the no-observed-adverse-effect level or NOAEL

$$MTD{=}exp\left[\frac{logNOAEL - a}{b}\right]. \tag{6.10}$$

```
*****************************************************;
***Obtaining Parameter Estimates                *****;
*****************************************************;
DATA beta1 (keep = estimate rename = (estimate = a))
     beta2 (keep = estimate rename = (estimate = b));
SET beta;
if effect = 'Intercept' then output beta1;
if effect = 'ldose'      then output beta2;
RUN;

*****************************************************;
***Obtaining Variance-Covariance Estimates       ****;
*****************************************************;
DATA covar1 (keep = col1 rename = (col1=vara))
     covar2 (keep = col1 rename = (col1=covarab))
     covar3 (keep = col2 rename = (col2=varb));
SET covar;
if effect = 'Intercept' then output covar1;
if effect = 'ldose'      then output covar2;
if effect = 'ldose'      then output covar3;
RUN;

DATA estcov;MERGE beta1 beta2 covar1 covar2 covar3;RUN;

*************************************;
***Estimating MTD with CI        ****;
*************************************;
DATA estcov1;
SET estcov;
lmtd = (log(400)-a)/b;
selmtd = SQRT((a**2*varb+b**2*vara-2*a*b*covarab)/b**4);
lowerlmtd = lmtd-1.64*selmtd;
upperlmtd = lmtd+1.64*selmtd;
mtd = exp(lmtd);
lower = exp(lowerlmtd);
upper = exp(upperlmtd);
RUN;

PROC print;VAR mtd lower upper;RUN;
```

Figure 6.19 SAS code for calculating MTD and confidence interval.

Suppose for our example that the NOAEL was set for the mean AUC to be below 400, so that if we do not wish to have the mean exposure exceed this value, we would choose

$$MTD = exp\left[\frac{log 400 + 0.2300}{1.0061}\right] = 484.79. \tag{6.11}$$

The variance for this is

$$Var(MTD) \approx \frac{a^2 Var(b) + b^2 Var(a) - 2ab Cov(a, b)}{b^4} \tag{6.12}$$

This is estimated from Var(a) = 0.02422, Var(b) = 0.001743 and Cov(a,b) = −0.00603, of the covariance matrix in the SAS output of Figure 6.16. These lead to a 90% CI (388.612 to 615.871).

Note Patterson and Jones (2006) recommend bootstrapping to calculate the CI, although Fieller's theorem could also be used.

Note too that these MTD calculations can involve extrapolating beyond the range of the data.

Example SAS code is given in Figure 6.19 for this analysis.

7 Bayesian and Frequentist Methods

7.1 INTRODUCTION

So far we have discussed very little statistical inference for early phase trials, as often these trials are exploratory in nature. In the context of succeeding chapters however it is now worth taking an aside to discuss Bayesian and frequentist inferential assessments in the framework of early phase trials.

7.2 FREQUENTIST APPROACHES

For late-phase development, frequentist methods are, and probably will remain, the main way for assessing evidence of benefit for a given regimen. In this context, trials are assessed through *a priori* declaring a null hypothesis, depending on the objective of the trial, and then formally testing this null hypothesis through the trial data obtained.

7.2.1 HYPOTHESIS TESTING AND ESTIMATION

Consider the hypothetical example of a study designed to examine the effectiveness of two treatments for migraine. In the study, patients are randomly allocated to two groups corresponding to either treatment A or treatment B. It may be that the primary objective of the trial is to investigate whether there is a difference between the two groups with respect to migraine outcome; in this case we could carry out a significance test and calculate a P-value (hypothesis testing). Alternatively it may be that the primary objective is to quantify the difference between treatments together with a corresponding range of plausible values for the difference; in this case we would calculate the difference in migraine response for the two treatments and the associated confidence interval for this difference (estimation).

7.2.2 HYPOTHESIS TESTING

Figure 7.1 reviews the essential steps in the process of hypothesis testing that we have discussed earlier. At the outset it is important to have a clear research question and identify the outcome variable to be compared. Once the research question has been stated, the null

An Introduction to Statistics in Early Phase Trials Steven A. Julious, Say Beng Tan and David Machin

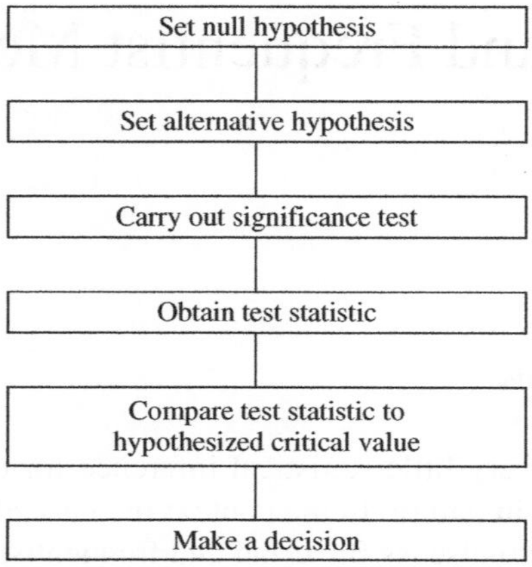

Figure 7.1 Hypothesis testing: the main steps.

and alternative hypotheses can be formulated. Here we will assume that the null hypothesis (H_0), as will often be the case, assumes that there is no difference in the outcome of interest between the study groups, and that the alternative hypothesis (H_1) states that there is a difference between the study groups.

A common misunderstanding about the null and alternative hypotheses is that, when carrying out a statistical test, it is the alternative hypothesis (that there is a difference) that is being tested. This is not the case – what is being examined is the null hypothesis, that there is no difference between the study groups; we conduct a hypothesis test in order to establish how likely (in terms of probability) it is that we have obtained the results that we have obtained, if there truly is no difference in the population.

For the migraine trial, the research question of interest is:

'For patients with chronic migraines, which treatment for migraine is the most effective?'

There may be several outcomes for this study, such as the frequency of migraine attacks, the duration of individual attacks or the total duration of attacks. Assuming we are interested in reducing the frequency of attacks, then the null hypothesis, H_0, for this research question is:

'There is no difference in the frequency of attacks between treatment A and treatment B groups.'

and the alternative hypothesis, H_1, is:

'There is a difference in the frequency of attacks between the two treatment groups.'

In general, the direction of the difference (for example: that treatment A is better than treatment B) is not specified, and this is known as a two-sided (or two-tailed) test. By specifying no direction we investigate both the possibility that A is better than B and the possibility that B is better than A. If a direction is specified, this is referred to as a one-sided test (one-tailed) and we would be evaluating only whether A is better then B, with the possibility of B being better than A of no interest. There will be further discussion of one-tailed and two-tailed tests when describing bioequivalence trials in Chapter 9.

Having set the null and alternative hypotheses, the next stage is to carry out a significance test. This is done by first calculating a test statistic using the study data. This test statistic is then compared to a theoretical value under the null hypothesis in order to obtain a P-value. The final and most crucial stage of hypothesis testing is to make a decision, based upon the P-value. In order to do this it is necessary to first understand what a P-value is and what it is not, and then understand how to use it to make a decision about whether to reject or not reject the null hypothesis.

So what does a P-value mean? A P-value is the probability of obtaining the study results (or results more extreme) if the null hypothesis is true. Common misinterpretations of the P-value are that it is either the probability of the data having arisen by chance, or the probability that the observed effect is not a real one. The distinction between these incorrect definitions and the true definition is the absence of the phrase: 'when the null hypothesis is true'. The omission of this phrase leads to the incorrect belief that it is possible to evaluate the probability of the observed effect being a real one. The observed effect in the sample is genuine, but what is true for the entire population is not known. All that can be known with a P-value is, if there truly is no difference in the population, how likely is the result obtained (from the sample). Thus a small P-value indicates that the difference we have obtained is unlikely if there genuinely was no difference in the population – it gives the probability of obtaining the difference between the two study samples observed (or results more extreme) if there is actually no difference in the population.

In practice, what happens in a trial is that the null hypothesis that two treatments are the same is stated, that is, $A = B$ or $A - B = 0$. The trial is then conducted and a particular difference, $d = A - B$, is observed. Due to pure randomness, even if the two treatments are the same you would seldom observe $d = 0$. Now if d is small (say a 1% difference in the frequency of migraine attacks), then the probability of seeing this difference under the null hypothesis is very high, say $P = 0.995$. If a larger difference is observed, say $d = 0.05$, then the probability of seeing this difference by chance is reduced and the P-value could be $P = 0.562$. As the difference increases, therefore, so the P-value falls, such that $d = 0.20$ may equate to $P = 0.021$. This relationship is essentially illustrated in Figure 7.2; as d increases then the P-value (under the null hypothesis) will fall.

It is important to remember that a P-value is a probability, and its value can vary between 0 and 1. A 'small' P-value, say close to zero, indicates that the results obtained are unlikely if the null hypothesis is true: consequently the null hypothesis is rejected. Alternatively, if the P-value is 'large', then the results obtained are likely when the null hypothesis is true and the null hypothesis is not rejected. But how small is small? Conventionally, the cut-off value or two-sided significance level for declaring that a particular result is statistically significant is set at 0.05 (or 5%). Thus if the P-value is less than this value the null hypothesis (of no difference) is rejected and the result is said to be statistically significant at the 5% or 0.05 level (Table 7.1).

For the example above, if the P-value associated with the mean difference in the number of attacks was 0.01, as this is less than the cut-off value of 0.05 we would say that there was a statistically significant difference in the number of attacks between the two groups at the 5% level.

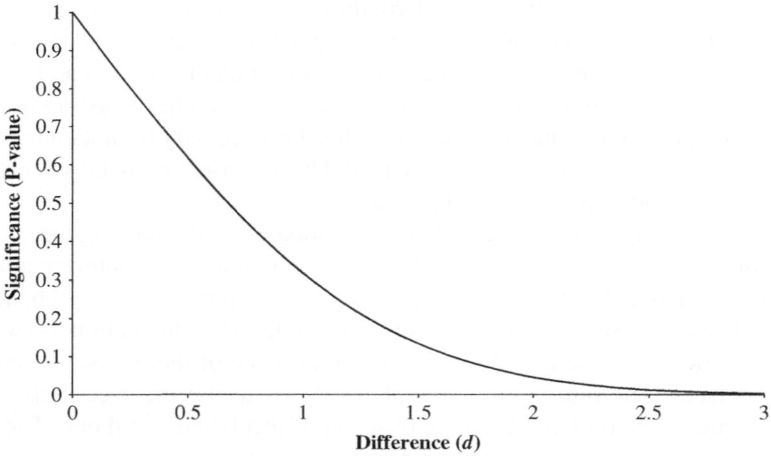

Figure 7.2 Hypothetical relationship between the observed difference and the P-value under the null hypothesis.

Table 7.1 Statistical significance.

	$P < 0.05$	$P \geq 0.05$
Result is	Statistically significant	Not statistically significant
Decide	That there is sufficient evidence to reject the null hypothesis and accept the alternative hypothesis	That there is insufficient evidence to reject the null hypothesis
	We say that our results are statistically significant if the P-value is less than the significance level (α), usually set at 5%	We can never say that the null hypothesis is true, only that there is not enough evidence to reject it

The choice of 5% is somewhat arbitrary, and though it is commonly used as a standard level for statistical significance, its use is not universal. Even where it is, one study that is statistically significant at the 5% level is not usually regarded as convincing enough to change practice; replication is required. For example, to get a regulatory license for a new drug, usually two statistically significant studies are required at the 5% level, which equates to a single study at the 0.00125 significance level. It is for this reason that larger 'super' studies are conducted to get significance levels that would change practice, that is, a lot less than 5%.

The significance level of 5% has, to a degree, become a 'tablet of stone'. To such a degree that it is not unknown for P-values to be presented as $P = 0.04999999$, as P must be less than 0.05 to be significant, and written to two decimal places $P = 0.05$ is considered to present far less evidence for rejection of the null hypothesis than $P = 0.04999999$.

7.2.3 ESTIMATION

Statistical significance does not necessarily mean the result obtained is clinically significant or of any practical importance. A P-value will only indicate how likely the results obtained are when the null hypothesis is true. It can only be used to decide whether the results are statistically significant or not, it does not give any information about the likely size of the clinical difference. Much more information, such as whether the result is likely to be of clinical importance, can be gained by calculating a confidence interval. This is particularly true for early phase trials which may not be sufficiently powered to detect a difference of clinical importance.

Technically, the 95% confidence interval is the range of values within which the true population quantity would fall 95% of the time if the study were to be repeated many times. Crudely speaking, the confidence interval gives a range of plausible values for the quantity estimated; although not strictly correct it is usually interpreted as the range of values within which there is 95% certainty that the true value in the population lies.

7.2.4 WORKED EXAMPLE 7.1

Suppose a Phase II trial is undertaken, where H_0 is that the prevalence (p) for a particular adverse event (AE) is greater than 10%, against the alternative H_1 that it is less than 10%. Formally this would be written as

$$H_0 : p \geq 0.10$$

$$H_1 : p < 0.10.$$

The hypothesis is to be investigated through constructing a 95% confidence interval and assessing if the upper tail for this is less than 10% (which is equivalent to undertaking a one-tailed test at the 2.5% level of significance). This is quite a simple example but is sufficient to illustrate both frequentist and Bayesian approaches.

Due to the low anticipated response rates, exact confidence intervals are applied that use the beta distribution, such that the lower confidence interval bound is defined as (Daly, 1992; Newcombe, 1998; Julious, 2005b)

$$1 - BETAINV(1 - \alpha/2, n - k + 1, k), \tag{7.1}$$

and upper as

$$BETAINV(1-\alpha/2, k+1, n-k). \tag{7.2}$$

Here, α is the level of statistical significance ($\alpha = 0.05$ would give 95% confidence intervals), k the number of AEs observed, and n the sample size in the investigation; and $BETAINV(\bullet)$ refers to the cumulative distribution function of a beta distribution.

Calculations using the beta distribution are referred to in some texts as Clopper–Pearson methods (Newcombe, 1998). The beta distribution and its link to the binomial distribution will be discussed in greater detail in Chapter 15 with a Go/No Go case study.

In the actual trial 223 subjects were enrolled on the active arm and 9 cases of the AE were observed. This gives an observed response rate of 4%. The 95% confidence interval is 1.8% to 7.5%. Hence as the confidence interval excludes 10% we reject the null hypothesis and accept the alternative, concluding that the true response is likely to be lower than 10%.

7.3 BAYESIAN APPROACHES

Our discussion so far in this chapter has been in the context of trials involving frequentist statistical approaches where a null hypothesis is first established; an experiment is conducted, and based on the strength of the evidence observed, the null hypothesis is 'accepted' or 'rejected'. The decision as to whether to accept or reject is based on the P-value and the confidence intervals.

However, the frequentist approach is somewhat naïve in some ways. For example, prior to the start of a (new) pivotal (basis for licence) Phase III trial, many earlier trials may have been initiated and/or completed. A frequentist approach excludes this pertinent work from consideration when the results of the pivotal trial are considered.

In simple terms, Bayesian approaches formally account for this related work (and/or of beliefs held by investigators) by setting *priors* before the start of a study. Once the trial has been completed, the observed data are combined with the priors to form a posterior distribution for the treatment response. This is done via the application of Bayes' theorem and the effects are best seen graphically. For example, Figure 7.3 shows the results from a study for the risk of a given event. From the figure, we see how the prior distribution has been 'superimposed' with the observed data (in the form of a likelihood distribution) to provide a posterior distribution. From this posterior distribution (95%) credibility intervals can then be calculated for the true value. This credible interval provides a range in which there is a 95% chance the true value of any difference will lie. (Note the difference between this definition and that for confidence intervals.)

Chapter 15 will give a detailed description of how to calculate credibility intervals and how different priors may affect the results.

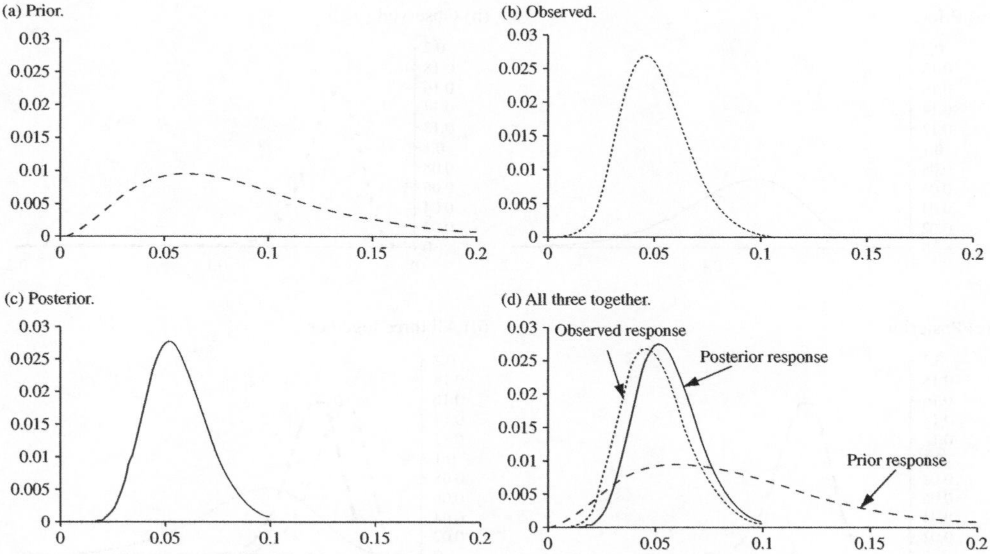

Figure 7.3 Prior distribution, observed and posterior distribution.

7.3.1 WORKED EXAMPLE 7.2

Repeating the earlier example where the observed AE rate was 9 / 223 subjects (4.0%). Suppose a pessimistic prior had been set *a priori*, and this specified that the most likely outcome was 7.5% subjects having an AE, together with a (at least) 90% certainty that the AE rate is less than 12.5%. Figure 7.4 gives the three distributions together. We can see how, with a pessimistic prior, the posterior distribution is centred around a higher risk than the observed response.

Hence, from the prior and the data, the anticipated posterior response rate is 5.2% (larger than 4.0% but smaller than 7.5%), with a credibility interval of 3.1 to 8.0%. The credibility interval still excludes 10%. Therefore, with this pessimistic prior, the posterior rate is higher than the observed likelihood distribution.

With a more optimistic prior that the most likely response is 2.5%, and at least 90% certain that it is less than 5%, Figure 7.5 gives the three distributions together. The prior now is centred around a slightly lower risk than observed. The effect would be that the point estimate and limits of the credibility interval will be less, and even further away from 10%.

Finally we have a noninformative prior, which corresponds to a uniform probability distribution over the whole range of possible values of 0 to 100%. Figure 7.6 gives the three distributions and we can see from this that the prior has little effect. Hence, the posterior response rate is 4.0%, with credibility interval of between 1.8% and 7.5% – about the same as that obtained for the confidence intervals previously.

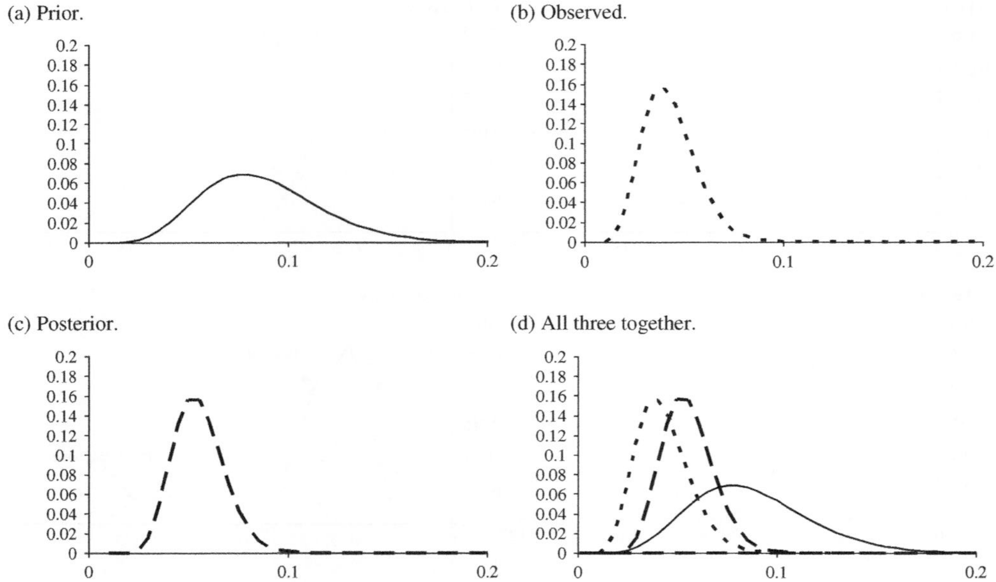

Figure 7.4 Prior distribution, observed and posterior distribution for a pessimistic prior.

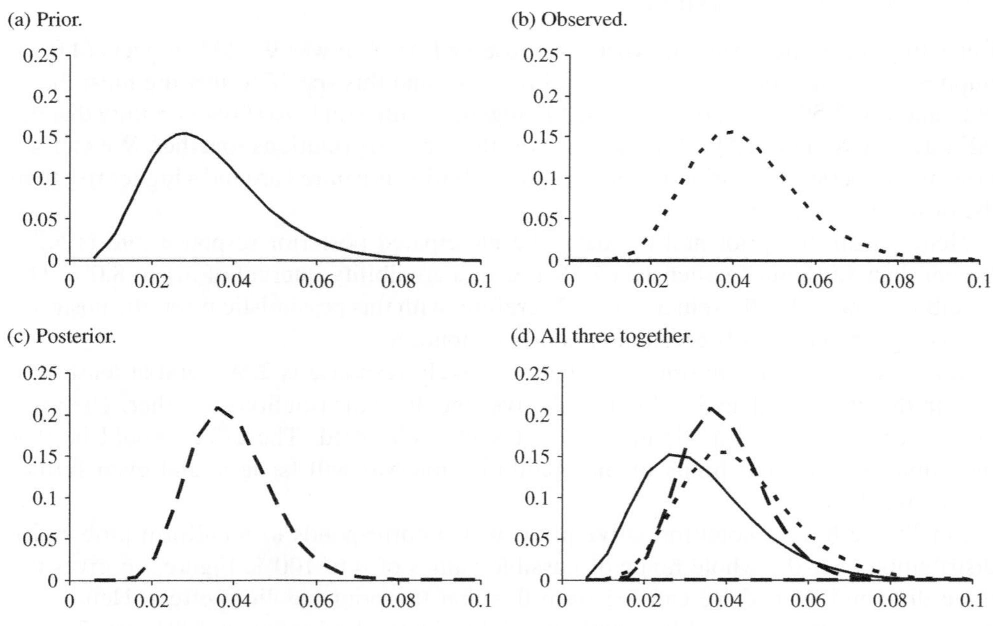

Figure 7.5 Prior distribution, observed and posterior distribution for an optimistic prior.

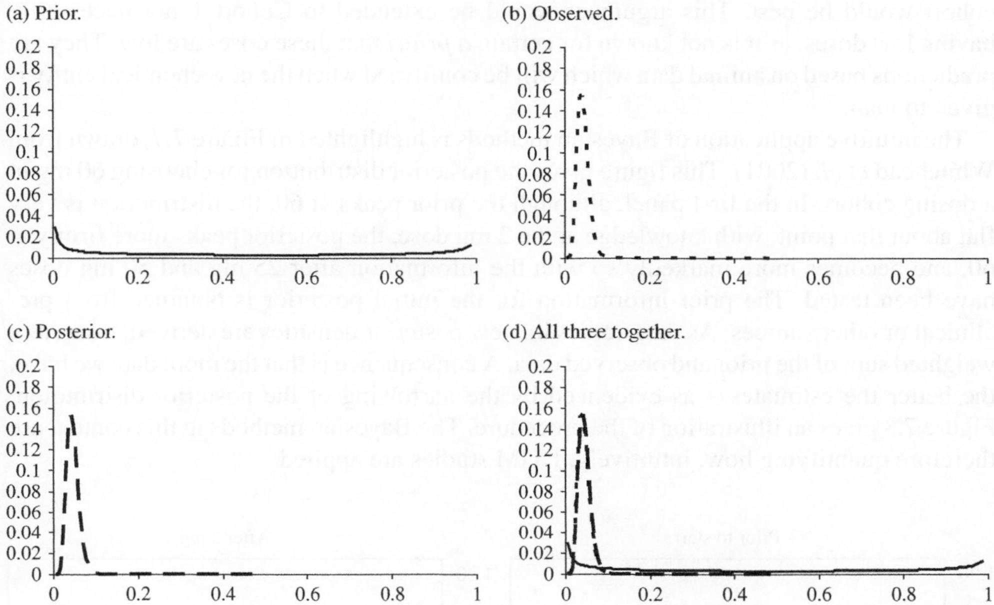

Figure 7.6 Prior distribution, observed and posterior distribution.

7.4 UTILITY OF BAYESIAN METHODS

First-time-into-man (FTIM) studies are good examples to illustrate the utility of Bayesian methods. Table 7.2 gives the scheduled doses for an escalating FTIM study across five cohorts.

If a person naïve to drug development was asked to select a cohort to enter the study, they would probably choose Cohort 1. When asked why, they would likely say because these are the lowest (and hence safest) doses. In contrast, someone familiar with drug development would choose Cohort 4 or even Cohort 5. When asked, they would say because the safety information for what is a completely new chemical entity in man would have been received from the other cohorts by then, so with this prior knowledge a later

Table 7.2 Scheduled doses in a hypothetical FTIM study.

Cohort	Scheduled doses
1	Placebo, 1, 2 or 5 mg
2	Placebo, 10, 20 or 40 mg
3	Placebo, 80, 150 or 300 mg
4	Placebo, 500, 750 or 1500 mg
5	Placebo, 2500, 5000 or 7500 mg

cohort would be best. This argument would be extended to Cohort 1 not necessarily having low doses, as it is not known for certain *a priori* that these doses are low. They are predictions based on animal data which will be confirmed when the new chemical entity is given to man.

The intuitive application of Bayesian methods is highlighted in Figure 7.7, drawn from Whitehead *et al.* (2001). This figure gives the posterior distribution for choosing 60 mg in a dosing cohort. In the first panel, although the prior peaks at 60, the distribution is very flat about that point; with knowledge at the 2 mg dose, the posterior peaks more firmly at 60, and becomes more markedly so with the information after 25 mg and 50 mg doses have been tested. The prior information for the initial posterior is obtained from pre-clinical or other sources. As data comes in, new posterior densities are derived, taken as a weighted sum of the prior and observed data. A consequence is that the more data we have, the better the estimates – as evidenced by the narrowing of the posterior distribution. Figure 7.8 gives an illustration of the procedure. The Bayesian methods in this context are therefore quantifying how, intuitively, FTIM studies are applied.

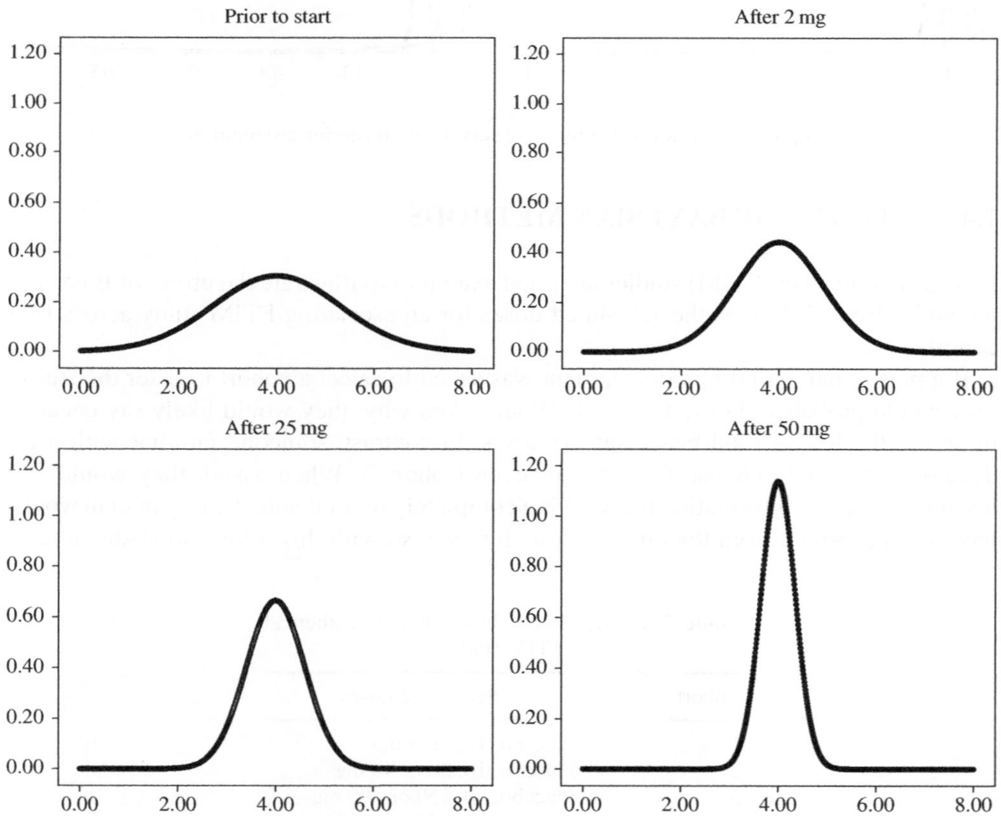

Figure 7.7 Posterior densities for $\log_e$ AUC for an untested subject administered a dose of 60 mg.

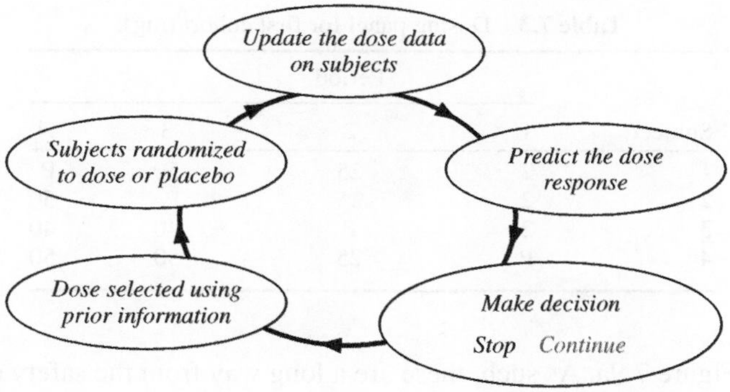

Figure 7.8 Assigning subjects to dose.

The utility of Bayesian methods is that they may allow for better assessment of dose response in the range where there is the most interest. For example, in Figure 7.9 the AUC may be assessed across the full dose profile, as in Figure 7.9a, in a FTIM study, when in actuality it is only the linear part (Figure 7.9b) where there is any interest. So what is required is a strategy to concentrate resources on this linear part most efficiently, such as in Figure 7.9c.

In truth there is nothing particularly clever about Bayesian methods, although they are quite intuitive in allowing information to be used to better inform decisions. Table 7.3 gives an example, from Whitehead *et al.* (2001), of possible doses in the first cohort, that may have been found to be at the bottom of the dose–response curve, such as in the first

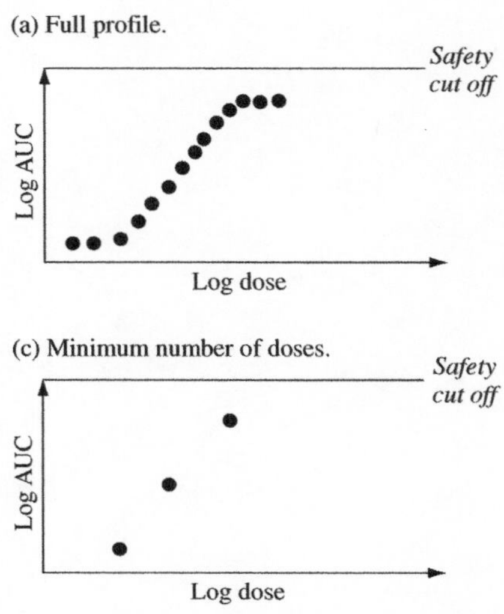

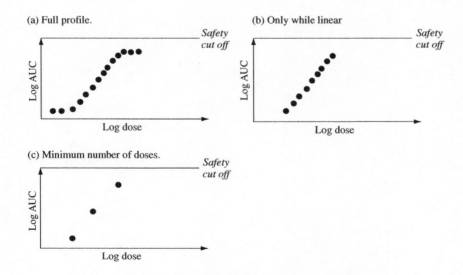

Figure 7.9 Illustration of possible dosing profiles.

Table 7.3 Dosing panel for first cohort (mg).

	Period			
Subject	1	2	3	4
1	2	25	50	P
2	2	25	P	50
3	2	P	40	40
4	P	25	50	50

three points of Figure 7.9a. As such, these are a long way from the safety cut off. In such circumstances, a recommendation after the first period could be to go from a dose of 2 mg to one of 25 mg in the next period. In reality, a jump from 2 mg to 25 mg may never happen, but would such a recommendation not give assurance that a dose of 4 mg is safe after giving 2 mg?

8 First-Time-into-New-Population Studies

8.1 INTRODUCTION

The chapters so far have concentrated on the design and analysis of studies that would be undertaken in healthy volunteers. Often it is not possible, however, to undertake trials in healthy volunteers, as the new chemical entity being investigated may be toxic. Hence, the trial designs discussed in Chapter 6 will not be appropriate as there would now be a necessity to investigate a new compound immediately in a patient population. This chapter describes the types of trial design for this situation.

8.2 BACKGROUND

For patients with a specific disease, one objective of treatment may be to reduce (ideally eradicate) the disease burden. However, it is recognized that any attack on the disease itself by an agent may bring collateral damage to normal tissue and vital organs. The usual strategy is to attempt to balance the two by first establishing the concept of dose-limiting toxicity (DLT) which then helps identify the maximum tolerated dose (MTD) of the drug concerned.

The aim of such a (Phase I) trial is to establish the MTD of a particular compound or treatment modality so that it can then be tested at that dose in a subsequent Phase II trial to assess activity. In some circumstances, the treatment under test may prove to be too toxic and so no MTD is established. In this case a Phase II trial would not be initiated for subsequent further testing. Overestimation of the MTD may lead to unacceptable toxicity (even death) in some patients at the later stages. On the other hand, underestimation of the MTD may lead to an apparent lack of efficacy. In either situation, a potentially useful compound may be shelved and opportunities for a therapeutic advance stalled.

In the designing of such trials, the number of patients to be recruited is often stated in advance. In many cases, like for first-time-into-man (FTIM) studies discussed in Chapter 7, there is often very little knowledge about the MTD, and there could only be a suggestion as to the starting dose based on animal studies. As with healthy volunteers, for FTIM studies the early doses are usually chosen to be conservative, hence most Phase I trials are larger than they would be if more was known about the MTD. Clearly, if there is some (previous) knowledge about the actual MTD, then fewer patients may be needed. The uncertainty with respect to the final study size makes planning these studies quite difficult.

An Introduction to Statistics in Early Phase Trials Steven A. Julious, Say Beng Tan and David Machin

8.3 ELIGIBILITY OF PATIENTS

As already indicated, 'first-time-into-new-population' studies often need to be carried out in patient populations rather than healthy volunteers. Indeed, for diseases such as cancer, they are typically carried out in patients without any established therapeutic alternatives. Although there may be exceptions, as indicated by the Committee for Medicinal Products for Human Use (CHMP, 2005a):

> Provided that safety is reasonably established and that there is a scientific rationale, it might be appropriate to conduct further dose and/or schedule finding studies also in patients for whom alternative therapies are available. This includes the neo-adjuvant setting in treatment naïve patients scheduled for surgery, provided that patient benefit has not been established for other neoadjuvant therapies and that delay in surgery cannot be detrimental to the patient. The safety and interests of the patient must always be guaranteed and a detailed justification should be provided in the study protocol. In these cases, the use of sensitive measures of anti-tumour activity is expected. Similarly, patients with diseases where the tumour activity is low (defined by minimal symptoms and expected slow progression) and where anti-tumour activity is easily measured and with no available curative treatment options may be included in this type of studies [sic]. An example could be clinically indolent, chronic lymphocytic leukaemia.

8.4 CHOOSING THE DOSES TO INVESTIGATE

In advance of the first patient being recruited in a Phase I trial, we first identify the range of the doses to consider and all the specific dose levels, within this range, to test. Thus, the first dose given to any patient, d_{START}, will be one of these options, and the ultimately identified MTD will also be one of these predefined doses.

The choice of the minimum dose to investigate, $d_{MINIMUM}$, is based on considerations from animal toxicity studies. In particular, the Committee for Proprietary Medicinal Products (CPMP) recommend a starting dose of 1/10 that of the corresponding MTD in rodents (CPMP, 1998b). Once $d_{MINIMUM}$ is determined then attention naturally turns to establishing what might be considered the therapeutic range, and the setting of the maximum dose, $d_{MAXIMUM}$, for the study. Once these are established then the remaining (intermediate) doses to investigate can then be determined.

For convenience we label the k doses finally chosen as $d_1 = d_{MINIMUM}$, d_2, d_3, ... , $d_k = d_{MAXIMUM}$. However, we still need to choose k and the specific values for each of the intermediate doses between the minimum and maximum values already defined. Statistical design considerations may suggest that these should be chosen equally spaced between $d_{MINIMUM}$ and $d_{MAXIMUM}$, on either a linear or a logarithmic scale. The doses chosen may depend on how the drug is 'packaged'; perhaps in tablet form or vial of a certain volume where dose choice may be limited, or in a powder or liquid more easily made up into any dose.

Table 8.1 Dose-escalation methods based on the Fibonacci series.

	Fibonacci ratio	
Dose	Full	'Modified'
d_1	1	1
d_2	2	2
d_3	1.50	1.67
d_4	1.67	1.50
d_5	1.60	1.40
d_6	1.63	1.33
d_7	1.62	1.33
⋮	⋮	⋮
d_∞	**1.33**	**1.33**

Practice has often revealed that as the dose increases in equal steps it may become sequentially more and more toxic, and hence possibly dangerous for the wellbeing of the patient. This caution has then led to designs which decrease the step sizes as the dose increases. One method uses the Fibonacci series: $a_0 = a_1 = 1$, then from a_2 onwards $a_{n+1} = a_n + a_{n-1}$. This gives the series: 1, 1, 2, 3, 5, 8, 13, 21, 34, and so on. There is no theoretical reason why this or any other mathematical series should be chosen for this purpose – they are merely empirical devices. The corresponding Fibonacci ratios of successive terms are: 1 / 1 = 1, 2/1 = 2, 3/2 = 1.5, 5/3 = 1.667, 8/5 = 1.600, 13/8 = 1.625, 21/13 = 1.615, 34/21 = 1.619, . . . , and eventually as n gets larger and larger this approaches $1.618 = (1 + \sqrt{5})/2$. These ratios are shown in Table 8.1 and, for relatively small n appropriate to the number of dose levels in a Phase I study, the ratio oscillates up and down. In mathematical terminology the series of ratios is not monotonically decreasing and so in fact does not provide successively decreasing step sizes.

Nevertheless, it is usually regarded as desirable that successive doses are a decreasing multiplier of the preceding dose and thus (often without a clear explanation provided) 'modified' Fibonacci multipliers like those of Table 8.1 are substituted in practice. However, it is usually pragmatic considerations that determine the modifications and no systematic rationale underlies the changes.

8.5 DESIGNS

8.5.1 C33D

A common Phase I design is termed the 'three-subjects-per-cohort design', or 'cumulative 3 + 3 dose' (C33D). This design gives successive (small) groups of patients increasing doses of the compound under investigation, and monitors the number who experience DLT with each dose. The next dose given depends on the experience of the immediately preceding patients with their corresponding administered dose; an unacceptable level of DLT in the group will lower the subsequent dose or stop the study, while an acceptable level will increase this dose.

The C33D chooses a 'low' starting dose, perhaps with $d_{\mathrm{START}} = d_{\mathrm{MINIMUM}}$, and a fixed number of replicates (by definition 3) at each dose. The choice of the next dose, d_{NEXT}, then depends on the number of patients (0, 1, 2 or 3) experiencing DLT. Clearly, if no patients experience DLT, then the subsequent dose to investigate will be higher than the one just tested. This process continues until either the stopping level of DLT is attained in the successive groups of 3 patients or d_{MAXIMUM} has been tested.

The MTD from this Phase I design is therefore established by adding cohorts of 3 patients at each dose level and observing the number of patients who present DLT. Although this process will (in general) establish the MTD, a pragmatic consideration dictates the Phase I trial should have tested at least 6 patients at d_{MTD}. This may mean that once first identified, extra patients are then recruited and tested at this provisional d_{MTD} until 6 patients in total have experienced this dose. It is also based on the premise that an acceptable probability of DLT will be somewhere between 1 in 6 (17%) and 1 in 3 (33%) of patients.

However, practical (and ethical) issues often constrain the size of Phase I trials, and a maximum size of up to 24 (8×3) is often chosen. This multiple of 3 arises from the use of the C33D design. This implies that if predetermined doses are to be used, and the final dose chosen will have 3 extra patients tested, then $k = 7$ dose options are the maximum that can be chosen for the design as $(k \times 3) + 3 = 24$ patients; although the precise numbers included will be dependent on the DLT experience observed.

Although the standard C33D specifies that groups of three patients are to be recruited at each dose level, the actual number chosen often differs from this. The basic design will function whatever the number of dose levels and/or cohort sizes chosen, although good design practice dictates that precise reasons for the specific choice made should be detailed in the trial protocol and its subsequent reporting. Figure 8.1 describes a commonly used version of the C33D design.

The C33D design, with or without the Storer (2001) modification (see Section 8.5.3), has no real statistical basis, and more efficient alternatives have been sought. Efficiency here can be thought of as achieving the right MTD and with as few patients as possible. However, the design is easy to implement and requires little (statistical) manipulation – only keeping a count of the number of patients experiencing DLT at each dose tested.

Commencing with the lowest dose, $h = 1$:
(**A**) Evaluate 3 patients at d_h:
- (**A1**) If 0 of 3 experience DLT, then escalate to d_{h+1}, and go to (**A**).
- (**A2**) If 1 of 3 experience DLT, then go to (**B**)
- (**A3**) If at least 2 of 3 experience DLT, then go to (**C**).

(**B**) Evaluate an additional 3 patients at d_h:
- (**B1**) If 1 of 6 experience DLT, then escalate to d_{h+1}, and go to (**A**).
- (**B2**) If at least 2 of 6 experience DLT, then go to (**C**).

(**C**) Discontinue dose escalation.

Figure 8.1 Establishing the MTD in a typical C33D design for a Phase I trial.

The lack of a firm statistical (design) basis clearly makes designing such Phase I trials somewhat problematic but perhaps unavoidable, since critically ill patients are often involved. Nevertheless, such difficulties imply that the results obtained need to be interpreted with due caution and carefully reviewed before taking the next step in the development process.

8.5.2 'BEST-OF-5'

A perhaps less commonly used Phase I design is termed the 'Best-of-5'. As with the C33D, this design gives successive (small) groups of patients increasing doses of the compound under investigation, and monitors the number who experience DLT with each dose. The next dose given depends on the experience of the immediately preceding patients with their corresponding administered dose; an unacceptable level of DLT in the group will lower the dose or terminate the study, while an acceptable level will increase the dose.

The 'Best-of-5' chooses a 'low' starting dose, perhaps with $d_{START} = d_{MINIMUM}$, and a fixed number of replicates (by definition 5) at each dose. The choice of the next dose, d_{NEXT}, then depends on the number of patients (0 to 5) experiencing DLT. If no patients experience DLT then the subsequent dose to investigate will be higher than the one just tested. This process continues until either the stopping level of DLT is attained in the successive groups of 5 patients, or $d_{MAXIMUM}$ has been tested. In circumstances where the first 3 (of 5) patients all experience DLT at a particular dose, it is not usual to give the fourth patient this same dose but to change the dose chosen to a lower one from the prespecified dose range. The MTD is therefore established by adding cohorts of 5 patients at each dose level and observing DLT (Figure 8.2).

Commencing with the lowest dose, $h = 1$:
(A) Evaluate 3 patients at d_h:
- **(A1)** If 0 of 3 experience DLT, then escalate to d_{h+1}, and go to **(A)**.
- **(A2)** If 1 or 2 of 3 experience DLT, then go to **(B)**.
- **(A3)** If 3 of 3 experience DLT, then go to **(D)**.

(B) Evaluate an additional 1 patient at d_h:
- **(B1)** If 1 of 4 experience DLT, then escalate to d_{h+1}, and go to **(A)**.
- **(B2)** If 2 of 4 experience DLT, then go to **(C)**.
- **(B3)** If 3 of 4 experience DLT, then go to **(D)**.

(C) Evaluate an additional 1 patient at d_h:
- **(C1)** If 2 of 5 experience DLT, then escalate to d_{h+1}, and go to **(A)**.
- **(C2)** If 3 of 5 experience DLT, then go to **(D)**.

(D) Discontinue dose escalation.

Figure 8.2 Establishing the MTD in a 'Best-of-5' design for a Phase I trial.

8.5.3 STORER DESIGN

This design gives successive (single) patients increasing doses of the compound under investigation, and monitors whether or not they experience DLT with each dose. The dose given depends on the experience of the immediately preceding patient; an absence of DLT will increase the dose for the next patient, while the presence of a DLT will suggest that the immediate prior (and lower) dose will be the starting dose of the full C33D, Best-of-5 or CRM (see Section 8.6) Phase I design to follow.

The strategy is essentially to enable the start of the 'full' Phase I designs to begin at a more informative dose than d_{MINIMUM}. This precursor design suggests recruiting (starting at d_{MINIMUM}) single individuals to successive doses, and moving up the dose escalation scale until a DLT is observed. Once this occurs, the next patient is recruited at the dose below that just tested. Once this dose is retested, the design moves into the 'full' Phase I design at this dose provided no DLT is observed. Alternatively, should a DLT be observed then d_{START} is taken as the dose below the level just tested. Clearly if a DLT occurs at d_{MINIMUM}, they would have to reconsider the whole dose-level choice strategy, as they would in the absence of a DLT at all doses up to and including d_{MAXIMUM}.

The design enters one patient at a dose at a time, and the presence or absence of DLT is assessed before determining the next dose to be given. Although this could be varied to, for example, two patients, this design then becomes close to C33D, and the point of the design as a precursor to C33D, Best-of-5 or CRM is then lost.

The strategy of a Storer-type precursor design is implemented by following the rules of Figure 8.3 to determine whether dose escalation should or should not occur. We have termed Storer a 'precursor' design as its objective is to determine a starting dose for other designs. Nevertheless, it may be used as a 'stand-alone' design examining a different dose range (perhaps wider or with intermediate steps)

First Stage - precursor
Commencing with the lowest dose, $h = 1$:
(**A**) Evaluate 1 patient at d_h:
(**A1**) If the first patient recruited experiences DLT the trial is stopped – in which case we need to reconsider the dose range.
(**A2**) If 0 patients have experienced DLT, then increase to d_{h+1}, and go to (A). (If all doses have been tested and no DLT, we need to reconsider the dose range.)
(**A3**) Once 1 patient has experienced DLT, then decrease to d_{h-1}, and go to (**A**).
(**A4**) Once the first patient has experienced DLT, and at least 1 of the prior patients has not, then decrease the dose to d_{h-1}, and go to (**B**).

Second Stage-C33D (or other)
(B) Evaluate 3 patients at d_h:
(B1) If 0 of 3 experience DLT, then escalate to d_{h+1}, and go to (B).
(B2) If 2 of 3 experience DLT, then go to (B).
(B3) If at least 2 of 3 experience DLT, then decrease the dose to d_{h-1}, and go to (B).

Figure 8.3 Establishing the starting dose using a Phase I precursor design of the Storer type.

than might have been considered if one of the 'full' designs had been initiated from the start. Conducted in this way, it may be used to guide the ultimate choice of the doses to be investigated in the more detailed study planned for the next stage of this Phase I investigation.

8.6 CONTINUAL REASSESSMENT METHOD (CRM)

This design gives successive (small) groups of patients changing doses of the compound under investigation, and monitors the number who experience DLT with each dose. The dose given to the next patient at any one time depends on the experience of all the preceding patients. In general an unacceptable level of DLT in the preceding group will lower the dose for the next cohort, while an acceptable level will increase the dose. The design starts with d_{START} chosen to be the dose which has a (subjective) probability of DLT closest to that which is deemed acceptable.

O'Quigley *et al.* (1990) and O'Quigley (2001) have proposed the continual reassessment method (CRM) with the goal to improve the (statistical) performance of dose escalation designs in determining the MTD.

8.6.1 DOSE–RESPONSE MODEL

CRM assumes a continuous dose–toxicity model such that as the dose increases the probability of DLT also increases. Such a model is illustrated in Figure 8.4 (with an illustration of an MTD with an associated probability of DLT of 0.2).

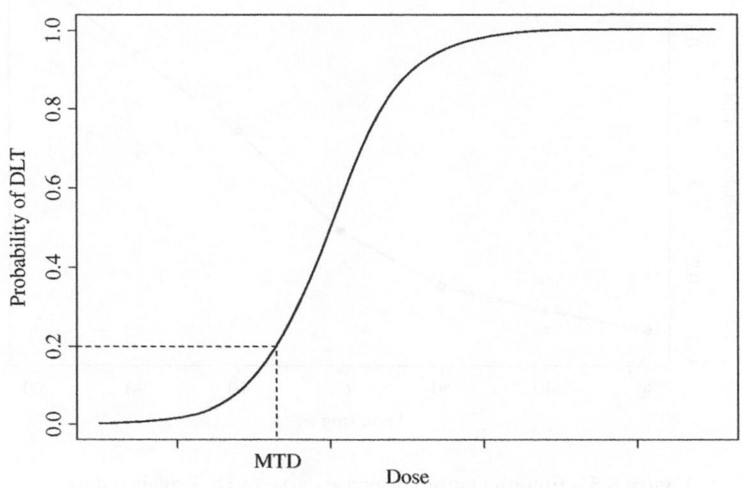

Figure 8.4 Hypothetical dose–response curve of the probability of DLT against received dose.

8.6.2 DETERMINING THE PROBABILITY OF DLT

The same process of selecting the range and actual doses for the C33D or Best-of-5 designs is necessary for the CRM design. In addition, however, to implement CRM it is necessary to attach to each of these doses the probability of patients experiencing DLT at that dose. We label these probabilities $\theta_1, \theta_2, \theta_3, \ldots, \theta_k$, as in Table 8.2.

Once the prior probabilities are attached to each dose that has been selected for investigation then this provides an empirical dose–response plot such as that of Figure 8.5.

It is implicit in the method of selecting these probabilities that, once they are assigned, then a 'reasonable' starting dose, d_{START}, would correspond to the dose that gives a value of θ_{START} close to some predefined 'acceptable' value, termed the target value and denoted θ_0. This probability is often chosen as less than 0.3, the 0.3 arising as a less than 1 in 3 chance; the '3' coming from history associated with the use of C33D. The chosen d_{START} would not usually correspond to the extremes $d_{MINIMUM}$ or $d_{MAXIMUM}$ of the dose range cited.

Table 8.2 Tabulation of the actual dose, corresponding working dose and probability of DLT.

Dose level, i	1	2	...	k
Actual dose, d_i	d_1	d_2	...	d_k
Working dose, z_i	z_1	z_2	...	z_k
Probability of DLT, θ_i	θ_1	θ_2	...	θ_k

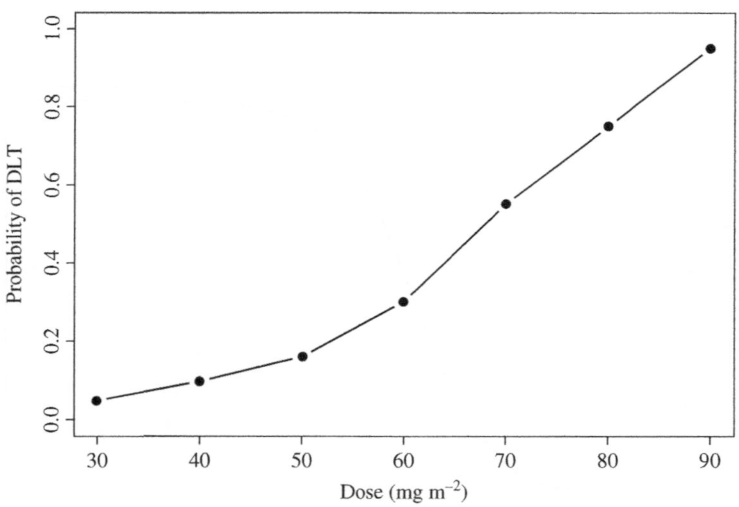

Figure 8.5 Empirical dose–response curve of DLT against dose.

As we have indicated, CRM uses a mathematical model for the idealized dose–response curve of the type in Figure 8.4 that is increasing with increasing dose.

One model for this defines the probability of severe toxicity, perhaps the DLT, at working dose z, using the tanh function, as

$$\mathrm{PT}(z, q) = \left(\frac{tanh\ z + 1}{2}\right)^q = \left(\frac{1}{1 + exp\ (-2z)}\right)^q, q > 0. \tag{8.1}$$

where

$$tanh\ z = \frac{e^z - e^{-z}}{e^z + e^{-z}}. \tag{8.2}$$

Thus $\mathrm{PT}(z, q)$ is the probability of DLT at 'working' dose z, and q is a parameter to be estimated. Remember that each probability of DLT, θ_i, has a dose, d_i (Table 8.2), 'attached' to it.

It is important to note that z does not correspond to the actual dose of the drug, d, but the so-called working dose level and, if (8.1) is chosen, the working doses, z, are determined by

$$z = \frac{1}{2}\ log\left(\frac{\theta^{\frac{1}{q}}}{1 - \theta^{\frac{1}{q}}}\right). \tag{8.3}$$

Thus from (8.3), for example: if $\theta = 0.5, z = 0$; $\theta = 0.025, z = -1.83$; whereas if $\theta = 0.975$, $z = +1.83$. An alternative model to that of (8.1) is the logistic function

$$\mathrm{PT}(z, q) = \frac{exp\ (qz + 3)}{1 + exp\ (qz + 3)}. \tag{8.4}$$

The choice, of the '3' in (8.4), follows from the empirical study conducted by Chevret (1993), who 'fine-tuned' the CRM model by examining a range of possible values that might be placed in the equation and opted for the value 3.

If (8.4) is chosen, the working doses z are determined by

$$z = \frac{1}{q}\left[log\left(\frac{\theta}{1 - \theta}\right) - 3\right]. \tag{8.5}$$

Thus from (8.3), for example: if $\theta = 0.5$, $z = -3$; $\theta = 0.025$, $z = -6.664$; whereas if $\theta = 0.975$, $z = +0.664$.

To begin the implementation of the CRM design, the parameter q is set to 1 in the chosen model of either (8.1) or (8.4). A tanh model 'fitted' to the 'subjective probability' data that were illustrated in Figure 8.5 is shown in Figure 8.6.

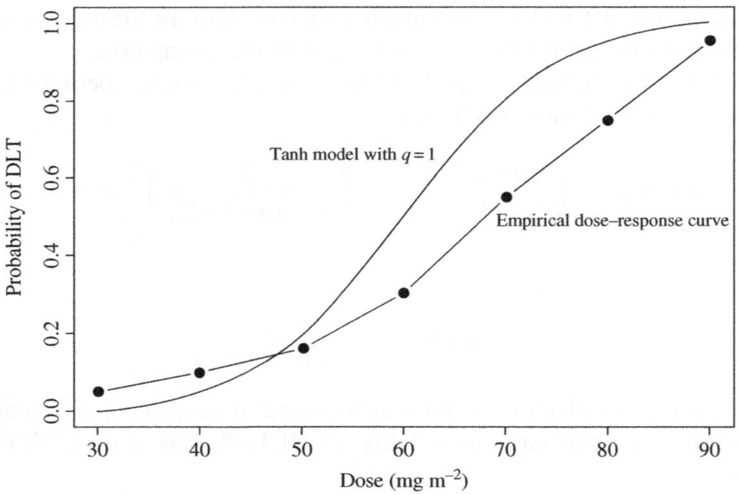

Figure 8.6 The first (no patient data – hence $q = 1$) model.

8.6.3 DETERMINING *Q*

The notion of uncertainty with respect to the value of q is expressed via a *prior* distribution, $g(q)$. There are several options which have been used for $g(q)$ and these are chosen to have the same mean for q but increasing uncertainty about the value of q as expressed through the variance. These distributions for q are summarized in Table 8.3. Thus, if we had a lot of 'experience' in similar patients with similar drugs to that under study, then the exponential distribution might be chosen. In the opposite extreme, gamma 2 might be chosen. In broad terms this would imply more patients would be needed to determine a suitable value for q.

Once this distribution has been selected, patients enter the trial and provide relevant toxicity data. From this information the value for q can be updated following each successive patient outcome. This then allows PT(z, q) to be calculated and 'fitted' onto the subjective probability data. Figure 8.6 shows one such example (compare with Figure 8.7), in which if the latest patient experiences toxicity the 'curve' moves 'up'

Table 8.3 Prior distributions for q.

Type of prior distribution	$g(q)$	Mean	Variance	Prior
Exponential[a]	$\lambda\, exp\ (-\lambda q)$	$\frac{1}{\lambda}=1$	$\frac{1}{\lambda^2}=1$	$\exp(-q)$
Gamma 1	$\frac{\lambda^r}{\Gamma(r)} q^{r-1}\, exp\ (-\lambda q)$	$\frac{r}{\lambda}=1$	$\frac{r}{\lambda^2}=5$	$\frac{0.2^{0.2}}{\Gamma(0.2)} q^{0.2-1}\, exp\ (-0.2q)$
Gamma 2	—	$\frac{r}{\lambda}=1$	$\frac{r}{\lambda^2}=10$	$\frac{0.1^{0.1}}{\Gamma(0.1)} q^{0.1-1}\, exp\ (-0.1q)$

[a] The gamma distribution with $r = 1$ is the exponential distribution.

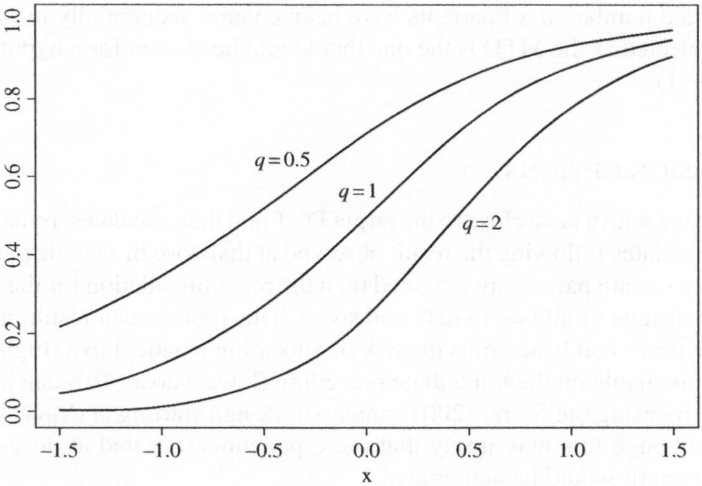

Figure 8.7 Updated working dose–response curves following a single observation investigating DLT (occurrence of DLT results in $q < 1$, no DLT results in $q > 1$).

otherwise 'down'. A move 'up' implies a more 'toxic' drug and hence we would move down the dose options for the next patient.

8.6.4 BAYES AND MAXIMUM LIKELIHOOD

The object of CRM is to estimate q and find the value of z, hence of d, which corresponds to $PT(z_{MTD}, q) = \theta_0$.

At the start of the trial, the first entered patient would be treated at a level chosen by the sponsor, believed in the light of all current available knowledge to be the dose, d_{START}, leading to the target probability of DLT level, θ_0. As indicated above, once given that dose, whether or not a DLT occurs is noted (we denote this as $y_1 = 0$ or 1). On the basis of this (single) observation, q (originally set equal to 1) is then estimated.

There are two methods by which this updating is carried out. One is by maximum likelihood and the other uses a Bayesian approach. Although we omit the details, to implement the likelihood method, a number of patients (at least 2) have to be recruited as the method intrinsically needs at least 1 patient to give $y = 0$ and one to give $y = 1$.

The Bayesian approach does not rely on this heterogeneity of responses and so will 'work' even for the first patient. After each patient is treated and the presence or absence of toxicity observed, the current (prior) distribution $g(q)$ is updated along with the estimated probabilities of toxicity at each dose level. The next patient is then treated at the dose level minimizing a measure of the distance between the current estimate of the probability of toxicity and θ_0.

After a fixed number, n, of patients have been entered sequentially in this fashion, the dose level selected as the MTD is the one that would be chosen for a hypothetical patient number $(n + 1)$.

8.6.5 DESIGN OPTIONS

The CRM starts with a dose close to the target DLT and then escalates, remains at the same dose or de-escalates following the result observed at that dose in a single patient. Once the results from a second patient are obtained then the recommendation for the third patient is based on the results of all two to date and so on. This process can result in jumping over intermediate doses and hence runs the risk of allocating a patient to a (high) dose with no information available on the immediate preceding (lower) dose. This can be overcome to some extent by using the Storer (2001) precursor design starting at d_{MINIMUM} as we have described, although this may imply that more patients are tested at doses for which no therapeutic benefit would be anticipated.

Alternatively, a modification to the CRM design itself by Goodman *et al.* (1995) suggests assigning more than one patient to each dose level chosen, and only allowing escalation by one dose level at a time. This is an attempt to limit having too extreme jumps/changes in dose levels, although it should of course be noted that whether a jump is ‘too extreme’ or not will depend also on how widely spaced the different levels were defined to be in the first instance. For de-escalation, the dose recommended by CRM is chosen.

8.6.5.1 Example 8.1

Suppose in a Phase I study of a new chemotherapy agent for the treatment of non-Hodgkin’s lymphoma, summarized in Table 8.4, a dose escalation strategy was utilized with decreasing multiples of the previous dose used. The design was based on the CRM of O’Quigley *et al.* (1990), incorporating some of the modifications of Goodman *et al.* (1995). Software to implement this design is available from various sources, including Machin *et al.* (2008).

Table 8.4 DLT observed in patients with advanced Non-Hodgkin’s Lymphoma.

Dose (mg m^{-2})	Dose escalation multiplier	Prior probability of DLT, θ	Number of patients recruited	Number of patients with DLT
40	—	0.10	—	—
50 (start)	1.25	0.20	2	0
60	1.20	0.30	8	0
70	1.17	0.40	9	2
80	1.14	0.50	1	1
90	1.13	0.65	—	—
100	1.11	0.80	—	—

Table 8.5 Updated values for z based on ($y_1 = 0$ or 1) at first working dose $z = -0.69$. If $y_1 = 0$ the dose is increased – panels with italics. If $y_1 = 1$ the dose is decreased – panels underlined.

Dose (mg m^{-2})	d	40	50	60	70	80	90	100
First patient								
Probability of DLT	θ	0.10	**0.20**	0.30	0.40	0.50	0.65	0.80
Start dose	d		**50**					
Start	z	<u>−1.10</u>	**−0.69**	*−0.42*	−0.20	0.00	0.31	0.69
(a) No DLT observed								
$y_1 = 0$, $q = 1.38$	z	−0.73	*−0.40*	−0.17	0.03	0.21	0.50	0.87
Next dose	d_{NEXT}			***60***				
(b) DLT observed								
$y_1 = 1$, $q = 0.72$	z	−1.57	<u>−1.06</u>	−0.73	−0.47	−0.24	0.10	0.51
Next dose	d_{NEXT}	<u>**40**</u>						

The prior probabilities, θ, attached to each dose are given in Table 8.4. As would be expected, as the dose is increased, the anticipated (subjective) prior probability of DLT increases, so that with dose 40 mg m^{-2}, θ is only 0.1 (or anticipated to be seen in 1 in every 10 patients with this dose), whereas at dose 100 mg m^{-2}, θ is 0.8 (4 in every 5 patients). The starting dose of 50 mg m^{-2} corresponds to a prior probability of toxicity, θ, of 0.2.

We have $\Pr(\text{DLT}) = \theta_{START} = 0.20$; then $d_1 = 50$ mg m^{-2}, and from equation (2.2), $z = -0.69$. If, once a patient is tested at this dose, $y_1 = 0$, then q (initially set to 1) is updated to 1.38 and the next dose is raised to $d_2 = 60$ mg m^{-2}. Whereas if $y_1 = 1$, then q is updated to 0.72 and the next dose is lowered to $d_2 = 40$ mg m^{-2} (See Table 8.5). In this manner, all subsequent patients are allocated to the appropriate dose level depending on the outcomes of the previous patients, with the accumulating information being used to provide better and better estimates of the probability of DLT associated with each dose level. This process continues until the prespecified maximum sample size is reached.

8.7 WHICH DESIGN?

Despite the fact that the traditional C33D (and implicitly the Best-of-5) method for dose escalation has been criticized by Heyd and Carlin (1999) and others, for the tendency to include too many patients at suboptimal dose levels and give a poor estimate of the MTD, it is still widely used in practice because of its algorithm-based simplicity.

Although the CRM method is more efficient than the C33D and Best-of-5 designs, it is considerably more difficult to implement, as the (statistical) manipulation required to determine the next dose to use is technically complex and requires specialist computer statistical

C33D	Best-of-5	CRM
Requires establishing the specific doses to be used at the design stage	Requires establishing the specific doses to be used at the design stage	Requires establishing the specific doses to be used at the design stage
		Requires clinical opinion of the associated probability of toxicity at each of the chosen doses
For each patient requires the presence of DLT to be determined	For each patient requires the presence of DLT to be determined	For each patient requires the presence of DLT to be determined
Dose for the next patient is easily established	Dose for the next patient is easily established	Dose for the next patient requires detailed calculation
		Dose for the next patient uses information on all those so far included in the study
Easy to explain	Easy to explain	Difficult to explain
Requires no specialist statistical software	Requires no specialist statistical software	Requires specialist statistical software
Requires the most patients	Requires intermediate number of patients	In general, will require the least number of patients

Figure 8.8 Basic features of the C33D, Best-of-5 and CRM designs

software. Although we have discussed these points previously, a review of the comparative features of the C33D, Best-of-5 and CRM designs are summarized in Figure 8.8.

The CRM design reduces the number of patients receiving the (very) low dose options. O'Quigley *et al.* (1990) argue that this avoids patients receiving doses at which there is little prospect of them deriving benefit, but the design has been criticized by Korn *et al.* (1994) for exposing patients to the risk of receiving potentially very toxic doses. However, using the Storer (2001) precursor prior to the original design allows both these difficulties (too low or too high) to be overcome. There have also been other variations to the CRM proposed, including the so-called time-to-event CRM (TITE-CRM), that allows patients to be entered in a staggered fashion (Cheung and Chappel (2000)).

Zohar and O'Quigley (2006) also proposed a design which focuses on finding the dose at which the 'overall success rate' (defined as the product of the rate of seeing 'nontoxicities' together with the rate of tumour response) is the highest.

Finally, it has to be recognized that such FTIM trials, however carefully designed, will include relatively few patients and so the corresponding level of uncertainty with respect to the true MTD will be high. It is also recognized that the designs do not (in one sense) estimate the MTD but rather choose one of the options. This implies that very careful consideration needs to be given to the dose options available within the design.

9 Bioequivalence Studies

9.1 INTRODUCTION

Bioequivalence trials are undertaken when the test and reference comparators are ostensibly the same. For example, the manufacturing site may have moved or a formulation been altered slightly for marketing purposes. Bioequivalence trials are also used for licensing applications for generic copies of licensed drugs, and in this context though termed 'early phase trials' they are really submittable licensing studies, and as such are one of the study types that do not fall within any specific phase of development.

Bioequivalence studies are conducted to demonstrate that two formulations of a drug have similar bioavailability, that is, to answer the question of whether the same amount of drug gets into the body irrespective of formulation. The assumption with bioequivalence trials therefore is that if the two formulations have equivalent bioavailability then we can infer that they have equivalent effect for both efficacy and safety. The pharmacokinetic bioavailability is therefore a surrogate for the clinical endpoints.

Equivalent bioavailability will be concluded if the drug concentration-by-time profiles for the test and reference formulations are superimposable; see Figure 9.1 for an example. By determining that the two profiles are superimposable we can conclude that the two formulations are clinically the same.

In bioequivalence studies, therefore, we can determine *in vivo* whether the two formulations are bioequivalent by assessing the concentration time profiles for the test and reference formulations. This is usually done by assessing if the rate and extent of absorption are the same, where the pharmacokinetic parameter AUC (area under the concentration curve) is used to assess the extent of absorption and the parameter C_{max} (maximum concentration) is used to assess the rate of absorption. Figure 9.1 gives a pictorial representation of these parameters.

9.2 BACKGROUND

As bioequivalence trials are submittable studies, there are regulatory guidelines which give definitions in the context of the trials. The FDA (2006b) defines pharmaceutical equivalents as the following:

An Introduction to Statistics in Early Phase Trials Steven A. Julious, Say Beng Tan and David Machin

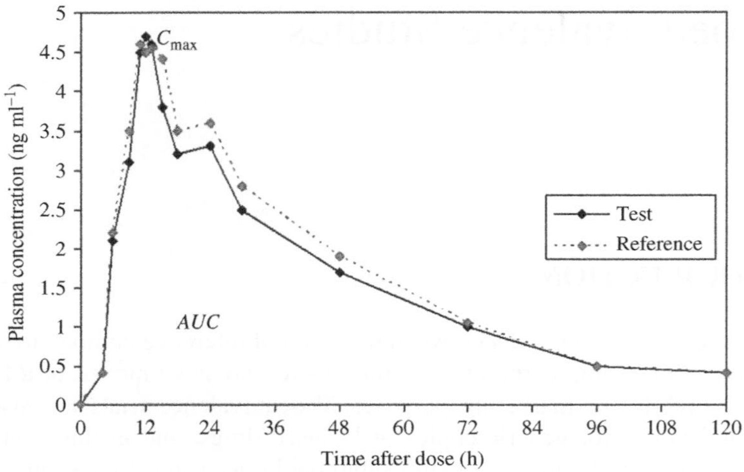

Figure 9.1 Pharmacokinetic profiles for two compounds which are bioequivalent.

> Drug products are considered pharmaceutical equivalents if they contain the same active ingredient(s), are of the same dosage form, route of administration and are identical in strength or concentration (e.g., chlordiazepoxide hydrochloride, 5 mg capsules). Pharmaceutically equivalent drug products are formulated to contain the same amount of active ingredient in the same dosage form and to meet the same or compendial or other applicable standards (i.e., strength, quality, purity, and identity), but they may differ in characteristics such as shape, scoring configuration, release mechanisms, packaging, excipients (including colors, flavors, preservatives), expiration time, and, within certain limits, labeling . . .

This refers to the comment at the start of the chapter that the two comparators are ostensibly the same, giving definition as to pharmaceutical equivalence, the first step in the process leading to a bioequivalence trial. Obviously, if there is a small tweaking in the trial formulations for marketing reasons or a change in the manufacturing site this definition may not be a concern. However, this definition may be an issue for generic copies of previously patented therapies.

A drug is considered a pharmaceutical alternative if it is defined as below (FDA, 2006b):

> Drug products are considered pharmaceutical alternatives if they contain the same therapeutic moiety, but are different salts, esters, or complexes of that moiety, or are different dosage forms or strengths (e.g., tetracycline hydrochloride, 250 mg capsules vs. tetracycline phosphate complex, 250 mg capsules; quinidine sulfate, 200 mg tablets vs. quinidine sulfate, 200 mg capsules). Data are generally not available for FDA to make the determination of tablet to capsule bioequivalence. Different dosage forms and strengths within a product line by a single manufacturer are thus pharmaceutical alternatives, as are extended-release products when compared with immediate-release or standard-release formulations of the same active ingredient.

Hence, as the definition states, a controlled-release or immediate-release formulation would be defined as a pharmaceutical alternative, as could a generic attempted copy of a drug if it failed to be defined as a pharmaceutical equivalent. Even if shown to be a therapeutic alternative, the bioavailability of a formulation may need to be assessed, where bioavailability is defined as (FDA, 2006b):

> The rate and extent to which the active ingredient or active moiety is absorbed from a drug product and becomes available at the site of action. For drug products that are not intended to be absorbed into the bloodstream, bioavailability may be assessed by measurements intended to reflect the rate and extent to which the active ingredient or active moiety becomes available at the site of action.

For a modified formulation, therefore, it could be through a bioavailability assessment that its properties are determined. For example: to delay t_{max} and lower C_{max} but maintain AUC for a modified formulation; or for AUC for a once-a-day formulation to be the same as that for two doses of a twice-a-day formulation. Here, the new formulation may not be equivalent to the comparator formulation but its new properties defined in terms of its bioavailability may be desirable.

For comparators that are ostensibly the same, the bioavailability of the compounds could be used to assess bioequivalence given as (FDA, 2006b):

> This term describes pharmaceutical equivalent or alternative products that display comparable bioavailability when studied under similar experimental conditions. ... shall be considered bioequivalent:
>
> The rate and extent of absorption of the test drug do not show a significant difference from the rate and extent of absorption of the reference drug when administered at the same molar dose of the therapeutic ingredient under similar experimental conditions in either a single dose or multiple doses.

Hence, as stated before, the pharmacokinetics of a compound are used as a surrogate for the clinical outcomes – in terms of safety and efficacy – to enable therapeutic equivalency to be declared under the following (FDA, 2006b):

> Drug products are considered to be therapeutic equivalents only if they are pharmaceutical equivalents and if they can be expected to have the same clinical effect and safety profile when administered to patients under the conditions specified in the labeling.
>
> FDA classifies as therapeutically equivalent those products that meet the following general criteria:
>
> - they are approved as safe and effective;
> - they are pharmaceutical equivalents in that they
>
> (a) contain identical amounts of the same active drug ingredient in the same dosage form and route of administration, and

   (b) meet compendial or other applicable standards of strength, quality, purity, and identity;
- they are bioequivalent in that
   (a) they do not present a known or potential bioequivalence problem, and they meet an acceptable *in vitro* standard, or
   (b) if they do present such a known or potential problem, they are shown to meet an appropriate bioequivalence standard;
- they are adequately labeled;
- they are manufactured in compliance with Current Good Manufacturing Practice regulations.

9.3 ESTABLISHING BIOEQUIVALENCE

Bioequivalence studies are conducted to show that two formulations of a drug have similar bioavailability, that is, similar rate and extent of drug absorption, with the assumption that equivalent bioavailability ensures equivalent therapeutic effect (both efficacy and safety). As stated, the concentration–time profiles for the test and reference formulations need to be superimposable, which is usually assessed by determining if the rate (C_{max}) and extent (AUC) of absorption are the same. Both AUC and C_{max} must be equivalent to declare bioequivalence. Hence, if we define

μ_T to be the average bioavailability of test formulation,

μ_R to be the average bioavailability of reference formulation,

then we need to the equivalence of μ_T and μ_R. Formally, the null and alternative hypotheses can be defined as

H_0: the test and reference formulations give different drug exposures ($\mu_T \neq \mu_R$).

H_1: the test and reference formulations give equivalent drug exposure ($\mu_T = \mu_R$).

In particular, the null and alternative hypotheses can be rewritten as

$$H_0 : \frac{\mu_T}{\mu_R} \leq 0.80 \text{ or } \frac{\mu_T}{\mu_R} \geq 1.25, \quad H_1 : 0.80 < \frac{\mu_T}{\mu_R} < 1.25.$$

Here we have the bioequivalence margin set to be 20%, which on the log scale is (0.80 to 1.25). A 20% margin is (0.80 to 1.25) on the log scale as these limits are invariant to the choice of reference; that is, they correspond to a constant difference on the log scale. The margin need not be 20%, and the following sections will discuss this.

Two comparator formulations can thus be declared bioequivalent within a 20% margin if it can be demonstrated that the mean ratio is wholly contained within 0.80 to 1.25. To test the null hypothesis, two one-sided tests at the 5% level are constructed to determine whether $\mu_T/\mu_R \leq 0.80$ or $\mu_T/\mu_R \geq 1.25$. If neither of these tests hold then the alternative hypothesis of $0.80 < \mu_T/\mu_R < 1.25$ can be accepted. As we are performing two simultaneous tests on the null hypothesis, both of which must be rejected to accept the alternative hypothesis, the Type I error is maintained at 5%. The convention is to represent the two one-sided tests as a 90% confidence interval around the mean ratio of μ_T/μ_R, which neatly summarizes the results of the two one-tailed tests.

9.3.1 STANDARD BIOEQUIVALENCE MARGINS

There are a number of regulatory guidelines from different international locations that give the definition of bioequivalence, which we will now summarize.

9.3.1.1 United States

To declare bioequivalence the FDA (2001, 2003b) recommend that both C_{max} and AUC bioequivalence be set at 20%, such that the 90% confidence interval should be wholly contained within (0.80 to 1.25).

9.3.1.2 Europe

For Europe, the Committee for Proprietary Medicinal Products (CPMP, 1998a) state that for AUC a margin of 20% (0.80 to 1.25) should be used although 'In rare cases a wider acceptance range maybe acceptable if it is based on sound clinical justification.' Likewise for C_{max} a margin of 20% is recommended, though 'In certain cases a wider interval may be acceptable. The interval must be prospectively defined e.g. 0.75–1.33 ...'

9.3.1.3 Canada

Canadian guidelines (Health Canada 1992, 1996) state that, for AUC, bioequivalence should be tested against a 20% (0.80 to 1.25) margin, while for C_{max} the only requirement is that the point estimate for C_{max} is contained within (0.80 to 1.25).

9.3.1.4 Japan

Like other regions, Japanese guidelines (NIHS, Japan, 1997) recommended 20% limits for both AUC and C_{max}. However, they also state that:

> ... even though the confidence interval is not in the above range, test products are accepted as bioequivalent, if the following three conditions are satisfied; 1) the total sample size of the initial bioequivalence study is not less than 20 ..., 2) the differences in average values of logarithmic AUC and C_{max} between two products are between log(0.9)–log(1.11), and 3) [the average amount dissolved from test product does not deviate by more than 10% from reference.]

where the final point refers to extensive *in vitro* dissolution work. Hence, if *in vitro* results demonstrate that the formulations are bioequivalent then it may be appropriate just to show the point estimate alone falls within the margin (0.9 to 1.11).

Note, though, there should still be some limited formal analysis when quoting just point estimates. In particular, it is important to perform a formal analysis especially if quoting arithmetic means, as these may be biased. This is because, from Chapter 2, the mean for each group is defined as

$$m_{\mathrm{T}} = e^{\left(\mu_{\mathrm{T}}+\sigma_{\mathrm{T}}^2/2\right)} \text{ and } m_{\mathrm{R}} = e^{\left(\mu_{\mathrm{R}}+\sigma_{\mathrm{R}}^2/2\right)}.$$

Hence, we could have the situation where $\mu_{\mathrm{T}}/\mu_{\mathrm{R}}$ falls just within (0.9 to 1.11) but $m_{\mathrm{T}}/m_{\mathrm{R}}$ does not because of chance differences in the variances σ_{T}^2 and σ_{R}^2.

9.3.2 NARROW THERAPEUTIC INDEX

In previous chapters we have discussed the importance of having wide safety and efficacy windows for a given compound. Having narrow windows affects how bioequivalence may be assessed. In terms of the safety window, the FDA (2005a, 2005b) gives the following definition:

> Evidence that the drug products exhibit a narrow therapeutic ratio, e.g., there is less than a 2-fold difference in median lethal dose (LD50) values, or have less than a 2-fold difference in the minimum toxic concentrations and minimum effective concentrations in the blood, and safe and effective use of the drug products requires careful dosage titration and patient monitoring . . .

while for the efficacy window we have (FDA, 2003b):

> This guidance defines narrow therapeutic range drug products as containing certain drug substances subject to therapeutic drug concentration or pharmacodynamic monitoring, and/or where product labeling indicates a narrow therapeutic range designation. Examples include digoxin, lithium, phenytoin, theophylline, and warfarin. Because not all drugs subject to therapeutic drug concentration or pharmacodynamic monitoring are narrow therapeutic range drugs, sponsors and/or applicants can contact the appropriate review division at CDER to determine whether a drug can or cannot be considered to have a narrow therapeutic range. This guidance uses the term narrow therapeutic range instead of narrow therapeutic index drug, although the latter is more commonly used . . .

Narrow safety and efficacy windows affect bioequivalence, as the margins that can be safely accepted as being bioequivalent may need to be tightened. With respect to narrow therapeutic index compounds and bioequivalence, different agencies have different recommendations:

- Health Canada (2006) recommends that for AUC we use a margin of 0.90 to 1.12 (sic), while for C_{max} a margin of 0.80 to 1.25 is recommended.

- Europe: the CPMP (1998a) state for both AUC and C_{max} '*In specific cases of a narrow therapeutic range the acceptance interval may need to be tightened.*' In draft guidelines the Committee for Medicinal Products for Human Use (CHMP, 2008) more specifically stated '*...the acceptance interval for concluding bioequivalence should generally be narrowed to 90–111%.*'
- The FDA (2003b) give the following guidance:

This guidance recommends that sponsors consider additional testing and/or controls to ensure the quality of drug products containing narrow therapeutic range drugs. The approach is designed to provide increased assurance of interchangeability for drug products containing specified narrow therapeutic range drugs. It is not designed to influence the practice of medicine or pharmacy.

Unless otherwise indicated by a specific guidance, this guidance recommends that the traditional BE limit of 80 to 125 percent for non-narrow therapeutic range drugs remain unchanged for the bioavailability measures (AUC and C_{max}) of narrow therapeutic range drugs.

9.3.3 HIGHLY VARIABLE DRUGS

A highly variable drug is defined as a drug with a within-subject coefficient of variation (CV_w) greater than 30% (FDA, 2000). Both the CHMP (2006b) and Health Canada (2003) have discussed this problem in terms of scaling. Basically, instead of investigating a mean difference

$$log_e \mu_T - log_e \mu_R,$$

we investigate something of the form

$$\frac{log_e \mu_T - log_e \mu_R}{\sigma}.$$

However, there are no formal guidelines beyond this for the rescaling. As discussed earlier in the chapter, a wide margin for C_{max} may be argued for particular instances in Europe. With respect to the FDA, the 20% margin still holds.

9.3.4 SUMMARY OF ASSESSING BIOEQUIVALENCE

With respect to the 'standard' bioequivalence criteria, we look to demonstrate that average drug exposure on the test is within 20% of the reference on the log scale. Thus, the null and alternative hypotheses can be rewritten as

$$H_0 : \frac{\mu_T}{\mu_R} \leq 0.80 \quad \text{or} \quad \frac{\mu_T}{\mu_R} \geq 1.25, \qquad H_1 : \; 0.80 < \frac{\mu_T}{\mu_R} < 1.25.$$

A test formulation of a drug can therefore said to be bioequivalent to its reference formulation if the 90% confidence interval for the ratio test : reference is wholly contained within the range 0.80 to 1.25, for both AUC and C_{max}. As both AUC and C_{max} must be equivalent to declare bioequivalence there is no need to allow for multiple comparisons.

For certain indications, other parameters, such as C_{min} (defined as the minimum concentration over a given period) or T_{mic} (defined as time above a minimum inhibitory concentration over a given period), may also need to be simultaneously assessed.

The methodology described in this section can also be applied to other types of *in vivo* assessment such as the assessment of a food–drug interaction, or special populations, which will be discussed in Chapter 10.

9.4 SAMPLE SIZE CALCULATIONS FOR BIOEQUIVALENCE STUDIES

In Chapter 3 we described the sample size calculations for early phase trials where the objective of the trial was to determine superiority or to estimate a response with a requisite precision. Here we will describe the calculations where the objective of the trial is to show that two formulations are bioequivalent.

9.4.1 GENERAL CASE OF RATIO NOT EQUALLING UNITY

We first consider the general case where we cannot assume that the mean ratio (μ_T/μ_R) will be unity. For this situation we cannot obtain a direct estimate of the sample size. Instead we must iterate until a sample size is reached which gives the required Type II error (and power). Thus, to calculate the power for the bioequivalence acceptance limits of (0.80, 1.25), the following result can be used

$$1-\beta=\Phi\left(\sqrt{\frac{(log_e(\mu_T/\mu_R)-log_e(1.25))^2 n}{2\sigma_w^2}}-Z_{1-\alpha}\right)$$
$$+\Phi\left(\sqrt{\frac{(log_e(\mu_T/\mu_R)-log_e(0.80)^2 n}{2\sigma_w^2}}-Z_{1-\alpha}\right)-1, \quad (9.1)$$

where σ_w^2 is the within-subject variability on the log scale and n is the total sample size. Note, it is important to highlight again that σ_w^2 is the within-subject variability taken from the residual line of an analysis of variance. The within-subject variance is introduced in Chapter 4.

As with superiority trials discussed in Chapter 3, although (9.1) is more straightforward to apply, a more precise calculation to estimate the power, and hence sample size, would be (Julious, 2004b)

$$1-\beta=\text{Probt}\left(-t_{1-\alpha,n-2},n-2,\tau_2\right)$$
$$-\text{Probt}\left(t_{1-\alpha,n-2},n-2,\tau_1\right), \quad (9.2)$$

where τ_1 and τ_2 are noncentrality parameters

$$\tau_1 = \frac{\sqrt{n}\left(log_e\left(\mu_T/\mu_R\right) - log_e(0.80)\right)}{\sqrt{2\sigma_w^2}} \quad \text{and} \quad \tau_2 = \frac{\sqrt{n}\left(log_e\left(\mu_T/\mu_R\right) - log_e(1.25)\right)}{\sqrt{2\sigma_w^2}}.$$

An estimate of the sample size for the case when μ_T/μ_R is greater than unity can be obtained from the following equation

$$n = \frac{2\sigma_w^2\left(Z_{1-\beta} + Z_{1-\alpha}\right)^2}{\left(log_e\left(\mu_T/\mu_R\right) - log_e(1.25)\right)^2}, \tag{9.3}$$

which can be used to provide an initial value for the iterations. This equation provides reasonable approximations for $\mu_T/\mu_R \neq 1$, especially when the mean ratio becomes large relative to (0.80 to 1.25), that is, greater than 1.05 or less than 0.95. This is because in such circumstances most of the Type II error comes from one of the two one-sided tests. For quick calculations (for 90% power and a Type I error of 5%), the following formula can be used

$$n = \frac{17\sigma_w^2}{\left(log_e(\mu_T/\mu_R) - log_e(1.25)\right)^2}. \tag{9.4}$$

Note that although we give the Normal approximation results they should be used with caution. For example, for a $CV_w \left(= \sqrt{e^{\sigma_w^2} - 1}\right)$ of 15% (mean ratio assumed to be unity), (9.2) gives the sample size as 12, whilst (9.1) returns a sample of 10. The sample size of 10 subjects equates, from (9.1), to a Type II error of 17%. For bioequivalence trials it is therefore strongly recommended that the more precise result is always used for final sample size estimation, with the quick results only used for early ball-park calculations.

Table 9.1 gives sample size estimates using (9.2) for different values of CV_w and mean ratios, and acceptance criteria 10% (0.90 to 1.11), 15% (0.85 to 1.18), 20% (0.80 to 1.25) and so on, for a Type I error rate of 5%, and 90% power.

9.4.2 SPECIAL CASE OF THE RATIO EQUALLING UNITY

For the special case where the true mean ratio is expected to be unity (μ_T/μ_R=1), the sample size can be derived directly from the following formula.

$$n = \frac{2\sigma_w^2\left(Z_{1-\beta/2} + Z_{1-\alpha}\right)^2}{\left(log_e(1.25)\right)^2}. \tag{9.5}$$

Table 9.1 Total sample sizes (n) for bioequivalence studies for different *CV*w, levels of bioequivalence and true mean ratios, for 90% power and Type I error of 5%.

		Levels of bioequivalence				
CV_w(%)	Ratio	10%	15%	20%	25%	30%
10	0.80				43	12
	0.85			48	13	7
	0.90		54	14	8	5
	0.95	60	16	8	6	5
	1.00	21	10	7	5	5
	1.05	55	15	8	6	5
	1.10		40	13	7	5
	1.15			26	10	6
	1.20			104	17	8
15	0.80				93	23
	0.85			106	26	12
	0.90		119	29	14	8
	0.95	132	33	15	9	7
	1.00	45	20	12	8	6
	1.05	121	31	15	9	7
	1.10		86	25	12	8
	1.15			57	19	10
	1.20			231	36	15
20	0.80				163	40
	0.85			185	45	20
	0.90		207	50	22	13
	0.95	232	56	25	14	10
	1.00	78	34	19	12	9
	1.05	212	54	24	14	10
	1.10		151	43	20	12
	1.15			99	33	16
	1.20			405	62	24
25	0.80				251	60
	0.85			284	68	30
	0.90		320	77	33	18
	0.95	357	86	37	21	14
	1.00	120	52	28	18	12
	1.05	326	82	36	21	14
	1.10		232	65	30	17
	1.15			151	49	24
	1.20			625	95	36
30	0.80				356	85
	0.85			403	96	41
	0.90		454	108	46	25
	0.95	507	121	52	29	18
	1.00	170	73	39	25	17
	1.05	463	116	51	28	18
	1.10		329	92	42	24
	1.15			214	69	33
	1.20			888	135	50
35	0.80				477	113
	0.85			540	128	54
	0.90		608	145	61	33

	0.95	679	162	69	38	24
	1.00	227	97	52	32	22
	1.05	620	155	67	37	24
	1.10		440	123	55	31
	1.15			287	92	44
	1.20			1190	180	67
40	0.80				612	144
	0.85			694	164	69
	0.90		780	185	78	42
	0.95	871	207	88	48	30
	1.00	291	124	66	41	27
	1.05	796	198	86	47	30
	1.10		565	157	71	39
	1.15			367	118	56
	1.20			1527	231	86
45	0.80				760	179
	0.85			861	203	86
	0.90		969	230	97	52
	0.95	1082	257	109	60	37
	1.00	361	153	82	50	33
	1.05	989	246	106	59	37
	1.10		701	195	87	48
	1.15			456	146	69
	1.20			1897	286	106

Estimating the power from a noncentral t-distribution, (9.5) can be rewritten to

$$1 - \beta = 2\mathrm{Probt}(-t_{1-\alpha,n-2}, n-2, \tau) - 1, \qquad (9.6)$$

where τ is the noncentrality parameter defined as

$$\tau = \frac{\sqrt{n}(\,log_e(0.8))}{\sqrt{2\sigma_w^2}}.$$

For the special case of the mean ratios equalling unity, (9.5) can be used to obtain initial estimates of the sample size to use in (9.6). For quick calculations for 90% power, 5% Type I error rate and a 20% acceptance criteria on the log scale we could use

$$n = 433\sigma_w^2. \qquad (9.7)$$

Note that although the calculations for the special case are more straightforward, it is recommended that, even if you expect *a priori* the mean ratio to be unity, where practical you should consider calculating sample sizes under the assumption of a small mean difference (of 5% say), as the power of a study is very sensitive to the assumption about the mean ratio. Indeed, in a review of over 1500 drug submissions between 1996 and 2005, Haidar *et al.* (2006) found the average mean difference to be 3.1% for AUC and 4.5% for C_{max}. So a small mean difference should be anticipated.

9.4.3 REPLICATE DESIGNS

For compounds with high variability, the standard AB/BA design can require relatively large sample sizes, especially if the mean ratio is not expected to be unity. Designs which can partially overcome this problem are replicate crossover designs. Through adding an extra period arm to the study, such that the sequences are say ABB/BAA, the sample size is reduced by 25% compared to a standard AB/BA design. An additional two periods and sequences, say of ABBA/BAAB, can reduce the sample size by 50% (Julious, 2004c). These reductions are possible due to the fact that the variances used in the contrast of the means in the final analysis are halved for a four-period replicate design, and reduced by 25% for a three-period replicate design.

Note, these reductions hold under the (reasonable) assumptions that there is no interaction between subject and formulation. Note also that replicate designs may not be practical for certain compounds, for example those with a long half-life, but they are a possible option for compounds with high pharmacokinetic variability.

9.4.4 WORKED EXAMPLE 9.1: SAMPLE SIZE CALCULATION

A bioequivalence trial to compare a test with reference formulation is to be designed. The standard bioequivalence criteria of 0.80 to 1.25 will be used to demonstrate that the average drug exposure on the test is bioequivalent to the reference. Two previous studies had been undertaken, and the summary of the variance data is given in Table 9.2.

The pooled within-subject coefficients of variation expected were estimated from the weighted sum of the variances on the log scale, with the degrees of freedom providing the weights – as described in Chapter 3.

The overall estimates for C_{max} and AUC respectively are 27% and 29%, and the mean ratio is expected to be unity ($\mu_T/\mu_R=1$). For this example, to be a little conservative, the CV_w is taken to be 30%, which equates to a within-subject SD of 0.294 ($=\sqrt{log\,(CV_w^2-1)}$). The study design is to be an AB/BA two-period crossover. From Table 9.1 it can be seen that one would need, at a minimum, a total sample size of 39 subjects. Practically this would equate to at least 20 subjects on each sequence (AB and BA).

Table 9.2 Within-subject coefficients of variability with their corresponding degrees of freedom (*df*) observed in two previous studies.

	AUC		C_{max}	
	CV_w (%)	*df*	CV_w (%)	*df*
Study 1	33	13	20	13
Study 2	24	15	23	15
Pooled	29	28	27	28

Note, using $CV_w = 29\%$ and result (9.2), the total evaluable sample size is estimated to be 37. However, the more conservative sample size of 40 will be used. To allow for a 20% dropout rate, 48 (= 40 / 0.80) subjects will be in enrolled.

Revisiting the calculations, suppose that the test formulation is expected, on average, to have exposures 5% greater than the reference so that $\mu_T/\mu_R = 1.05$), then the total evaluable sample size would increases to 51 subjects (or 26 per sequence).

To mitigate the increase in sample size to 52, suppose instead of an AB/BA design a replicate ABB/BAA or ABBA/BAAB design was being considered for the case where exposures were expected to be 5% greater on test compared to reference. If we adopted a four-period replicate design then one would multiply the total sample size calculated earlier by 0.50 to get $52 \times 0.5 = 26$ evaluable subjects in total required. If we adopted a three-period replicate design then the total sample size calculated earlier should be multiplied by 0.75 to get $52 \times 0.75 = 39$ or 40 evaluable subjects in total required.

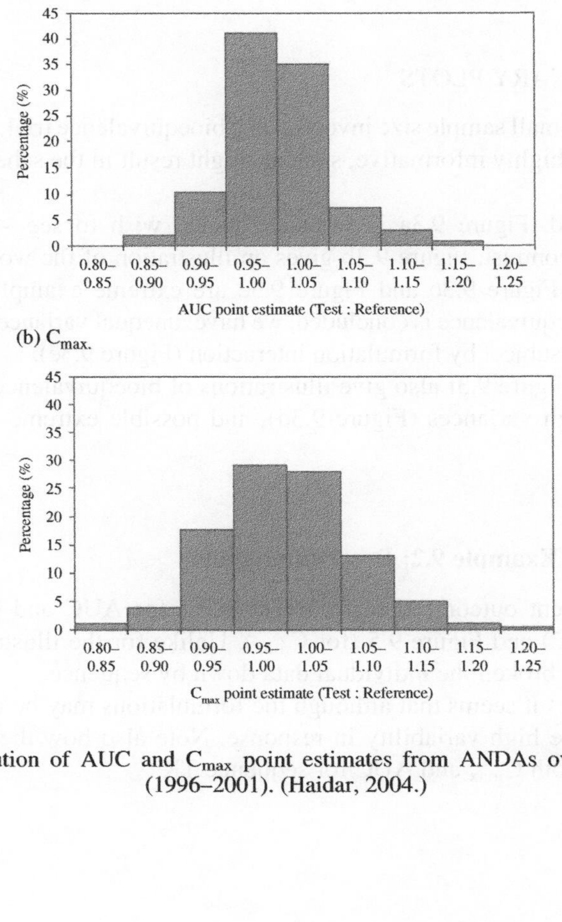

Figure 9.2 Distribution of AUC and C_{max} point estimates from ANDAs over a five-year period (1996–2001). (Haidar, 2004.)

9.4.5 COMMENT ON SAMPLE SIZE CALCULATIONS

In Worked Example 9.1, it was AUC which had the largest variance and so was the endpoint that drove the sample size calculations. This usually is not the case, as highlighted in Figure 9.2, taken from Haidar (2004). This gives the distribution of point estimates from abbreviated new drug applications (ANDAs). As is evidenced from this figure, it is apparent that it is C_{max} that tends to have the highest variability and tends to drive the calculations.

9.5 ANALYSIS OF BIOEQUIVALENCE STUDIES

To illustrate the statistical analysis of a bioequivalence study, we use data from a trial taken from Patterson and Jones (2006) and given in Table 9.3, for which the sample size was calculated in Worked Example 9.1. To begin with we will describe some descriptive plots for bioequivalence trials, followed by methods for formal statistical analysis and assessment.

Note that although described here in the context of bioequivalence studies, these plots can also be applied to any crossover trial such as described in Chapter 4.

9.5.1 PRELIMINARY PLOTS

With the relatively small sample size involved in a bioequivalence trial, plots of individual subject data can be highly informative, such as might result in the schematized format of Figure 9.3.

In an ideal world, Figure 9.3a is what we would wish to see – an illustration of bioequivalence. In contrast, Figure 9.3b gives an illustration of the worst case scenario – nonbioequivalence. Figure 9.3c and Figure 9.3e are extreme examples of situations of where, although bioequivalence is concluded, we have: unequal variances on the treatments (Figure 9.3c), and a subject by formulation interaction (Figure 9.3e).

Figure 9.3d and Figure 9.3f also give illustrations of bioequivalence but for situations where we have: high variances (Figure 9.3d), and possible extreme values in the data (Figure 9.3f).

9.5.1.1 Worked Example 9.2: Descriptive Plots

The individual patient outcome data from Table 9.3 for AUC and C_{max} are given in Figure 9.4 (for AUC) and Figure 9.5 (for C_{max}). Unlike for the illustrative examples in Figure 9.3, we have broken the individual data down by sequence.

From these figures it seems that although the formulations may be averagely bioequivalent, there may be high variability in response. Note also how there seems to be an extreme value for both C_{max} and AUC for sequence TR.

Table 9.3 Data from a bioequivalence trial.

Sequence RT					Sequence TR				
Subject	Period	Formulation	*AUC*	C_{max}	Subject	Period	Formulation	*AUC*	C_{max}
1	2	T	79.34	2.827	2	1	T	150.12	5.145
1	1	R	58.16	2.589	2	2	R	142.29	3.216
3	2	T	85.59	4.407	4	1	T	36.95	2.442
3	1	R	69.68	2.480	4	2	R	5.00	0.498
5	2	T	.	.	6	1	T	24.53	1.442
5	1	R	121.84	5.319	6	2	R	26.05	2.728
8	2	T	377.15	11.808	7	1	T	22.11	2.007
8	1	R	208.33	9.634	7	2	R	34.64	3.309
10	2	T	14.23	1.121	9	1	T	703.83	15.133
10	1	R	17.22	1.855	9	2	R	476.56	11.155
11	2	T	750.79	6.877	12	1	T	217.06	9.433
11	1	R	1407.90	13.615	12	2	R	176.02	8.446
13	2	T	21.27	1.055	14	1	T	40.75	1.787
13	1	R	20.81	1.210	14	2	R	152.40	6.231
15	2	T	8.67	1.804	16	1	T	52.76	3.570
15	1	R	.	0.995	16	2	R	51.57	2.445
18	2	T	269.40	9.618	17	1	T	101.52	4.476
18	1	R	203.22	7.496	17	2	R	23.49	1.255
20	2	T	412.42	12.536	19	1	T	37.14	2.169
20	1	R	386.93	16.106	19	2	R	30.54	2.613
21	2	T	33.89	2.129	22	1	T	143.45	5.182
21	1	R	47.96	2.679	22	2	R	42.69	3.031
24	2	T	32.59	1.853	23	1	T	29.80	1.714
24	1	R	22.70	1.727	23	2	R	29.55	1.804
26	2	T	72.36	4.546	25	1	T	63.03	3.201
26	1	R	44.02	3.156	25	2	R	92.94	5.645
27	2	T	423.05	11.167	28	1	T	.	0.891
27	1	R	285.78	8.422	28	2	R	.	0.531
31	2	T	20.33	1.247	29	1	T	56.70	2.203
31	1	R	40.60	1.900	29	2	R	21.03	1.514
32	2	T	17.75	0.910	30	1	T	61.18	3.617
32	1	R	19.43	1.185	30	2	R	66.41	2.130
36	2	T	1160.53	17.374	33	1	T	1376.02	27.312
36	1	R	1048.60	18.976	33	2	R	1200.28	22.068
37	2	T	82.70	6.024	34	1	T	115.33	4.688
37	1	R	107.66	5.031	34	2	R	135.55	7.358
39	2	T	928.05	14.829	38	1	T	17.34	1.072
39	1	R	469.73	6.962	38	2	R	40.35	2.150
43	2	T	20.09	2.278	40	1	T	62.23	3.025
43	1	R	14.95	0.987	40	2	R	64.92	3.041
44	2	T	28.47	1.773	41	1	T	48.99	2.706
44	1	R	28.57	1.105	41	2	R	61.74	2.808
45	2	T	411.72	13.810	42	1	T	53.18	3.240
45	1	R	379.90	12.615	42	2	R	17.51	1.702
47	2	T	46.88	2.339	46	1	T	.	1.680
47	1	R	126.09	6.977	46	2	R	.	.
50	2	T	106.43	4.771	48	1	T	98.03	3.434
50	1	R	75.43	4.925	48	2	R	236.17	7.378
2	1	T	150.12	5.145	49	1	T	1070.98	21.517
2	2	R	142.29	3.216	49	2	R	1016.52	20.116

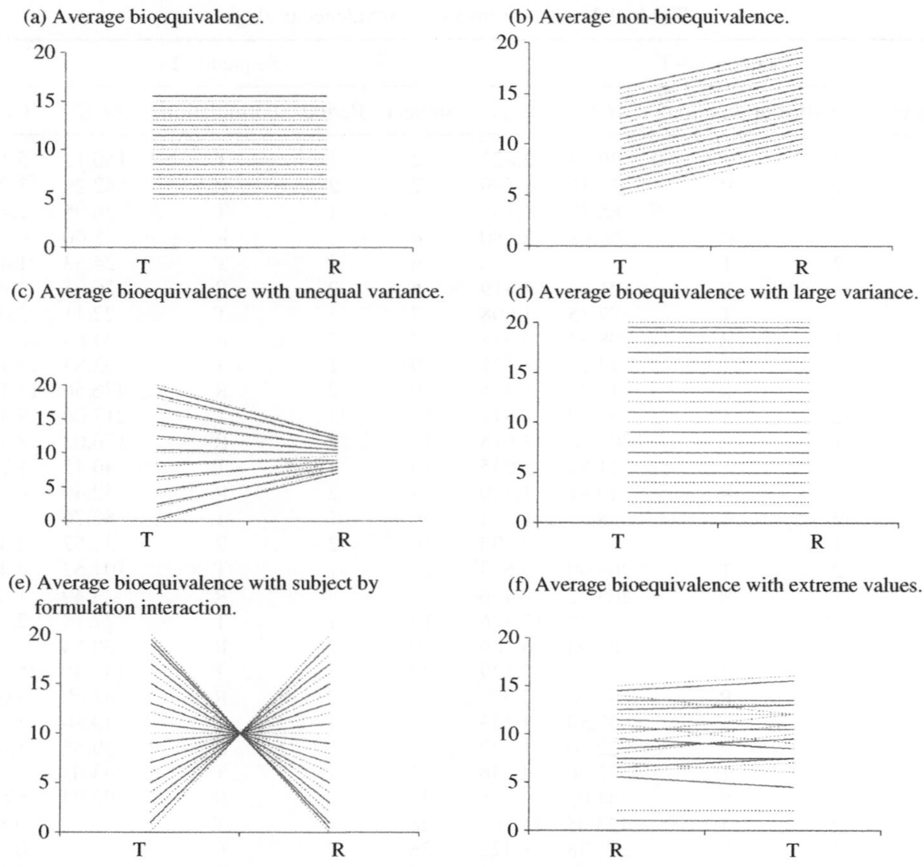

Figure 9.3 Illustration of possible outcomes from a bioequivalence trial. (Patterson and Jones, 2006.)

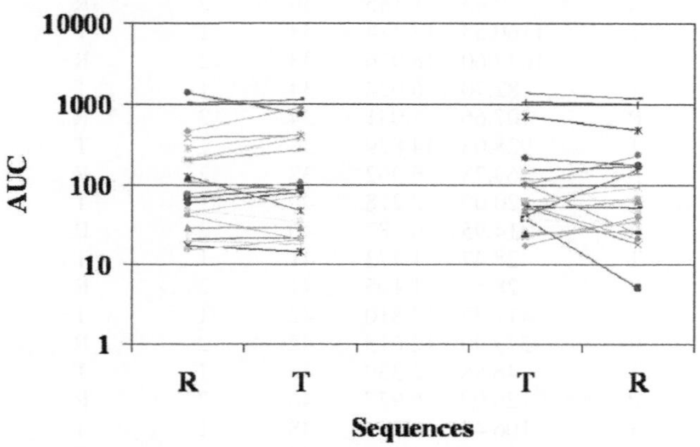

Figure 9.4 Individual patient outcomes for AUC for a bioequivalence study.

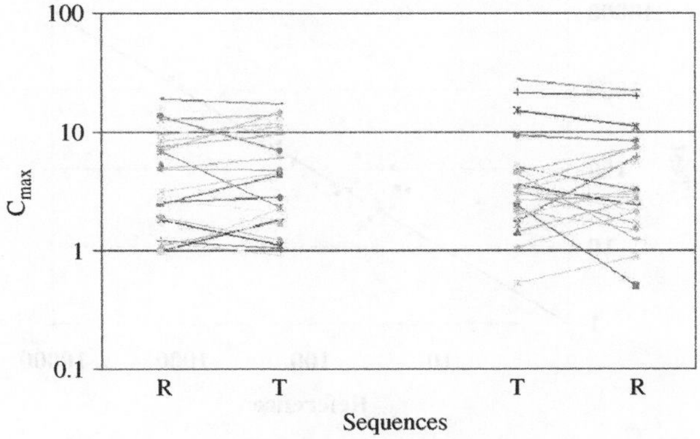

Figure 9.5 Individual patient outcomes for C_{max} for a bioequivalence study.

9.5.2 PAIRED AGREEMENT PLOTS

An illustration of possible outcomes from paired agreement plots is given in Figure 9.6. The line in each graph is the line of unity, while the data from each sequence are given a different symbol. Figure 9.6a gives an ideal situation of perfect agreement between

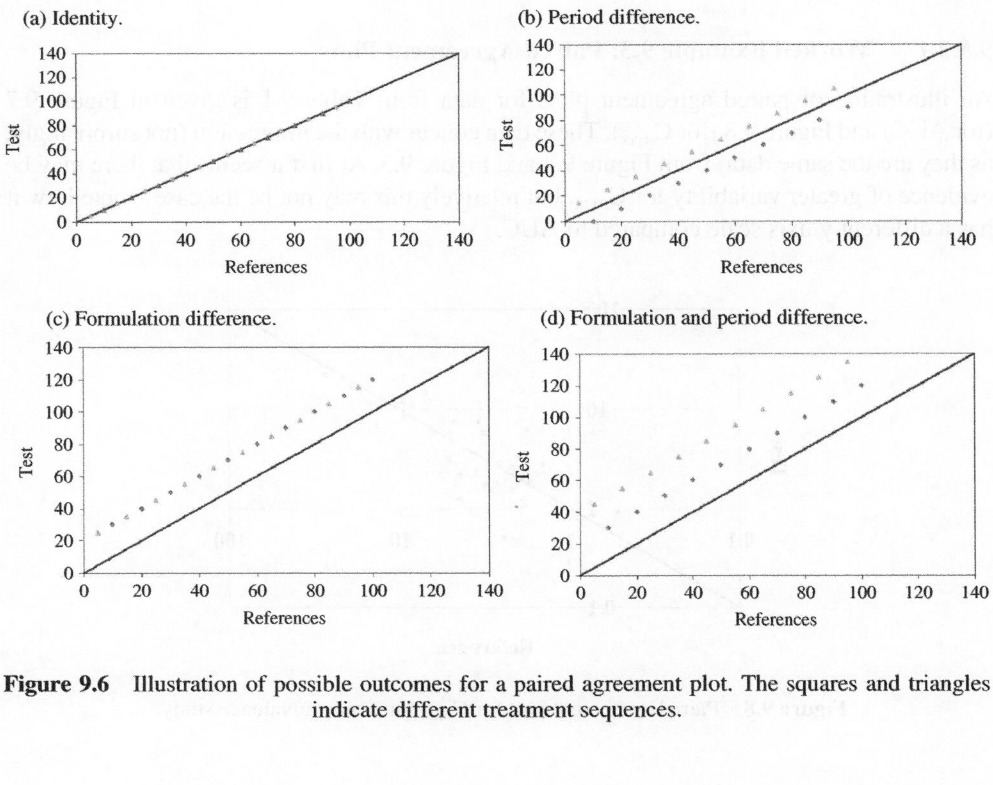

Figure 9.6 Illustration of possible outcomes for a paired agreement plot. The squares and triangles indicate different treatment sequences.

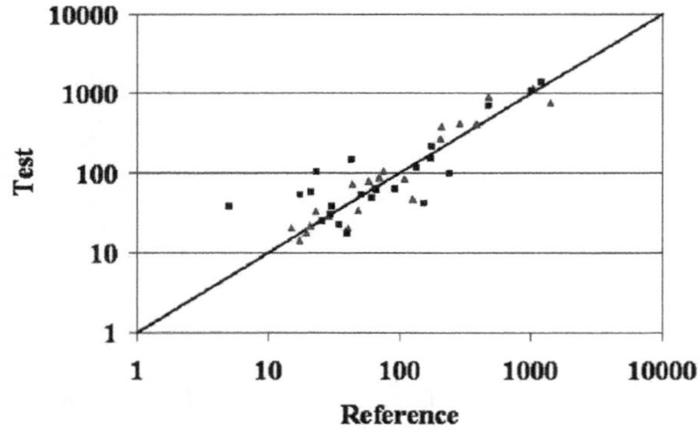

Figure 9.7 Paired agreement plot for AUC for a bioequivalence study.

formulations; that is, bioequivalence, while Figure 9.6b also gives an illustration of agreement but with a possible period effect.

Figure 9.6c and Figure 9.6d give examples of the non-ideal perspective – from the trialist's perspective. Figure 9.6c illustrates a formulation difference, while Figure 9.6d shows a situation with a formulation and period difference.

Note, as with Figure 9.3, paired agreement plots can be applied generally to any crossover trial.

9.5.2.1 Worked Example 9.3: Paired Agreement Plots

An illustration of paired agreement plots for data from Table 9.1 is given in Figure 9.7 (for AUC) and Figure 9.8 (for C_{max}). These data concur with the impression (not surprisingly, as they are the same data) from Figure 9.4 and Figure 9.5. At first it seems that there may be evidence of greater variability for C_{max}, but relatively this may not be the case – note how it has a different y-axis scale compared to AUC.

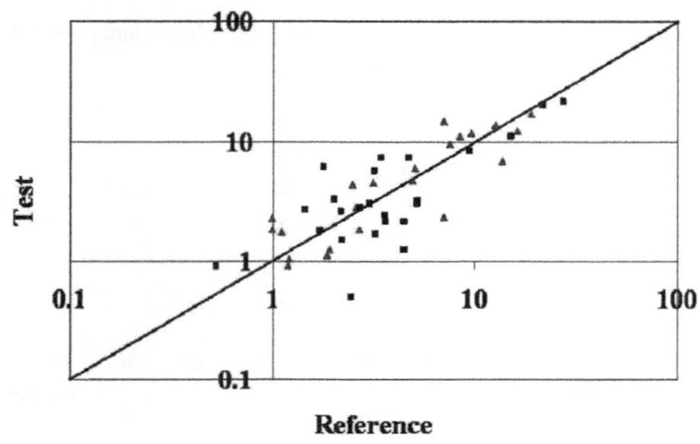

Figure 9.8 Paired agreement plot for C_{max} for a bioequivalence study.

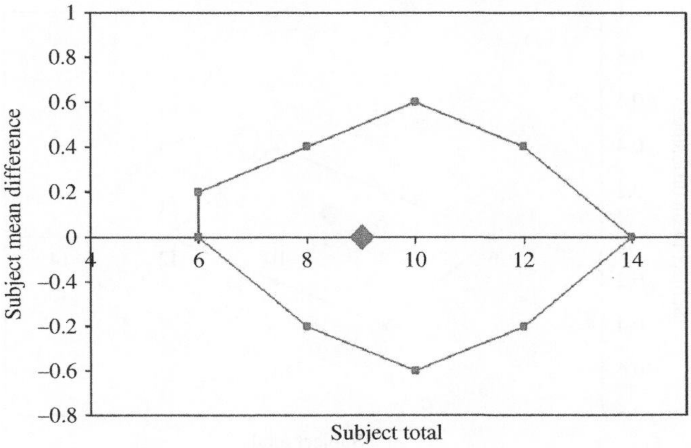

Figure 9.9 Illustration of mean-difference-versus-total plot.

9.5.3 MEAN-DIFFERENCE-VERSUS-TOTAL PLOTS

The final plot to be described is one which graphs the totals $(T+R)$ against mean differences, $(T-R)/2$, where T and R are the respective pharmacokinetic measures for the test and reference drugs respectively, measured on the logarithmic scale.

Figure 9.9 gives an illustration of a mean-difference-versus-total plot. Note that here the small square corresponds to overall mean on each axis; while the larger loop is the boundary formed by linking the most extreme observations and is an indication of the extent of the variability.

A more informative plot when investigating two formulations would be to work in terms of the periods, so for the y-axis take Period 1 away from Period 2 and divide the difference by 2, while the x-axis would be Period 1 added to Period 2. Then plot subjects separately for each sequence, such that for half the subjects we would use $T-R$, and for half, $R-T$.

In Figure 9.10 we illustrate two sequences in the same graph. The differences in the circumferences of the loops for the two sequences would indicate variance differences for the two sequences, while the mean difference on the y axis between boxes gives the period-adjusted mean difference between the two formulations (described in Chapter 3).

Conversely, the difference between the boxes on the x-axis indicates differences in carryover effect. As discussed in Chapter 4, it is not recommended to test for carryover in crossover trials.

9.5.3.1 Worked Example 9.4: Mean-Difference-versus-Total Plots

Examples of the mean-difference-against-total plots are given for AUC in Figure 9.11 and for C_{max} in Figure 9.12, for the trial data of Table 9.3. In these plots the individual data points are also given.

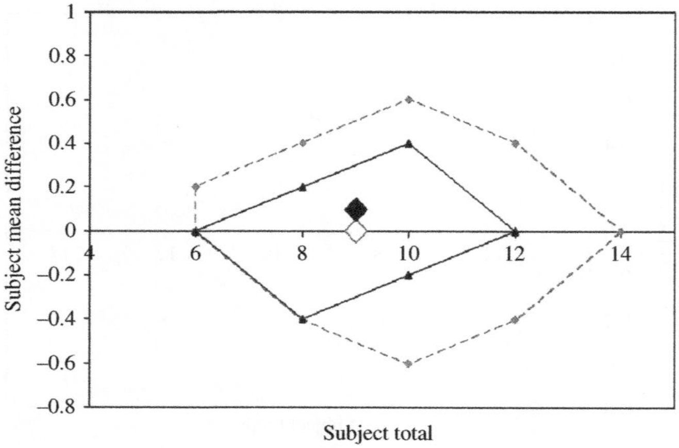

Figure 9.10 Illustration of mean-difference-versus-total plot by sequence.

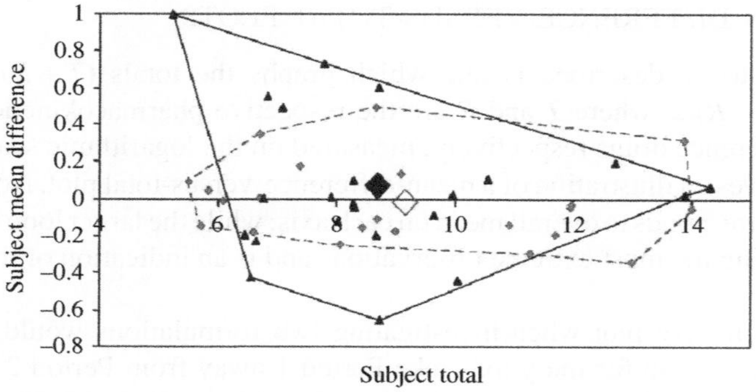

Figure 9.11 Illustration of mean-difference-versus-total plot by sequence for $\log_e$AUC.

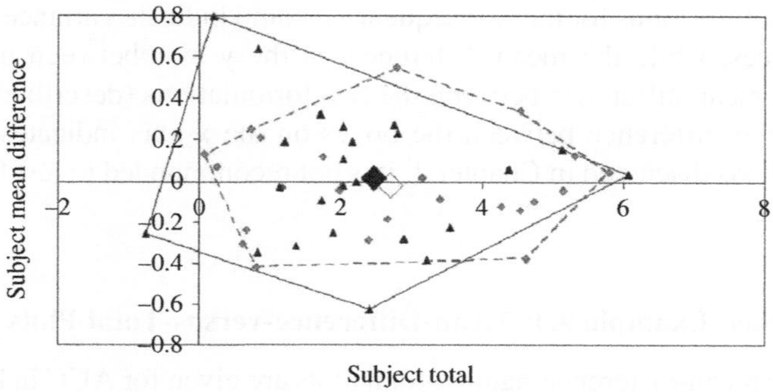

Figure 9.12 Illustration of mean-difference-versus-total plot by sequence for $\log_e C_{max}$.

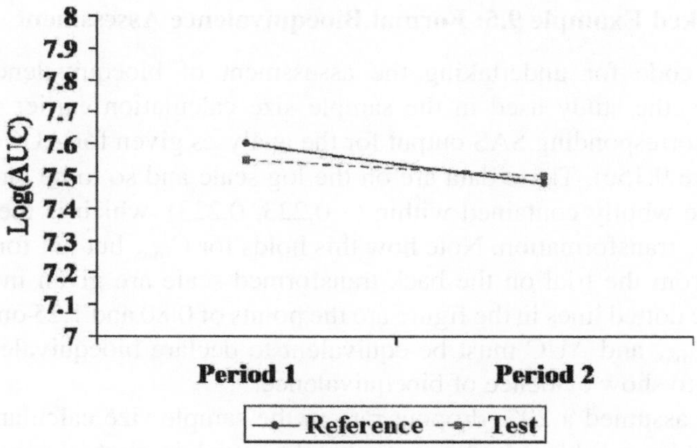

Figure 9.13 Mean plot for $\log_e$AUC by period.

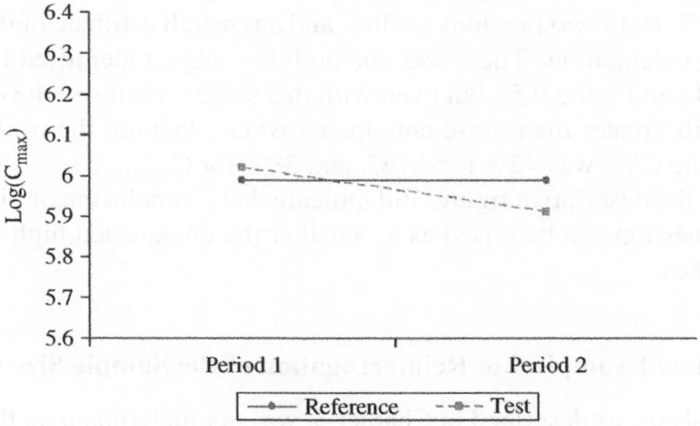

Figure 9.14 Mean plot for $\log_e C_{max}$ by period.

The final plots are Figure 9.13 and Figure 9.14, which give means for AUC and C_{max} for the data from Table 9.3, by period.

9.5.4 FORMAL ASSESSMENT OF BIOEQUIVALENCE

In Chapter 4 the analysis of crossover trials was described, which is now used for bioequivalence studies. Hence, to formally assess bioequivalence, the log-transformed AUC and C_{max} (and any other outcomes that are appropriate) are analysed by an analysis of variance (ANOVA) with appropriate terms for a crossover trial. The adjusted means are calculated on the log scale along with their corresponding 90% confidence intervals. These are then back-transformed to get ratio estimates and their corresponding 90% CI.

To be able to declare bioequivalence both AUC and C_{max} must be equivalent.

9.5.4.1 Worked Example 9.5: Formal Bioequivalence Assessment

Example SAS code for undertaking the assessment of bioequivalence is given in Figure 9.15a for the study used in the sample size calculation earlier in the chapter, along with the corresponding SAS output for the analyses given for AUC (Figure 9.15b) and C_{max} (Figure 9.15c). These data are on the log scale and so to be bioequivalent the 90% CI must be wholly contained within (−0.223, 0.223), which is the margin (0.80, 1.25) after a $\log_e$ transformation. Note how this holds for C_{max} but not for AUC.

The results from the trial on the back-transformed scale are given in Table 9.4 and Figure 9.16. The dotted lines in the figure are the points of 0.80 and 1.25 on the mean ratio axis. As both C_{max} and AUC must be equivalent to declare bioequivalence, this study therefore failed to show evidence of bioequivalence.

Note that we assumed a 20% dropout rate in the sample size calculation in Worked Example 9.1, but from Table 9.4 we can see that the actual dropout rate observed was a lot less than this.

One thing to highlight here is the relatively large estimates of the CV_w for the study, of 47% and 41% for AUC and C_{max} respectively. To design the study, variance estimates, given in Table 9.2, from two previous studies, and an overall estimate of the CV_w of 30%, were used in the calculations. There was one outlying subject identified from descriptive plots (Figure 9.4 and Figure 9.5), but even with this subject removed the observed values of CV_w were still greater than those anticipated when planning the trial; excluding the extreme value, the CV_w was 42% for AUC, and 38% for C_{max}.

Nevertheless, the descriptive figures did indicate that a conclusion of bioequivalence is possible but a question can be raised as to whether the unexpected high variances could have been foreseen.

9.5.4.2 Worked Example 9.6: Reinterrogation of the Sample Size Calculations

A sensitivity analysis, as described in Chapter 3, was not undertaken on the study sample size assumptions *a priori*, but retrospectively we now undertake this.

From the pooled estimates and their corresponding degrees of freedom given in Table 9.2, Table 9.5 could have been constructed, and the maximum plausible estimate for the CV_w, taken as the 95th percentile, would have been 38%. If this CV_w for the AUC was observed and not the 30% used in the calculations then the study would still have had 70% power. Thus, the study was reasonably robust to deviations about the variance estimate.

There are a couple of points worth noting. First, the actual CV_w observed in the study was greater than that estimated as the 95th percentile from the sensitivity analysis. Indeed, the variance estimates for C_{max} and AUC, excluding the outlying subject, fell on the 99th percentile based on the previous studies. This fact demonstrates that, although it would be nice to be wise after the event, no one has a crystal ball and that, by definition, unanticipated variances are indeed unanticipated.

The second point to highlight is that although the planned study was robust to deviations in the assumptions about the variance it was hit with the double whammy of an unexpected large variance and an unexpectedly large regimen difference (compared to the initial sample size assumption of a ratio of unity). This double whammy greatly impacted on the study.

(a) SAS code.

```
OPTIONS nodate nonumber;
TITLE 'AUC';
PROC mixed DATA = aucdat METHOD = reml ITDETAILS maxiter = 200;
CLASS sequence subject period formula;
MODEL lauc = sequence subject(sequence) period formula /outp = out;
LSMEANS formula;
ESTIMATE 'T-R' formula -1 1 /cl alpha = 0.10;
RUN;
```

(b) Log_e AUC output.

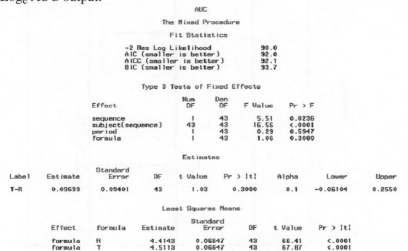

```
                              AUC

                      The Mixed Procedure

                        Fit Statistics

              -2 Res Log Likelihood            90.0
              AIC (smaller is better)          92.0
              AICC (smaller is better)         92.1
              BIC (smaller is better)          93.7

                 Type 3 Tests of Fixed Effects

                              Num     Den
         Effect               DF      DF     F Value    Pr > F

         sequence              1      43        5.51    0.0236
         subject(sequence)    43      43       16.56    <.0001
         period                1      43        0.29    0.5947
         formula               1      43        1.06    0.3080

                             Estimates

                      Standard
Label   Estimate       Error     DF   t Value   Pr > |t|   Alpha      Lower     Upper

T-R      0.09699     0.09401     43      1.03     0.3080     0.1   -0.06104    0.2550

                        Least Squares Means

                                          Standard
     Effect     formula    Estimate          Error    DF    t Value    Pr > |t|

     formula    R            4.4143        0.06647    43      66.41      <.0001
     formula    T            4.5113        0.06647    43      67.87      <.0001
```

(c) Log_e C_{max} output.

```
                              Cmax

                      The Mixed Procedure

                        Fit Statistics

              -2 Res Log Likelihood            83.7
              AIC (smaller is better)          85.7
              AICC (smaller is better)         85.8
              BIC (smaller is better)          87.5

                 Type 3 Tests of Fixed Effects

                              Num     Den
         Effect               DF      DF     F Value    Pr > F

         sequence              1      45        1.84    0.1815
         subject(sequence)    45      45       10.21    <.0001
         period                1      45        0.11    0.7456
         formula               1      45        0.38    0.5390

                             Estimates

                      Standard
Label   Estimate       Error     DF   t Value   Pr > |t|   Alpha      Lower     Upper

T-R      0.05083     0.08211     45      0.62     0.5390     0.1   -0.08707    0.1887

                        Least Squares Means

                                          Standard
     Effect     formula    Estimate          Error    DF    t Value    Pr > |t|

     formula    R            1.2619        0.05806    45      21.73      <.0001
     formula    T            1.3128        0.05806    45      22.61      <.0001
```

Figure 9.15 Example SAS code and SAS output for $\log_e$ AUC and $\log_e$ C_{max} for bioequivalence assessment.

Table 9.4 Summary of results of bioequivalence trial.

	n	Ratio	90% CI	$CV_w\%$
AUC	45	1.10	0.94 to 1.29	47
$\mathbf{C_{max}}$	47	1.05	0.92 to 1.21	41

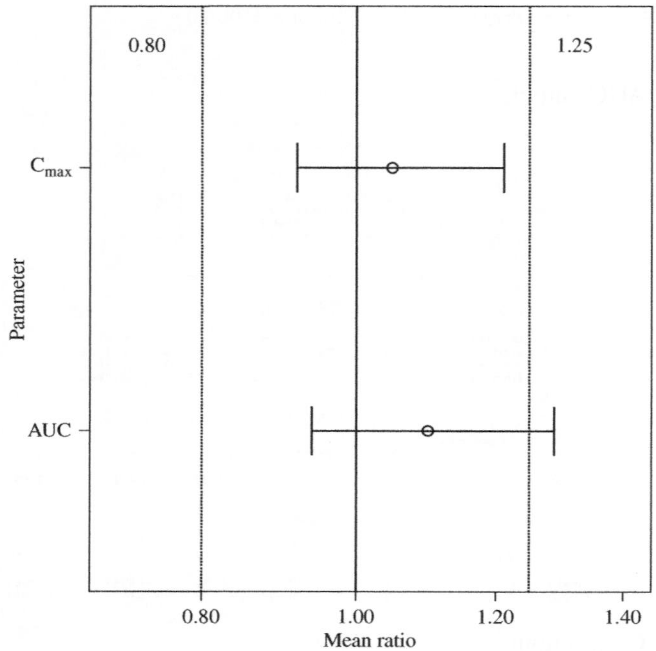

Figure 9.16 Summary of results, point estimates and 90% confidence intervals for the bioequivalence trial.

Table 9.5 Sensitivity analysis about the coefficients of variability (%) observed in two previous studies.

	CV_w (%)	95th (%)	Power for 95th (%)
AUC	29	38	70
$\mathbf{C_{max}}$	27	35	76

As stated, however, a sensitivity analysis was not undertaken *a priori* with this study. However, this study was the motivation for the discussion and work on sensitivity analysis given in Chapter 3, and led to the recommendation for sensitivity analyses to be prospectively applied (Julious, 2004a).

9.6 ADAPTIVE DESIGNS IN BIOEQUIVALENCE ASSESSMENT

One solution to the problem of having an uncertain estimate of the variability is to adopt an adaptive design approach (Julious, 2004a). The advantage of being adaptive is that it allows us to alter or stop the course of a study during its actual conduct. In this way, any unexpected occurrences are not encountered for the first time when the study has been completed and the final analysis is being undertaken. There are three approaches that can be adopted for such designs:

1. Apply a group sequential design where the sample size in each group is fixed but interim analyses are undertaken to investigate the null hypothesis, with a decision made at each analysis to stop the trial for success or failure or to enrol another cohort. The sample size is not re-estimated.
2. A design is applied where, at fixed interim analyses, the parameters used in the estimation of the sample size are re-estimated, such as the variance for Normal data, and the sample size is adjusted accordingly. The null hypothesis is not investigated.
3. A combination of (1) and (2), where at the interim analyses both the null hypothesis is investigated and the sample size is re-estimated – conditional on whether the trial is stopped for success or failure.

The first two approaches are relatively straightforward but the third is more complex, as the sample size re-estimation depends on a decision on the null hypothesis. Here we will concentrate on group sequential designs, on which the CHMP (2008) state:

> It is acceptable to use a two-stage approach when attempting to demonstrate bioequivalence. An initial group of subjects can be treated and their data analysed. If bioequivalence has not been demonstrated an additional group can be recruited and the results from both groups combined in a final analysis. If this approach is taken appropriate steps must be taken to preserve the overall Type I error of the experiment. The analysis of the first stage data should be treated as an interim analysis and both analyses conducted at adjusted significance levels (with the confidence intervals accordingly using an adjusted coverage probability which will be higher than 90%). The plan to use a two-stage approach must be prespecified in the protocol along with the adjusted significance levels to be used for each of the analyses.

To highlight the utility of adaptive designs in bioequivalence, a worked example will be described.

9.6.1 WORKED EXAMPLE 9.7: GROUP SEQUENTIAL

In this example the trial is not actually a bioequivalence study but a drug interaction study. These studies will be described in Chapter 10, but it is a good example to introduce the principles of group sequential approaches. In terms of statistical principles, the two types of study are the same.

In this particular example, *a priori* it was believed that the investigative compound (I) may interact, from a pharmacokinetic point of view, with desipramine (D), leading to the plan to conduct an *in vivo* study. The no-effect criteria, used to determine if adding the investigative compound had any effect on the drug exposure of the probe drug desipramine (μ_{D+I}) compared to desipramine alone (μ_D), was 24% on the log scale. Thus, the null and alternative hypotheses for the trial were

$$H_0: \frac{\mu_{D+I}}{\mu_D} \leq 0.76 \text{ or } \frac{\mu_{D+I}}{\mu_D} \geq 1.30, \qquad H_1: 0.76 < \frac{\mu_{D+I}}{\mu_D} < 1.30.$$

Here, the 'standard' 20% bioequivalence limits were not used as, *a priori*, it was believed that the wider margin of (0.76, 1.30) was sufficient to declare no effect. Likewise it was believed that only the AUC had to fall within the no-effect margin for 'no effect' to be declared. The study followed the drug regulatory guidelines for drug interaction studies (FDA 1999a, CPMP 1997).

One issue that became apparent when designing the study was that the variability observed in the pharmacokinetics of desipramine in previous studies varied quite markedly, with three studies on file having CV_w for AUC of 14%, 27% and 39%. There was no apparent rationale for the diverse variabilities observed, and so none of them could be discounted. This led to the issue of what variance to use to estimate the sample size, as the $CV_w = 39\%$ would lead to a sample size estimate approaching five times that of a $CV_w = 14\%$.

To overcome this particular problem a two-stage group sequential design was used. The advantage of this approach is that group sequential methodologies allow an interim analysis to be carried out on data from one cohort of subjects – where a decision can be made whether to stop the trial for success or failure or to enrol a second cohort of subjects. To allow for the fact that an interim analysis is made the overall Type I error rate of the study should be maintained at 5% by the use of appropriate statistical methods. The concept of the group sequential trial is captured in Figure 9.17.

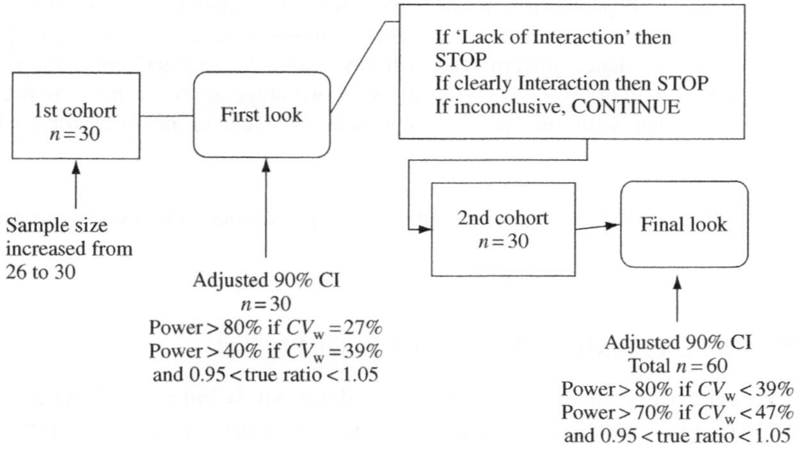

Figure 9.17 Group sequential trial illustration.

One issue to highlight with such trials is that it is essential that the stopping rule applied at the interim analysis be prespecified.

For the worked example, therefore, calculations were based on two one-sided tests, a Type I error rate of 5% and a no-effect range of 24%, that is, (0.76, 1.30). The group sample sizes were calculated assuming a true mean ratio of unity and CV_w values of 27% and 39%, which gave a sample size of 30 subjects in each cohort. To ensure 30 subjects completed it was planned to have 34 subjects start in each cohort.

An equal allocation, 2.5%, of the Type I error was spent in each cohort using a simple Bonferroni correction of dividing the test size by 2. This α-spending allocation is a little conservative but it was a pragmatic allocation given the equal cohort sample sizes. Thus, with the Bonferroni correction, the 90% confidence intervals were presented so that the overall Type I error was maintained at 5%.

Another pragmatic decision was the choice of CV_w for sample size calculations. The pooled estimate of the CV_w from the previous three studies was 28.5%; however, for this study it was decided just to use the two observed values of 27% and 39%.

Figure 9.17 gives a description of the study design and Table 9.6 gives the breakdown of the sensitivity of the study to deviations in the assumptions about the variability and the mean difference. This table appeared in the protocol of the study. As can be seen, the study was quite robust to most deviations.

The following stopping rules were applied at the interim analysis:

1. Lack of interaction: the 90% confidence interval for the ratio (D + I) : D of AUCs for desipramine falls within (0.76, 1.30).
2. Clear interaction: the ratio (D + I) : D of AUCs for desipramine falls outside (0.76, 1.30).
3. Otherwise: recruit a further 30 subjects.

A total of 34 subjects were included in the interim analysis. In the actual study the 90% confidence interval for the ratio was (D + I) / D = 0.94 (0.89, 1.00) with $CV_w = 11.7\%$ – a lower than expected variability. Therefore 'lack of interaction' of the compound on desipramine was demonstrated, and the study stopped.

Table 9.6 Sample size and sensitivity of the sample size to assumptions about the variability and mean ratio.

CV_w (%)	Cohort	n	Power (%) for true ratio of		
			1.00	1.05	1.10
14	1	30	99	99	99
	2	60	99	99	99
27	1	30	90	83	60
	2	60	99	99	90
39	1	30	42	38	28
	2	60	90	82	60

Had the study continued to a second cohort, the plan was to perform a 'fixed sample size' analysis in each cohort separately and then to combine the two cohorts using the method described by Gould (1995). With this approach the overall response of the log formulation difference is estimated by a weighted sum of the differences observed in each part of the trial; that is

$$\hat{d} = \frac{\sum_{i=1}^{k} w_i d_i}{\sum_{i=1}^{k} w_i}. \tag{9.8}$$

For the Gould method the weights are proportional to the group cohort sample size; that is, $w_i = n_i$. Here the differences d_i are the log mean ratios. Thus, the larger the cohort sample size proportional to the total sample size, the greater weight that cohort has.

The corresponding variance of the estimated difference, $d_{k-1} - d_k$ of interest, is given by

$$var(\sigma_w) = \frac{(n_{k-1} - 1)\sigma_{k-1}^2 + n_k\sigma_k^2 + \left(\frac{1}{n_{k-1}} + \frac{1}{n_k}\right)^{-1}(d_{k-1} - d_k)^2}{(n_{k-1} + n_k)(n_{k-1} + n_k - 1)} \tag{9.9}$$

Here, k refers to the group, n_k are the sample sizes in each group and σ_k are the within-subject standard deviations for each group.

9.6.2 UTILITY OF ADAPTIVE DESIGNS IN THE ASSESSMENT OF BIOEQUIVALENCE

The worked example highlights the key advantages in applying adaptive designs to bioequivalence studies. In the example, recruitment was controlled by the sponsor in that subjects were recruited and enrolled into a single centre and at a rate fixed by the sponsor. A consequence was that planning for the analyses was straightforward, as they were performed following preset timelines; that is, it was known when the subjects would be recruited and when the analyses would be undertaken.

As recruitment was controlled by the sponsor it was temporarily halted until the interim analysis was completed. If recruitment is not halted, but continues while the interim analysis is being conducted, then logistical and statistical issues are raised. In addition the endpoint in the interim analysis was the same as in the final analysis. Obviously there is a level of complication if this is not the case, for example if a surrogate was used or perhaps the same primary outcome measure but assessed at a different time point.

A disadvantage comes from the exact application of the science of hindsight. When everything goes to plan – we see the mean difference and variance as expected – there is an argument that there might have been an unnecessarily large sample size recruited – maybe 30% larger for the worked example. It should be noted though that across a large number of studies this saving may not be applicable, as failed studies from a nonadaptive design may have to be repeated, while with an adaptive design there is the option to enrol the second cohort.

10 Other Phase I Trials

10.1 INTRODUCTION

In this chapter we describe other trials which we group under the general banner heading of 'Phase I Trials'. However, as discussed in Chapter 1, although the label may be Phase I for the trials, the actual timing of these studies could be anywhere in the drug development process. This is due to the fact that, although many of these trials need to be done prior to a submission, many of them are enabling studies which can be performed in parallel with other critical-path activities, and so could take place while a compound is nominally in Phase II or Phase III.

10.2 DOSE PROPORTIONALITY

10.2.1 INTRODUCTION

Dose proportionality is one of the most important assumptions in drug development. For example it enables the prediction of repeat-dose pharmacokinetics from single doses, as well as facilitating straightforward dose adjustment for subpopulations. However, in spite of its importance, there are no formal guidelines on the design and conduct of dose-proportionality studies

A definition of dose proportionality for two dose-normalized doses is that the pharmacokinetic profiles of the doses are superimposable. This means that the pharmacokinetics of any dose are predictable due to the proportional increase in exposures. Hence, for example, if you double the dose you double the exposures.

The utility of this can be highlighted in Figure 10.1, particularly if there is a wide safety and efficacy window. Hence, with dose-proportional pharmacokinetics we can adjust a dose for a given subgroup and be confident that a subject would still fall within the safety and efficacy window.

Although dose proportionality is an important feature of a new chemical entity and an assessment usually should be made prior to any submission, dose-proportionality studies are usually not on the critical path and are completed in parallel with other activities.

An Introduction to Statistics in Early Phase Trials Steven A. Julious, Say Beng Tan and David Machin

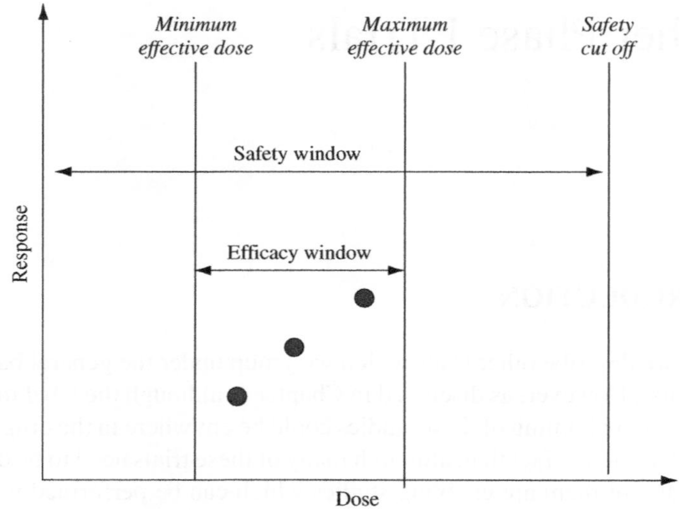

Figure 10.1 Illustration of safety and efficacy windows.

Dose proportionality is also referred to as dose linearity. This is due to the following result for extravascular dosing, which we derived in Chapter 2

$$c(t) = \frac{\lambda_2 F \cdot Dose}{V(\lambda_2 - \lambda_1)}\left(e^{-\lambda_1 t} - e^{-\lambda_2 t}\right), \tag{10.1}$$

which defines drug concentration ($c(t)$) at a given time for a given dose in terms of the clearance (Cl); the distribution volume (V); the elimination rate (λ_1), absorption rate (λ_2) and the bioavailability (F). Thus, for linear pharmacokinetics, in the context of a compartmental model, λ_1 and λ_2 should remain constant in (10.1) for any dose, such that exposures can be estimated at a given time simply from the dose.

A given compound does not need to have dose-proportional pharmacokinetics, but it does help in drug development. For example, bioequivalence studies would need to be undertaken only at a single dose, and not at several doses as would be the case if the pharmacokinetics were not dose proportional (CHMP, 2008). In addition, dose adjustments for subgroups are more straightforward.

10.2.2 DESIGN OF DOSE-PROPORTIONALITY STUDIES

In Chapter 6, for first-time-into-man (FTIM) studies, exploratory assessments of dose proportionality were described. The graphical and summary measures can also be applied to definitive assessments here. A main difference now, though, is that dose is no longer confounded with period, and so for a three-dose study plus placebo, a Williams square, as described in Chapter 5, can be derived with four treatment sequences. For example, subjects are then randomized to each of the following sequences. Here, the different subjects are in the rows and treatment periods in columns.

P	D1	D2	D3
D1	D2	D3	P
D2	D3	P	D1
D3	P	D1	D2

To make a formal assessment, three doses would first need to be selected that span the therapeutic range as illustrated in Figure 10.1. The sample size calculation will depend on the analysis approach to be applied: analysis of variance (Section 10.2.3.1) or the power method (Section 10.2.3.2). Senn (2007) describes their analysis in detail.

10.2.3 SAMPLE SIZE FOR DOSE-PROPORTIONALITY STUDIES

10.2.3.1 Analysis 1: Analysis of Variance

For the analysis of variance (ANOVA) approach, the design and analysis would be very similar to the methodology described for bioequivalence studies in Chapter 9. As two dose-normalized doses need to be superimposable the sample size would need to be calculated as for a bioequivalence study for each dose-normalized dose compared to the reference dose.

The reference dose is usually taken as either the lowest or highest dose and although there are no regulatory guidelines, the limits of (0.80, 1.25) could be used within which each pair-wise 90% confidence interval must be wholly contained (assuming there are three doses).

Here there are no issues with multiplicity as both comparisons must hold to declare dose proportionality.

A study design suggestion is to replicate the reference dose twice, so that for example a Williams square is built such that all subjects receive the reference dose D1 on two occasions. For example:

P D1 D3 D2 D1

As with other replicate designs, this design has the potential to reduce the sample size by 25%.

10.2.3.2 Analysis 2: Power Method

In Chapter 12 we will discuss the sample size calculations for a linear regression in the context of designing a study to assess dose response. On the log scale, the calculation of the sample size is equivalent to that for a linear regression.

A main consideration in the design and analysis of dose-proportionality studies is how to make the assessment of dose proportionality. For example, suppose that the doses were

1, 2 and 4. If we designed the study under the assumption that the analysis and assessment would be based on 2^{b-1}, then we would have a much smaller sample size compared to an assessment based on 4^{b-1}, where b is the slope of the response for the power model described in Chapter 6. For this example, 2^{b-1} would be an assessment per doubling of dose, while 4^{b-1} would be an assessment across the dose range.

Suppose the assessment is of r^{b-1}, where r is the log dose increment, and we wish to demonstrate that this is wholly contained within (0.80, 1.25). Then this is the same as showing that the slope b is wholly contained within

$$\left(-\frac{log_e 1.25}{log_e r}, \frac{log_e 1.25}{log_e r}\right). \tag{10.2}$$

From (10.2) therefore we can define the limit size as

$$l = \frac{log_e 1.25}{log_e r}. \tag{10.3}$$

Hence, under the assumption that $b=0$, the sample size can be calculated from (Sethuraman *et al.*, 2007)

$$n = \frac{\sigma_w^2 \left(Z_{1-\frac{\beta}{2}} + Z_{1-\alpha}\right)^2}{l^2 \sigma_x^2} \tag{10.4}$$

where σ_w^2 is the variance about the dose response and σ_x^2 is the design variance on the x-axis (i.e. between the chosen $\log_e$ doses).

For the special case of just two active doses, (10.4) becomes

$$n = \frac{2\sigma_w^2 \left(Z_{1-\frac{\beta}{2}} + Z_{1-\alpha}\right)^2}{(log_e 1.25)^2}. \tag{10.5}$$

This is the approximate sample size for a bioequivalence study with just two arms, given in Chapter 9. Hence, with just two doses the power method and the analysis of variance (ANOVA) approach are equivalent.

Note if, for example, the analysis of variance (ANOVA) approach is specified as the primary analysis, then the power model could be supporting, and vice versa.

10.3 REPEAT-DOSE ASSESSMENT

10.3.1 INTRODUCTION

For regimens that are to be administered chronically there is a need to assess the repeat-dose pharmacokinetics. This is usually at steady state.

The study design within a subject usually takes the form:

- An assessment of the pharmacokinetic profile of a single dose is made.
- Subjects are then 'washed out' for this dose.
- Repeat doses are then given until steady state is achieved, as in Figure 10.2.

The pharmacokinetic profiles are then assessed at steady state and compared to the single-dose pharmacokinetics for each subject. Trough pharmacokinetic samples may also be taken before each dose during the accumulation phase of study. The assessment of pharmacokinetic accumulation is therefore made within subject.

Repeat-dose studies for chronically administered drugs would be on the critical path as obviously there would need to be a repeat-dose assessment of a new chemical entity for safety and tolerability prior to it being administered in a patient population.

10.3.2 DESIGN OF REPEAT-DOSE STUDIES

An example design for a repeat-dose study is given in Figure 10.3, where each row refers to a different subject.

The study designs are usually therefore parallel group – in the sense that subjects are randomized to placebo or active, though the comparison of single to repeat-dose pharmacokinetics is made within subject – with each dosing cohort of subjects assigned to dose or placebo in a 2 : 1 or 3 : 1 ratio. More than one dose may be given to an individual, but usually different doses are assessed in separate dosing cohorts with different subjects.

The placebos here are usually not to facilitate formal comparisons to the active doses but to assist in the assessment and interpretation of subjective adverse events.

The sample size required is based primarily on feasibility, although the precision of the estimates can be assessed as described in Chapter 3.

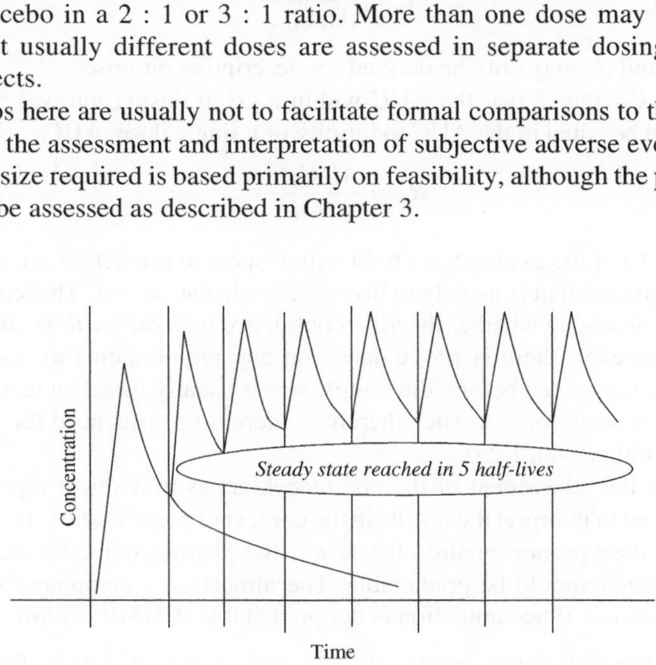

Figure 10.2 Repeat-dose pharmacokinetic profile to achieve steady state.

Cohort 1																	
D1	D1	D1	D1	D1	D1	D1	D1	D1	D1	D1	D1	P	P	P	P	P	P
Cohort 2																	
D2	D2	D2	D2	D2	D2	D2	D2	D2	D2	D2	D2	P	P	P	P	P	P
Etc.																	

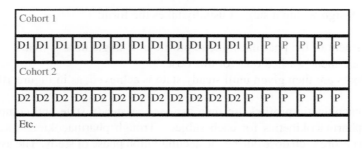

Figure 10.3 A repeat-dose assessment study design with allocation to placebo in a 2 : 1 ratio.

10.3.3 ANALYSIS OF REPEAT-DOSE STUDIES

With the single- and repeat-dose pharmacokinetics a number of assessments can be made. We can determine the predicted accumulation from the single-dose pharmacokinetics from

$$R_{\text{p}} = \frac{AUC_{0-\infty}}{AUC_{0-t}}, \tag{10.6}$$

while the observed accumulation ratio is

$$R_{\text{o}} = \frac{AUC_{0-\tau}}{AUC_{0-t}}. \tag{10.7}$$

In practice, R_{p} and R_{o} may only be derived for descriptive purposes.

We stated in Chapter 2 that the AUC within a given dosing interval at steady state, $\text{AUC}_{0-\tau}$, should be equal to the AUC to infinity of a single dose, $\text{AUC}_{0-\infty}$. Their ratio is

$$R_{\text{s}} = \frac{AUC_{0-\tau}}{AUC_{0-\infty}}, \tag{10.8}$$

and should equal 1 if the assumptions hold with respect to predictive accumulation.

The primary assessment is usually to investigate whether $R_{\text{s}} = 1$. This could be accomplished through assessing whether the 90% confidence interval for R_{s} is contained within (0.80, 1.25). However, there is no guidance on any requirements to assess predictive accumulation and, as stated before, the sample size is usually based on feasibility with no formal power considerations. As such therefore, there is no strict need for the confidence interval to be within (0.80, 1.25).

In addition to the assessment of the pharmacokinetics in a single repeat-dose study, there is also a need to interpret the results in the context of other studies. The most obvious study is that of dose proportionality, because if the pharmacokinetics are dose proportional, accumulation should be predictable. The impact on a compound's development could be quite marked if accumulation is not predictable (CHMP, 2008):

> . . . in case of dose or time-dependent pharmacokinetics, resulting in markedly higher concentrations at steady state than expected from single dose data, a potential difference in AUC between formulations may be larger at steady state than after single dose. Hence, a multiple dose

study may be required in addition to the single dose study to ensure that the products are bioequivalent regarding AUC also at steady state. However, if the single dose study indicates very similar PK profile for test and reference (the 90% confidence interval for AUC is within 90–111), the requirement for steady-state data may be waived.

Hence, with no predictable accumulation there may be a necessity to complete bioequivalence studies both at steady state and with a single dose, or at the very least at a single dose with narrower limits than the standard (0.80, 1.25).

10.4 DRUG INTERACTION

10.4.1 INTRODUCTION

Recall from Chapter 2 that for a single dose the pharmacokinetic profile could resemble Figure 10.4, where there is both an absorption and elimination phase. So although the body will be absorbing and eliminating the drug throughout the profile, there is a phase where the amount of drug in the body is increasing (absorption phase) and a phase where it is decreasing (elimination phase).

Due to the way a drug is eliminated in the body there may be a question as to whether the drug may interact with others that follow the same elimination pathway. A simple way of thinking of this is to think of a tap pouring into a sink with the plug open, as in Figure 10.5.

With just one tap turned on, the water will rise to a certain level while being eliminated through the plug hole. With two taps turned on, however, the finite capacity of the elimination through the plug will mean that the water in the sink will rise higher (analogous to C_{max}) and also reach a higher volume (analogous to AUC).

Drug interactions, actual or potential, emphasize the importance of having wide safety and efficacy windows, as with narrow margins there would need to be close monitoring of concomitant interactive medicines.

Drug interaction studies tend not to be on the critical path and are usually enabling studies done in parallel with other activities. As enabling studies they can have a major impact on inclusion and exclusion criteria such that, without *in vivo* assessment, certain

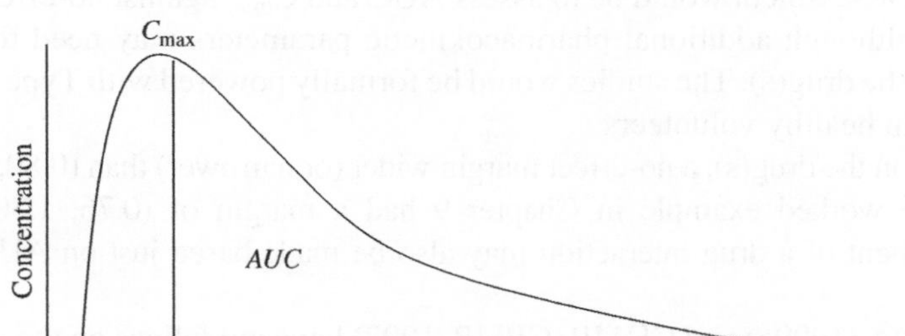

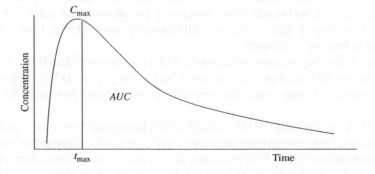

Figure 10.4 Example of a pharmacokinetic profile.

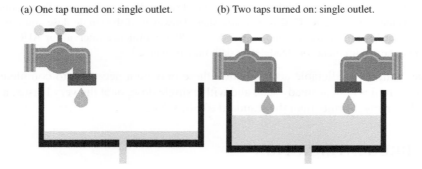

Figure 10.5 Simple pictorial of a drug interaction.

concomitant therapies may be precluded from being used in a trial. This may have a detrimental effect on recruitment rates in late-phase trials if a large portion of the patient population receives these treatments.

10.4.2 DESIGN AND ANALYSIS OF DRUG INTERACTION STUDIES

A standard drug interaction design would be two-period crossover, where the arms are substrate (S) and substrate with investigative drug (S + I), and the objective is to examine the effect of the investigative drug on the substrate. It is also possible that an assessment is also required of the substrate on the investigative drug, such that a drug–drug interaction design is planned, which would be a three-period crossover where the arms are S, S + I, I.

The null hypothesis and alternative hypotheses and sample size calculations are as with a bioequivalence assessment, as described in Chapter 9. It should be noted however that the statistical variability of S may increase when given with I, and so this may need to be allowed for in any sample size calculation.

The default assessment would be to assess AUC and C_{max} against no-effect margins of (0.80, 1.25), although additional pharmacokinetic parameters may need to be assessed depending on the drug(s). The studies would be formally powered with Type I error of 5%, and assessed in healthy volunteers.

Depending on the drug(s), a no-effect margin wider (or narrower) than (0.80, 1.25) may be justified – the worked example in Chapter 9 had a margin of (0.76, 1.30) – although formal assessment of a drug interaction may also be made based just on AUC, depending on the drug.

Both the FDA (1999a) and CHMP (CPMP, 1997) have guidelines on the assessment of drug interactions. Drug interactions may also be investigated in later-phase studies using population approaches (FDA, 1999b). Although it should be noted that when a population approach is applied, as discussed in Chapter 2, the assessment of effect should be made in terms of confidence intervals and not P-values.

10.5 FOOD-EFFECT STUDIES

Again, the null hypothesis, design and sample size calculations are similar to those for bioequivalence studies described in Chapter 9.

A standard food-effect study would be a two-period crossover where the two arms are drug alone, and drug with food. The food effect is assessed through AUC and C_{max} against no-effect margins of (0.80, 1.25). The FDA (2002a) has guidelines for these studies.

The studies should be formally powered with Type I error of 5% and assessed in healthy volunteers. As with drug interaction studies, the effect of food may be to increase the statistical variability of the pharmacokinetics and this would need to be considered when designing a study.

Food is also often assessed in 'first-look' early multiperiod studies, and the possible increase in statistical variability needs to be considered here. This may be particularly the case if other comparisons in the study are assessments of bioavailability of different formulations, as the FDA (2003b) state:

> If the sponsor chooses, a pilot study in a small number of subjects can be carried out before proceeding with a full BE study. The study can be used to validate analytical methodology, assess variability, optimize sample collection time intervals, and provide other information... A pilot study that documents BE can be appropriate, provided its design and execution are suitable and a sufficient number of subjects (e.g., 12) have completed the study.

Hence, the food arm may adversely affect the overall variability used in contrasts of other arms in multiperiod studies, and adversely affect the conclusion of bioequivalence. A recommendation therefore is to exclude the data from the food arm, when comparing the other arms in multiperiod studies.

10.6 HEPATIC OR RENAL IMPAIRMENT

10.6.1 HEPATIC IMPAIRMENT

Using the Child–Pugh classification, subjects are classified as having mild, moderate or severe impairment. 'Matched' controls are also included, who are similar in terms of age, gender and weight. A degree of adaptivity could be included in the design; for example to investigate 'moderate' subjects and controls first; if no effect is observed then do not recruit 'mild' subjects.

Both the CHMP (2005b) and the FDA (1999b) have guidelines for these studies, and they both recognize that the sample size for such studies is based primarily on feasibility, with the CHMP stating:

> The number of subjects enrolled should be sufficient to detect clinically important differences...

While the FDA state:

> A sufficient number of subjects should be enrolled in the study such that evaluable data can be obtained from at least 6 subjects in each arm...

```
PROC mixed DATA data;
CLASS subject treatment;
MODEL outcome = treatment / DDFM = SATTERTH;
REPEATED /SUBJECT = subject GROUP = treatment;
ESTIMATE 'A - B' treatment 1 -1 0 ;
ESTIMATE 'A - C' treatment 1 0 -1 ;
ESTIMATE 'B - C' treatment 0 1 -1 ;
LSMEANS treatment /DIFF;
RUN;
```

Figure 10.6 SAS code for a nonrandomized between-group comparison.

Population pharmacokinetics could also be considered in Phase II/III (FDA, 1999c).

A recommendation for any nonrandomized between-group comparisons – for hepatic here or later for renal, age or gender – is to use the code of Figure 10.6, as with this analysis the assumption of equality of variance (which may not be appropriate for nonrandomized comparisons; Julious, 2005c) is not made. For two groups this code gives the same result as an unpooled variance t-test.

10.6.2 RENAL IMPAIRMENT

Using estimated creatinine clearance rates, subjects are classified as having mild, moderate or severe impairment. End-stage renal disease patients may also be considered if these patients are to be in the final treatment population. 'Matched' controls are also included – similar in terms of age, gender and weight.

As with hepatic impairment studies, a degree of adaptivity could be included in the design – for example, include severe and controls first and if no effect observed, then do not recruit mild and moderate.

Both the CHMP (2004) and the FDA (1998a) has guidelines on these studies, and they both recognize that the sample size will be based primarily on feasibility considerations, with the CHMP stating:

> The number of subjects enrolled should be sufficient to detect clinically important differences . . .

While the FDA states:

> The number of patients enrolled should be sufficient to detect PK differences large enough to warrant dosage adjustments . . .

Population pharmacokinetics could also be considered in Phase II/III (FDA, 1999c).

10.7 AGE OR GENDER COMPARISON STUDIES

Remember from previous chapters that the pharmacokinetics for a compound can be used as a surrogate for safety and efficacy. Hence, if a no-effect assessment can be made in various subgroups in terms of the pharmacokinetics then appropriate inference can be drawn with respect to the safety and efficacy and recommendations as to dosage and posology made.

10.7.1 AGE COMPARISONS

The study design would typically be that of parallel groups of healthy young and healthy elderly volunteers. There is an ICH guideline (Topic E7) for studies in geriatric populations (ICH, 1994b).

10.7.2 GENDER COMPARISONS

A gender comparison could be included within an age comparison study. An ideal study would be elderly females; young females; elderly males and young males, but as discussed in Chapters 1 and 6 it is some time into a drug development programme before women of fertile potential may be included in a trial. Hence, if the study falls within this window it may be confined to elderly females, elderly males and young males.

Note, a logical covariate to fit in an age and gender study is creatinine clearance, but be aware that creatinine clearance is defined as

$$\frac{(140 - \text{age}) \times \text{weight}}{72 \times \text{serum creatinine}} (\text{multiply by } 0.75 \text{ for females}). \qquad (10.9)$$

Hence, there is a degree of confounding between this covariate and age and gender. The FDA has issued a guideline for gender studies (FDA, 2003c).

10.8 BRIDGING STUDIES

10.8.1 INTRODUCTION

Bridging is a rationale to get drugs and medicines to patients in new geographical locations based in part on clinical data used for the original licence. The objective is not to repeat entire programmes in new regions. Rather the wish is to extrapolate safety and efficacy findings from the original study region to the new region. There are intrinsic and extrinsic factors which could assist in the determination of whether bridging is appropriate, as given in Figure 10.7 (ICH Topic E5 – ICH, 1998c).

ICH Topic E5 (ICH, 1998c) identifies the following properties of a compound that make it less likely to be sensitive to ethnic factors:

- Dose-proportional pharmacokinetics (PK)
- A flat pharmacodynamic (PD) (effect–concentration) curve for both efficacy and safety in the range of the recommended dosage and dose regimen (this may mean that the medicine is well tolerated)
- A wide therapeutic dose range (again, possibly an indicator of good tolerability)
- Minimal metabolism, or metabolism distributed among multiple pathways
- High bioavailability, thus less susceptibility to dietary absorption effects
- Low potential for protein binding
- Little potential for drug–drug, drug–diet and drug–disease interactions
- Nonsystemic mode of action
- Little potential for inappropriate use.

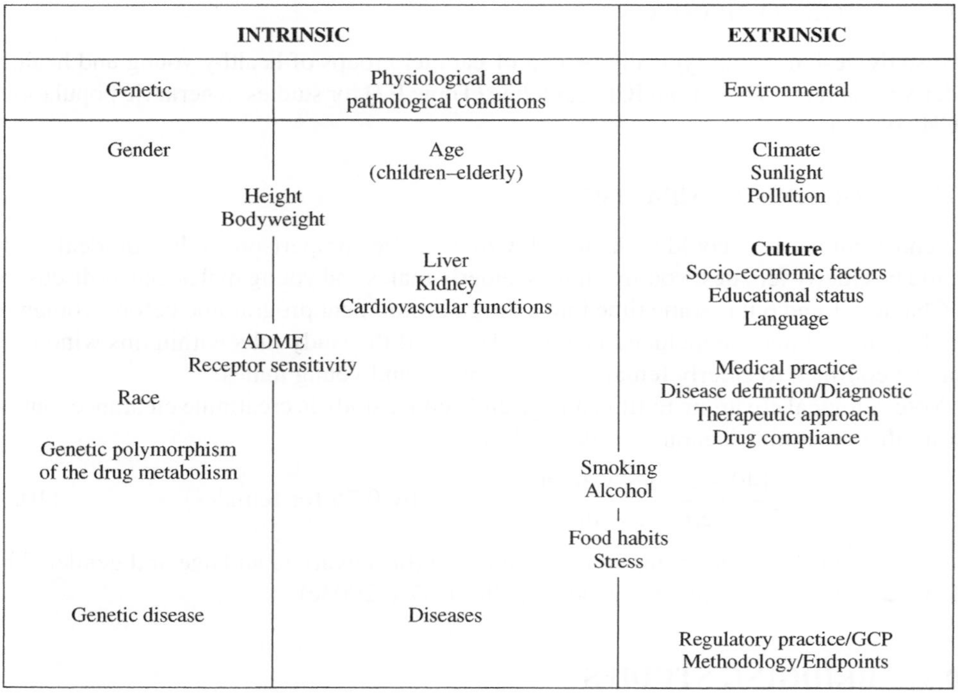

INTRINSIC
EXTRINSIC
Genetic
Physiological and pathological conditions
Environmental
Gender
Age (children–elderly)
Climate
Sunlight
Pollution
Height
Bodyweight
Culture
Socio-economic factors
Educational status
Language
Liver
Kidney
Cardiovascular functions
ADME
Receptor sensitivity
Medical practice
Disease definition/Diagnostic
Therapeutic approach
Drug compliance
Race
Genetic polymorphism of the drug metabolism
Smoking
Alcohol
Food habits
Stress
Genetic disease
Diseases
Regulatory practice/GCP
Methodology/Endpoints

Figure 10.7 Intrinsic and extrinsic ethnic factors (ICH, 1998c). ADME – absorption/distribution/metabolism/excretion; GCP – Good Clinical Practice.

10.8.2 STUDY DESIGN

Recommendations for bridging could be made through an assessment of the pharmacokinetics. The study design could take the form of two groups: original region and new region (not necessarily measured concurrently in the same study) and three doses. The doses themselves could be assessed either by within-subject (in a crossover) or between-subject (parallel-group) designs.

A comparison could be made of overall differences between the new and original region. For more discussion see Patterson and Jones (2006).

10.9 PAEDIATRIC STUDIES

An assessment of the effect of a drug in a paediatric population is one which will not be conducted in isolation. Such an assessment will hinge on studies of the types we have described in this chapter and previously in the book. There are a number of published guidelines for these trials, such as ICH guidelines (Topic E11 – ICH, 2001), and regional guidelines including those from both Europe (CHMP, 2006c) and the USA (FDA, 1998b), as well as more specific guidance from Europe in neonates (CHMP, 2007b). Reference should also be made to the guidelines on implementation of EU directive 2001/20/EC on ethics of trials in children (European Commission, 2006), and the European guideline for small trials (CHMP, 2006d).

It should also be noted that the European Medicines Agency has established a list of medical conditions that do not occur in children (EMEA, 2007) and indicated that medicines developed for treating any condition on the list will be granted a waiver from the requirement to submit results of paediatric studies in compliance with an agreed paediatric investigation plan when seeking a marketing authorization for their product.

In truth, trials in this specific population are very complex and the individual trial or plan of trials should be considered on a case-by-case basis with appropriate interaction with key stakeholders and agencies, usually through review and approval of a paediatric investigation plan.

Some basic principles do apply however, as for other forms of pharmacokinetic assessment. For example, if similar exposure in adult and paediatric patients can be assumed to have similar clinical effect then the pharmacokinetics may be used to extrapolate safety and efficacy from an adult population to a paediatric one, with the CHMP stating (CHMP, 2006c):

> An application for paediatric use of a medicinal product should include sufficient information to establish efficacy and safety. Paediatric patients have the same right to well investigated therapies as adults. There are, however, several reasons why it is more difficult to study a medicinal product in paediatric patients, particularly in very young patients. Hence, it is often unrealistic to expect the applicant to fully demonstrate efficacy and safety in paediatric patients in clinical studies. In such a situation pharmacokinetic data may be used to extrapolate efficacy and/or safety from data obtained in adults or in paediatric age groups other than the age groups applied for.
>
> ...
>
> Even if clinical efficacy and safety have been sufficiently documented for the paediatric population as a group, the clinical studies may not have sufficient power to detect differences in efficacy and safety in subgroups within the studied age interval. Pharmacokinetic data will then be important for identification of subgroups in which the exposure differs from the overall study population to a clinically relevant extent

If an assumption of similar relationship between concentration and clinical efficacy cannot be assumed then the situation is a little more complex and an evaluation of a dose–response relationship, maybe linking response with the pharmacokinetics, may be required for a given development programme. Also, there is an issue if the pharmacokinetics are not linked to efficacy (ICH, 2001 – Topic E11):

> An approach based on pharmacokinetics is likely to be insufficient for medicinal products where blood levels are known or expected not to correspond with efficacy or where there is concern that the concentration–response relationship may differ between the adult and paediatric populations. In such cases, studies of the clinical or the pharmacological effect of the medicinal product would usually be expected.

10.9.1 DESIGN

The following age classifications are suggested both by the ICH (2001 – Topic E11) and CHMP (2006c):

- Preterm newborn infants
- Term newborn infants (0–27 days)
- Infants and toddlers (28 days – 23 months)
- Children (2–11 years)
- Adolescents (12–17 years).

The FDA (1998b) guidelines have similar age groupings apart from the last category, which they define as 12–15 years. They also state that:

> In general, pharmacokinetic studies in the pediatric population should determine how the dosage regimen in the pediatric population should be adjusted to achieve approximately the same level of systemic exposure that is safe and effective in adults. Depending on the intended use of a drug in the pediatric population, studies should be performed in all pediatric age groups to allow dose adjustment within an individual over time. For drugs with linear pharmacokinetics in adults, single-dose studies often allow adequate pharmacokinetic assessment in the pediatric population.

Hence supporting the importance of dose proportionality in paediatric assessment. The CHMP make similar comments about using a range of age groups, while also stating (CHMP, 2006c):

> . . . effort should be made to balance the study population for factors predicted to affect the pharmacokinetics of the specific drug e.g. age/weight, renal or hepatic function or disease state . . .

Depending on the drug there may be concentration on the age groups where the greatest pharmacokinetic differences are expected relative to the adult population, particularly if certain age intervals can be reliably predicted (CHMP, 2006c). *A priori*, the greatest difference may be predicted to exist in children aged 2–4 years, while adolescents aged 12–17 years may be expected to have pharmacokinetics more similar to adults. For this group, puberty would be a factor to consider and there would need to be stratification by gender. Thus, pharmacokinetic data can be used to identify age groups with dissimilar exposure and dose need. It is also recommended to include measures of relevant pharmacodynamic variables as these can help in the determination of the pharmacokinetic toxicity–efficacy relationship, with the knowledge being used to guide dose selection in later phases of the clinical trials programme (CPMP, 2003).

A practical consideration for paediatric investigations is that, for ethical reasons, paediatric pharmacokinetic studies are usually performed in patients who may potentially benefit from the treatment, or other persons within the same age category with the same condition (European Commission, 2006):

Exceptionally and under the protective conditions prescribed by law, where the research has not the potential to produce results of direct benefit to the health of the person concerned, such research may be authorized subject to . . . the following additional conditions:

(1) The research has the aim of contributing, through significant improvement in the scientific understanding of the individual's condition, disease or disorder, to the ultimate attainment of results capable of conferring benefit to the person concerned or to other persons in the same age category or afflicted with the same disease or disorder or having the same condition;
(2) The research entails only minimal risk and minimal burden for the individual concerned.

10.9.2 SUPPORTING STUDIES

As already stated, many of the studies in the adult clinical programme would support the paediatric programme, but some specific considerations may also apply. There may be a need for special paediatric formulations with, for example, specific flavours, colours or suspensions, to assist compliance. It is generally preferable that the bioequivalence studies for these paediatric formulations are conducted in adults.

There is also a consideration if the paediatric population studies are from a specific geographical region. In which case, the arguments related to bridging described earlier would need to be considered to extrapolate these data to other regions.

10.9.3 SAMPLE SIZE

There is only general guidance as to what an appropriate sample size should be, beyond that it should be sufficient to provide appropriate estimates of the inter- and intrasubject variability and also to have appropriate precision to make dosage recommendations. The population sample to make these estimates, however, can be taken from either a single study or from several studies, especially to get an appropriate age distribution. The EU ethics guidelines state (European Commission, 2006):

> The size of the trial conducted in children should be as small as possible to demonstrate the appropriate efficacy with sufficient statistical power. Adaptative, Bayesian or other designs may be used to minimise the size of the clinical trial.

While the FDA (1998b) state:

> The standard pharmacokinetic approach is the usual approach for pharmacokinetic evaluation. It involves administering either single or multiple doses of a drug to a relatively small (e.g., 6–12) group of subjects with relatively frequent blood and sometimes urine sample collection.

10.9.4 DATA ANALYSIS

A general objective of a paediatric pharmacokinetic study is to make an assessment of the appropriate paediatric doses to achieve comparable systemic exposure measures to that seen in adults. To achieve this objective the analysis should make an assessment

- Of pharmacokinetics for rate (C_{max}) and extent of exposure (AUC)
- Of the relationship between different covariates and parameters such as C_{max} and AUC.

Given these objectives however, the analysis approaches are similar to other pharmacokinetic assessments.

10.10 RELATIVE POTENCY

10.10.1 INTRODUCTION

A relative-potency study fits more into discussions of Chapter 12 and an assessment of dose response, but it has been brought forward into this chapter due to its utility in the context of the studies described thus far.

Figure 10.8 gives an illustration of a relative-potency assessment. Here, the two lines equate to two assessments of dose response from two treatment groups. These groups might be, for example, two routes of administration for the same therapy, with subjects in each group randomized to a particular route and a dose level. Alternatively, the two groups may represent male and female participants or groups from two geographical regions.

10.10.2 ANALYSIS

The dose–response relationships summarized in Figure 10.8 are linear and parallel. Thus the overall difference in response between two groups is a – this would equate to the adjusted mean difference from an analysis of variance. The response measure could be

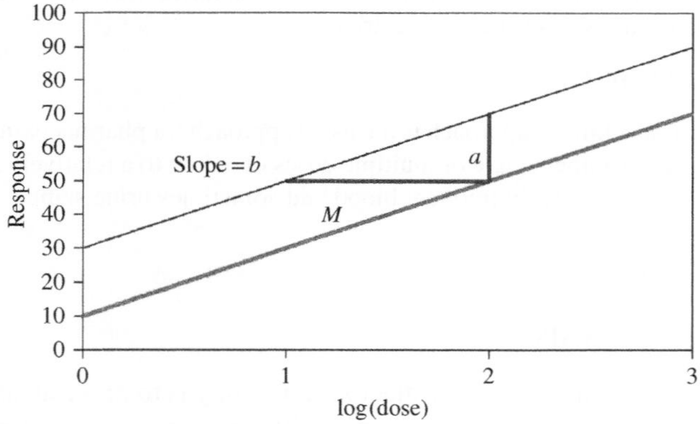

Figure 10.8 Assessment of relative potency.

clinical (Chapter 12) or a measure of bioavailability (Chapter 9). The term b is the slope for the dose response. Hence we have that

$$M = a/b, \tag{10.10}$$

which is the log(dose) required to have the same effect in the two groups. Thus exp(M) gives the relative dose adjustment required to obtain the same clinical effect. The variance of $\log_e M$ is estimated by

$$\mathrm{Var}(log_e M) \approx \frac{a^2\mathrm{Var}(b) + b^2\mathrm{Var}(a) - 2ab\mathrm{Cov}(a, b)}{b^4}, \tag{10.11}$$

and hence its confidence interval. As with estimating the maximum tolerated dose (MTD) in Chapter 6, a confidence interval can also be assessed through bootstrapping or through Fieller's theorem (Peace, 1988).

For bioavailability assessments this could be used to establish any necessary adjustments for different formulations, routes or different patient population groups. For clinical assessments (see Chapter 11), this could be used to evaluate dose adjustments to maintain the same clinical benefit for different patient groups.

For both types of assessment, if the pharmacokinetics are dose proportional we determine whether the confidence interval for exp(M) is wholly contained within some no-effect margin such as (0.80, 1.25).

An assessment of relative potency could also be used in trials to determine the dose adjustment requirements for (say) age, gender or for bridging.

11 Phase II Trials: General Issues

11.1 OVERVIEW

Although there is some variation in terminology and objectives depending on the disease or condition in question, Phase II trials are usually studies with the objective to investigate the therapeutic benefit of a proposed new therapeutic regimen. Most of these trials evaluate at least one new treatment relative to some form of standard. So they are inherently comparative, even though the assessment may not be formally factored into the power of the design. As with all clinical trials they should be undertaken under the principals of Good Clinical Practice (ICH, 1996a – Topic E6).

Phase II trial designs seek to detect a possible clinical signal for a new regimen over and above the variability or noise in the population being investigated. Factors that contribute to this variability include patient type, definition of response, interobserver differences in response evaluation, drug dosage and schedule, reporting procedures and sample size. With Phase II trials, the sample size may be less than in later phases but the noise can be reduced by having tighter control on enrolment – for example by having narrower inclusion criteria and being conducted in a smaller number of centres or even a single centre.

Phase II trials may be the first time assessments of both safety and efficacy of the new therapeutic regimen in a patient population are made. Safety is usually assessed in terms of adverse event rates but this aspect is not often part of the formal design considerations. Efficacy is typically measured using a disease-related response. This may not be the same response used in later-phase development but should provide sufficient confidence in any signal detected.

11.2 PLANNING

11.2.1 CHOICE OF ENDPOINT

As already indicated, Phase II trials seek to assess whether a new regimen is active enough to warrant a comparison of its efficacy in a large, and usually expensive, Phase III trial. Thus, appropriate endpoints need to be chosen to allow for such an assessment to be made. For example, in HIV research, suitable endpoints might include measures of viral load or immune function. In cardiovascular disease, we might look at blood pressure or lipid levels. While in oncology, tumour response (shrinkage) would often be used as the primary endpoint.

An Introduction to Statistics in Early Phase Trials Steven A. Julious, Say Beng Tan and David Machin

Sometimes it may be that the true endpoint of interest is difficult to assess, for whatever reason, in a Phase II trial context. Thus the chosen endpoint in Phase II may be one of shorter duration than that of primary interest in later-phase development, or it may be a surrogate or biomarker. If a surrogate or biomarker is to be used, then there is a real need to ensure that it is an appropriate surrogate for the (true) endpoint of concern (ICH, 1998b – Topic E9):

... the strength of the evidence for surrogacy depends upon (i) the biological plausibility of the relationship (ii) the demonstration in epidemiological studies of the prognostic value of the surrogate for the clinical outcome and (iii) evidence from clinical trials that treatment effects on the surrogate correspond to effects on the clinical outcome.

11.2.2 ELIGIBILITY

Common to all phases of clinical trials is the necessity to define precisely who the eligible subjects are. This definition may be relatively brief or complex depending on the regimen under investigation.

At the very early stages of the process great care must be taken in subject and particularly patient choice. In these situations, when relatively little is known about the compound, all the possible adverse eventualities have to be considered. Also, particularly in early Phase II, some of the enabling studies, for example drug interaction studies, may not have been conducted, excluding groups of subjects from the inclusion criteria. All these factors can result in quite a restricted definition as to those that can be recruited.

Once the possibility of some activity (and hence potential efficacy) is indicated, then there is at least a prospect of therapeutic gain for the patient. In this case, the sponsor may expand the horizon of eligible patients but simultaneously confine them to those in which a measurable response to the disease can be ascertained.

In addition, in Phase II it may be the first instance that certain patient subgroups have been investigated, such as the elderly, or women, as highlighted in Figure 11.1. So as well as having relatively tight inclusion criteria in comparison to Phase III, the inclusion criteria may still be wider than in previous studies.

11.2.3 CHOICE OF DESIGN

There are a relatively large number of alternative designs for Phase II trials, with disease area being the main influence on choice. Some of the more common designs will be discussed in Chapters 12 and 13, while the general sample size issues have been discussed in Chapter 3.

With such a plethora of different options for Phase II designs, it is clearly important that the sponsor chooses a design which is best for their purpose. In some cases the choice will be reasonably clear, while in other circumstances, the patient pool may be very limited and a key consideration will be the maximum numbers of patients that could feasibly be recruited within a reasonable period of time.

In general, factors which will need to be considered when designing a Phase II trial are given in Figure 11.1

Inclusion criteria	The inclusion criteria may be tighter than for a late-phase trial. This may be by choice – to use a narrow population most likely to give a signal – or by necessity, or because enabling studies such as Phase I drug interaction studies may not have been undertaken, requiring the exclusion of patients with certain concomitant therapies.
Exclusion criteria	For similar arguments as for the inclusion criteria, the exclusion criteria may be wider.
Gender	The trials to date may have been predominantly in males and so inclusion of females may be particularly important.
Special populations	As with gender, a Phase II trial may be the first time specific special populations may have been investigated in any number – e.g. ethnic groups, age groups.
Number of centres	The trials may be in a finite number of centres, but the number of centres in total will need to be considered.
Number of countries	The location of the centres – especially if using specialist centres – may influence the choice countries, but consideration would need to be given to countries chosen.
Covariates	Selection of covariates is an important consideration. In late-phase trials covariates should be prespecified, but in a Phase II trial there may be scope to select certain covariates based on the data – maybe with the selection undertaken prior to the randomization being revealed.

Figure 11.1 Selected key items to be considered when designing a Phase II trial.

11.2.4 STATISTICAL ANALYSIS

Prespecification is one of the central tenets of clinical research. This is particularly true for statistical analyses where different analyses may produce slightly different P-values which could affect inference. In its guidelines for Phase I, the Association of the British Pharmaceutical Industry state for the statistical analysis (ABPI, 2007):

There should be a statistical analysis plan (SAP) for each trial. A statistician should:

- Write and sign the SAP before the trial is unblinded and data analysis begins;
- Describe in the SAP the analyses that will be done, the procedures for dealing with missing data, and the selection of subjects to be included in the analyses;
- Put sample tables and listings in the SAP, to show how data will be presented;
- Include any planned interim analyses in the SAP;
- Describe and justify in the trial report any deviations from the SAP;
- Test and validate all software for data analysis;
- Validate the data analysis programs by at least running them on dummy or actual data, checking the program log for errors, checking the output against the source data and saving the final validated programs and output; and
- Check, or get someone else to check, all final tables and listings.

Although not specifically for Phase II trials, this guidance would be consistent with them, and could be generalized to such trials.

For a Phase II trial there may be instances where the trials themselves are exploratory in nature, with an exploratory analysis planned and undertaken in a data-driven way. It should still be prespecified that an exploratory analysis will be undertaken in the analysis plan, as this would affect the inference that can be drawn.

11.3 POTENTIAL PITFALLS

It should be emphasized that Phase II trials should never be seen as an alternative to well-designed (large) randomized Phase III trials. This is because the generally small sample sizes in Phase II trials give rise to estimates with very wide confidence intervals (that is, a high level of uncertainty). Moreover the trials may have a restricted randomization (see Chapters 12 and 13), in which case any conclusions drawn from them cannot be regarded as confirmatory.

11.4 TRIAL REPORTING

All clinical trials need reporting, but not all trials require a full report. Depending on the study, an abbreviated report or a shorter synopsis may be appropriate if the trial is to be included in a submission to a regulatory agency. ICH Topic E3 details the contents required in a full study report (ICH, 1996b), while the FDA has draft guidelines on abbreviated reports (FDA, 1998c).

11.4.1 FULL STUDY REPORT

In Phase III trials, much emphasis has been placed on developing standards for the good conduct and reporting of clinical trials. Among the aspects looked at are issues relating to informed consent, registration of subjects, monitoring the trial, and common standards for the reporting of trials. The FDA (1998c) recommended that for regulatory submissions:

Full study reports (i.e., the complete ICH E3) should ordinarily be submitted for all studies from clinical investigations of drugs or biological products that are the subject of very limited clinical development programs (i.e., programs with fewer than six clinical trials from any phase of drug development designed to determine effectiveness, including dose-comparison trials).

In addition, full study reports should be submitted for clinical effectiveness studies that (a) evaluate a dose, regimen, patient population, and indication for which marketing approval is sought, and (b) are capable by design, conduct, and enrollment of assessing the effectiveness of the product. Full study reports are expected for these studies whether or not they demonstrate a treatment effect. Examples include:

- Studies providing the basis for dose recommendations (e.g., dose-comparison studies).
- Controlled studies identified by the applicant as contributing directly to substantial evidence of effectiveness.
- Controlled studies that support an intended comparative claim.
- Controlled studies considered supportive of effectiveness (e.g., studies believed to show a favorable trend, possible effect in a subgroup).
- Controlled studies of different indications (stages of disease, different study populations) or dosage forms or regimens if they are intended to provide support for approval.
- Controlled studies evaluating effectiveness for the indication that failed to show an effect.

Considerable effort is required in order to conduct a clinical trial of whatever type and size, and this effort justifies reporting of the subsequent trial results with careful detail. In clinical trials, major strides in improving the quality have been made. Pivotal to this has been ICH Topic E3 (ICH, 1996b), which describes the structure and content of a study report, and the consolidation of the standards of reporting trials (CONSORT) statement described by Begg *et al.* (1996) and amplified by Moher *et al.* (2001). CONSORT describes the essential items that should be reported in a trial publication in order to give assurance that the trial has been conducted to a high standard.

The conduct and reporting of all trials should meet the same high standards demanded of the Phase III randomized controlled trial. All phases of the clinical trials process crucially affect the final conclusions made regarding the usefulness of new treatments and so, early phase trials, of whatever design, also need to be conducted and reported to the highest standards. Thus we advocate that the standards applied to Phase III trials should also be extended to early development wherever appropriate.

Figure 11.2 highlights some of the items from ICH E3 (1996b) that should be included in a full clinical trial report.

ICH E3 (1996b) recommends that a graphic along the lines of Figure 11.3 be produced to describe the disposition of patients. These are often referred to as CONSORT diagrams. The essential features of the diagram can be applied to all trials of whatever design and purpose.

11.4.2 ABBREVIATED STUDY REPORT

It is recognized that a full study report may not be appropriate for all studies in a regulatory review and in certain instances an abbreviated study report may be appropriate (ICH E3, 1996b):

Depending on the regulatory authority's review policy, abbreviated reports using summarised data or with some sections deleted, may be acceptable for uncontrolled studies or other studies not designed to establish efficacy (but a controlled safety study should be reported in full), for seriously flawed or aborted studies, or for controlled studies that examine conditions clearly unrelated to those for which a claim is made. However, a full description of safety aspects should be included in these cases. If an abbreviated report is submitted, there should be enough detail of design and results to

Figure 11.2 Items to be included in a full clinical trial report.

allow the regulatory authority to determine whether a full report is needed. If there is any question regarding whether the reports are needed, it may be useful to consult the regulatory authority.

In the context of a regulatory review, the FDA state that an abbreviated study report may be appropriate for the situation when (FDA, 1998c):

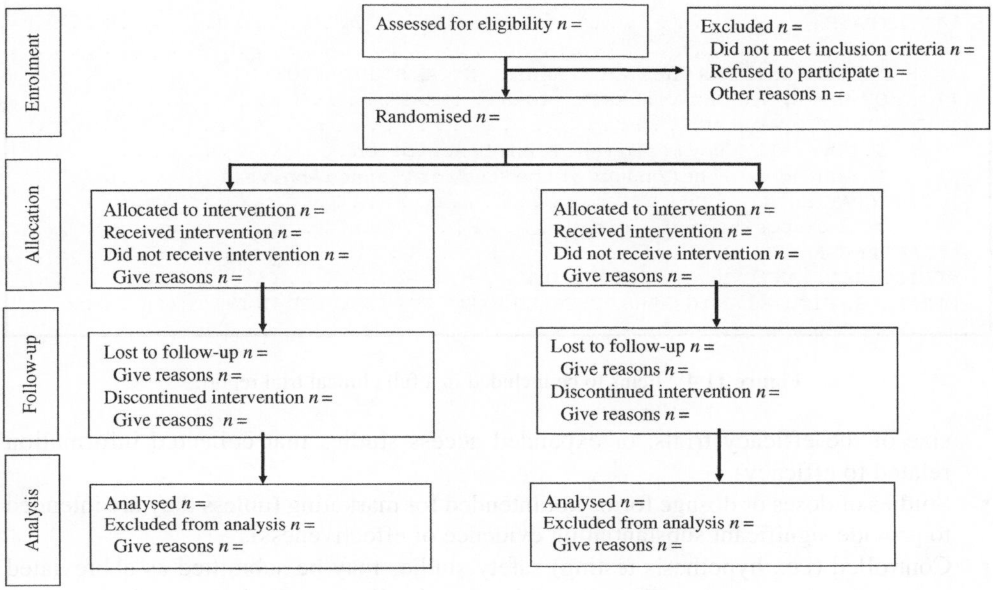

Figure 11.3 Template of the diagram showing the flow of participants through a single-arm Phase II trial.

(1) The studies are not intended to contribute to the evaluation of product effectiveness, but (2) the reviewer needs sufficient information about the studies to determine that their results do not cast doubt on the effectiveness claims for the product. Abbreviated reports should also be submitted for studies that do not fall under . . . [list of situations needing full study reports], but that contribute significantly to the safety database. Abbreviated reports should contain a full safety report.

Examples of studies that should be submitted as abbreviated reports include:

- Studies with active controls that do not provide the primary or substantiating evidence of effectiveness (e.g., active-controlled equivalence trials from clinical development programs in which the primary evidence of effectiveness is contributed by placebo-controlled, dose-controlled, or other superiority designs). Active-controlled trials in which differences were observed or that support a claim in labeling should be submitted as full study reports.
- Studies of related indications for which marketing approval is not being sought (unless they are intended to provide significant substantiating evidence of effectiveness for the indications being sought).
- Studies not designed as efficacy studies or designed as efficacy studies for different indications that contribute significant information about product safety (e.g., large, randomized or nonrandomized trials where enrollment approached or exceeded the

1 TITLE PAGE . . . .
2 SYNOPSIS . . . .
3 TABLE OF CONTENTS FOR THE INDIVIDUAL CLINICAL STUDY REPORT . .
4 LIST OF ABBREVIATIONS AND DEFINITIONS OF TERMS . . . .
9 INVESTIGATIONAL PLAN . . . .
    9.1 Overall Study Design and Plan: Description . . . .
    9.8 Changes in the Conduct of the Study or Planned Analyses . . . .
10 STUDY PATIENTS . . . .
    10.1 Disposition of Patients . . . .
12 SAFETY EVALUATION . . . .
13 DISCUSSION AND OVERALL CONCLUSIONS . . . .
14 TABLES, FIGURES AND GRAPHS REFERRED TO BUT NOT INCLUDED IN THE TEXT . . . . . .

Figure 11.4 Items to be included in a full clinical trial report.

size of the efficacy trials, or expanded access studies that collected information related to efficacy).

- Studies of doses or dosage forms not intended for marketing (unless they are intended to provide significant substantiating evidence of effectiveness).
- Controlled (i.e., hypothesis testing) safety studies may be submitted as abbreviated reports; however, as for all studies, adequate detail on study design and conduct to permit complete analysis of safety should be provided.

Specifically, from Figure 11.2 the FDA recommends that an abbreviated study report should contain the contents given in Figure 11.4. It should be noted, however, that a full report may be required from which to draw the abbreviated review for a submission to an agency.

11.4.3 STUDY SYNOPSES

Both abbreviated and full reports have study synopses as part of their contents. However, in the context of a regulatory review, only a study synopsis may be required (FDA, 1998c):

Some studies are generally only examined in sufficient depth to assess if they cast doubt on the safety of the product for the proposed indication. For these studies, complete safety information should be included in the ISS [integrated summary of safety] or, for biological products not containing an ISS, the safety information should be appended to the synopsis. Examples of studies that should be submitted as synopses include:

- Studies of unrelated indications for which marketing approval is not being sought (unless they form a significant portion of the safety database, in which case they should be submitted as abbreviated reports).
- Studies evaluating routes of administration for which marketing approval is not being sought.
- Incomplete studies, defined for the purpose of this guidance as enrolling fewer than one-third of intended patients, unless stopped for safety reasons or for futility

Name of Sponsor Company:	Individual Study Table Referring to Part of the Dossier Volume: Page:	*(For National Authority Use only)*
Name of Finished Product:		
Name of Active Ingredient:		
Title of Study:		
Investigation:		
Study centre(s):		
Publication (reference):		
Studied period (years): (date of first enrolment) (date of last completed)	Phase of development:	
Objectives:		
Methodology:		
Number of patients (planned and analysed):		
Diagnosis and main criteria for inclusion:		
Test product, dose and mode of administration, batch number:		
Duration of treatment:		
Reference therapy, dose and mode of administration, batch number:		

Name of Sponsor Company:	Individual Study Table Referring to Part of the Dossier Volume: Page:	*(For National Authority Use only)*
Name of Finished Product:		
Name of Active Ingredient:		
Criteria for evaluation: Efficacy: Safety:		
Statistical methods		
SUMMARY – CONCLUSIONS Efficacy results: Safety results: Conclusion: Date of the report:		

Figure 11.5 Items to be included in a synopsis (ICH, 1996b).

(inability to show efficacy). Those studies stopped for safety reasons or due to futility should be submitted as abbreviated reports.

- Uncontrolled studies not specifically identified as needing abbreviated or full study reports.
- Early safety-tolerance studies in Phase 1, but not specific toxicity studies (e.g., dermatotoxicity studies), which ordinarily should be submitted as full reports.

Figure 11.5 gives details of the contents of a synopsis taken from ICH E3 (1996b). It should be noted, however, that a full report may be required from which to draw the synopsis for a submission to an agency.

12 Dose–Response Studies

12.1 INTRODUCTION

The assessment of dose response, and consequent dose selection, is one of the most important aspects of drug development. Figure 12.1 gives an illustration of a possible dose response to highlight the importance of proper assessment. If you select a dose that is too small then it may have suboptimal efficacy. While if you selected a dose that is too high, although efficacious, it may have associated with it excessive (compared to lower doses) adverse events.

These points are recognized by the ICH in Topic E4 (ICH, 1994a), where the importance of quantifying the dose–response curve is highlighted:

> What is most helpful when choosing the starting dose is knowing the shape and location of the population (group) average dose–response curve for both desirable and undesirable effects. . . .a relatively high starting dose might be recommended for a drug with a large demonstrated separation between its useful and undesirable dose ranges. A high starting dose, however, might be a poor choice for a drug with a small demonstrated separation . . .

An assessment of a dose response is not something a particular study achieves in isolation. Previous studies, perhaps a first-time-into-man (FTIM) study (discussed in Chapter 8), may have helped to determine the maximum tolerated dose (MTD) and the safety window for a given compound. However, in Phase II we tend to move away from assessing the MTD and begin assessing the efficacy dose response and determining, for example, the minimum effective dose and the maximum effective dose. Hence, emphasis is on establishing the efficacy window as highlighted in Figure 12.2

There is a push for many development programmes to get to Phase III evaluation and hence to launch them as soon as possible. ICH E4 (ICH, 1994a) recognizes this push:

> Assessment of dose–response should be an integral . . . part of establishing the safety and effectiveness of the drug. If the development of dose–response information is built into the development process it can usually be accomplished with no loss of time and minimal extra effort compared to development plans that ignore dose–response.

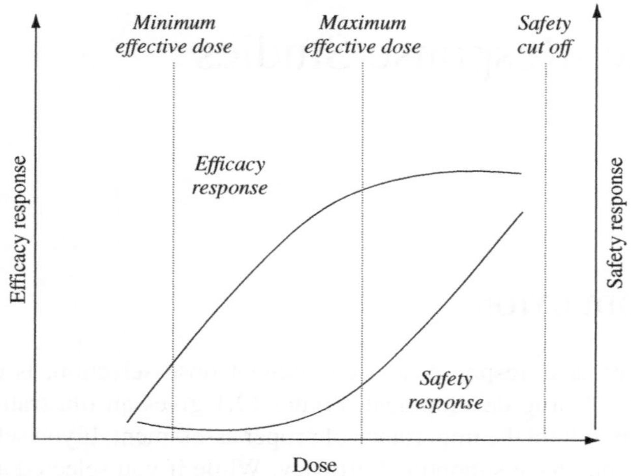

Figure 12.1 Dose–response profile.

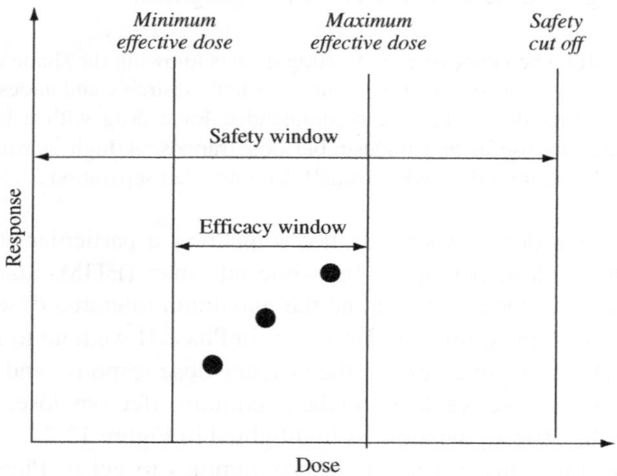

Figure 12.2 Dose–response profile with emphasis on the efficacy window.

Hence, adequately assessing dose response does not have to adversely affect timelines. However, adequately assessing dose response in early phase trials may save carrying forward more than one dose to the late-phase trials – with the consequential requirement of having to drop needless doses maybe through interim analyses. Thus, though it may take longer getting to the late-phase trials, these late-phase trials may be as a result be completed more quickly.

Even when overall drug development is longer, the danger of not adequately assessing dose response could be that a product may be launched with a suboptimal target product profile. For example, too high a dose with a correspondingly worse adverse event profile, as well as of being of suboptimal benefit to patients, will, from a commercial point of view, likely also have an impact on value.

We describe the main principles of dose response and introduce different types of dose–response designs including titration studies, studies based on estimation, and powered dose–response quantification.

12.2 DOSE ESCALATION STUDIES

Often the MTD in patients is many times higher than that in healthy volunteers. The rationale for this is easy to imagine. Suppose a new regimen's mechanism works by suppressing or raising levels of a factor associated with a condition. For a healthy volunteer with normal levels of this factor, being given the regimen may mean tolerability issues at relatively low subtherapeutic doses. This would mean their MTD being many times lower than in the patient population.

Studies could still be conducted in healthy volunteers to assess pharmacokinetics in the subtherapeutic doses. This could assist in pharmacokinetic predictions in the patient population. Drug interaction and food interactions could also be assessed, but perhaps not at therapeutic doses.

To assess the MTD, a single-dose-escalation study may be required in a patient population to ascertain a dose range for the safety window. Such studies would be parallel-group ascending-dose designs, usually undertaken in single or very limited number of centres. Subjects may be assigned to active or placebo in an allocation ratio of 2:1 or 3:1 in panels similar in form to Figure 12.3

As with repeat-dose studies, discussed in Chapter 10, the placebos in Figure 12.3 are usually not to facilitate formal comparisons to the active doses (in terms of an efficacy or other pharmacodynamic endpoint) but rather to assist in the assessment and interpretation of adverse events.

Sample size for such studies would primarily be based on feasibility considerations, with the study mainly designed to assess preliminary safety and (usually) pharmacokinetics. In addition, pharmacodynamic data may also be collected. Assessment of efficacy could also be made, although this would be on relatively very few subjects and probably not at the primary time endpoint for the ensuing Phase III trial.

Cohort 1

D1	D1	D1	D1	D1	D1	D1	D1	D1	D1	D1	D1	P	P	P	P	P	P

Cohort 2

D2	D2	D2	D2	D2	D2	D2	D2	D2	D2	D2	D2	P	P	P	P	P	P

etc.

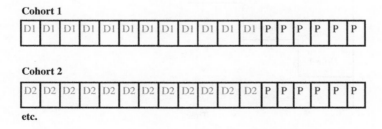

Figure 12.3 Possible dosing panels for a dose escalation study.

Table 12.1 Sample size required for different correlation coefficients: two-sided 5% significance level and 90% power.

	Correlation coefficient				
	0.4	0.5	0.6	0.7	0.8
n	61	37	25	17	12

If there is limited information available for sample size calculation purposes, then it may be important to consider the potential correlation between the outcome and the dose levels to be investigated. This is a rather crude approach but could be a useful calculation in a preliminary trial. Table 12.1 gives the sample size required for different anticipated correlations. Hence, with a total sample size of 37 (for example, 3 dose cohorts of 12 subjects in each) it would be possible to detect a correlation between dose levels and response of 0.5.

The utility of this calculation is not to say that in the final analysis a correlation will be calculated, but to give some indication of the relationship that can be assessed between dose and response. As sample size is based on feasibility with limited information for sample size purposes, this calculation may be useful. Obviously if there is more information other calculations could be undertaken.

12.3 TITRATION STUDIES

As previously mentioned, many early phase trials are 'enabling trials', undertaken to facilitate planned studies in a clinical programme. Titration studies fall under this heading as they facilitate later-phase dose titration, if the final dosing regimen requires titration to reach the required dose(s).

In titration studies each subject receives successively increasing doses of the drug from within a given dosing schedule. Thus, as in Figure 12.4, the subject begins with a particular starting dose chosen by the design. Once ready for the second dose, this is

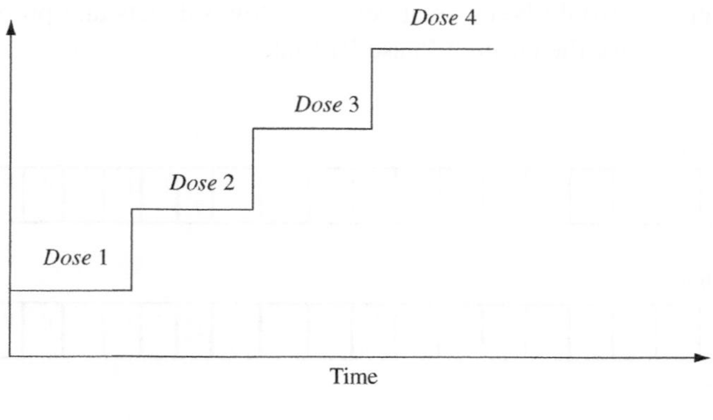

Figure 12.4 Successively increasing doses for a titration study in an individual.

given at a level higher than the preceding (first) dose. This process continues over subsequent doses until a preset maximum dose is achieved.

Titration studies are usually parallel-group, placebo-controlled trials in single or multiple cohorts, although different cohorts may have distinct dosing schedules, for example to escalate through doses more quickly.

Titration studies may assess doses (and possibly safety, efficacy and other responses) across a wide range, but the interpretation of any data would need to be made with caution; ICH E4 (1994a):

> Such titration designs, without careful analysis, are usually not informative about dose-response relationships. In many studies there is a tendency to spontaneous improvement over time that is not distinguishable from an increased response to higher doses . . . This leads to a tendency to choose, as a recommended dose, the highest dose used in such studies . . . that [is] well in excess of what [is] necessary, resulting in increased undesirable effects . . .

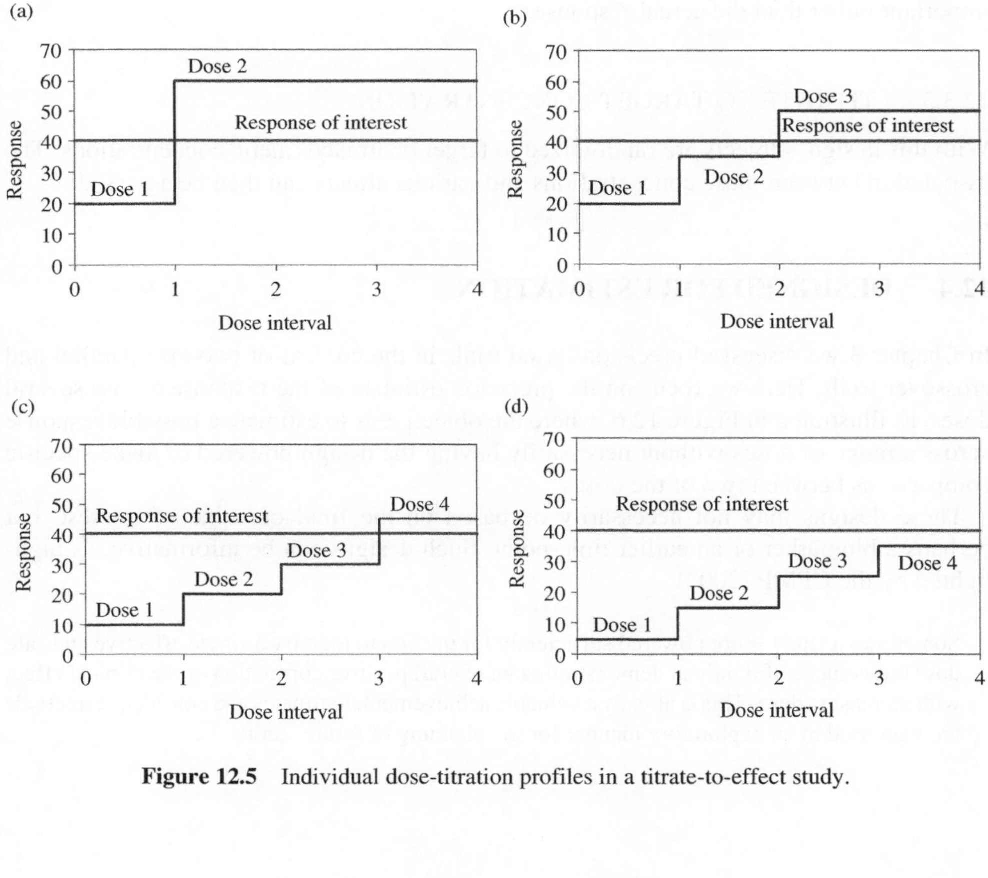

Figure 12.5 Individual dose-titration profiles in a titrate-to-effect study.

12.3.1 TITRATE TO EFFECT

With 'titrate-to-effect' studies, as the title suggests subjects are titrated until a given effect is observed. This effect could be determined by tolerance, a pharmacodynamic response or efficacy. Figure 12.5 shows how individuals in the study may reach the same effect but by different routes. Even within one study there may be a range of doses administered across individuals.

From this design, the average dose across the subjects could be determined, as well as limited efficacy, tolerance and other pharmacodynamic factors. In addition the pharmacokinetics can be assessed, together with the link between these and the response(s) of interest.

12.3.2 FORCED TITRATION

With this design all patients are given rising doses until a prespecified maximum dose or the MTD has been reached for an individual. The designs and endpoints are similar to the titrate-to-effect studies discussed in Section 12.3.1 and can be used, for example, to assess different dosing schedules to reach particular target doses.

As with the other titration studies discussed earlier, these studies can be used to assess different dosing schedules; however, with these studies it is the schedule that is most important rather than the actual response.

12.3.3 TITRATE TO TARGET CONCENTRATION

With this design, subjects are randomized to target pharmacokinetic concentrations. The association between these concentrations and various effects can then be assessed.

12.4 DESIGNED FOR ESTIMATION

In Chapter 3 we discussed precision-based trials in the context of two-arm parallel and crossover trials. Here we focus on the precision estimate of the response across several doses, as illustrated in Figure 12.6, where the objective is to estimate a possible response across a range of doses without necessarily having the design powered to make specific comparisons between two of the doses.

These designs may not necessarily be based on the final outcome of interest, but perhaps a biomarker or an earlier time-point. Such designs can be informative, as highlighted by the CPMP (2002):

> Sometimes a study is not powered sufficiently for the aim to identify a single effective and safe dose but is successful only at demonstrating an overall positive correlation of the clinical effect with increasing dose. This is already a valuable achievement. Estimates and confidence intervals are then used in an exploratory manner for the planning of future studies . . .

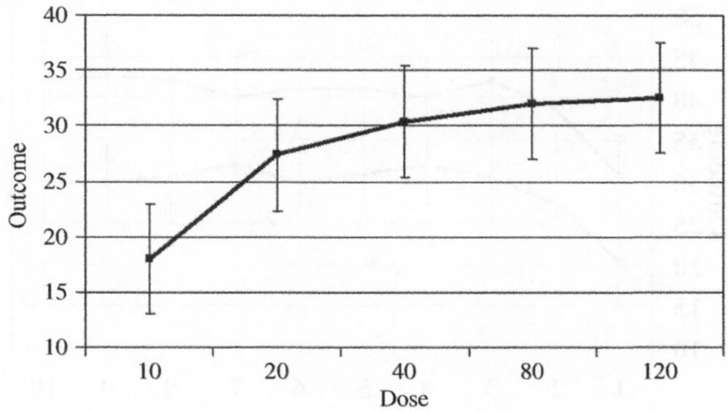

Figure 12.6 Results of a dose–response estimation study with means and 95% confidence intervals at each dose.

While the FDA (2006a) in their *Critical Path Opportunities Report* note that:

> Learning trials have a different underlying conceptual framework and require a statistical approach different from empirical trials. One type of trial in use today is the dose- or concentration-controlled trial, which uses biomarkers or other intermediate measures as endpoints to explore dose– or concentration–response relationships.

12.4.1 OVERLAPPING CONFIDENCE INTERVALS

A common figure used in comparative dose–response studies plots individual means for each treatment group against time with the associated 95% confidence intervals, as in Figure 12.7. These are often referred to as 'zipper' plots. This is an informative graph which helps in the assessment of trends over time, and from these an attempt at inference is made to help determine, for example, where the effects may be emerging.

Two common questions that are often asked when such exploratory plots are presented:

(1) If two 95% confidence intervals do not overlap does that imply there is a statistically significant difference, with $P < 0.05$, between the two groups?
(2) If two 95% confidence intervals do overlap does that imply there is not a statistically significant difference, that is, $P \geq 0.05$, between the two groups?

The answer to question 1 is 'Yes' but to question 2 is 'No' or at least 'Not necessarily', as some situations with overlapping confidence intervals will give a statistically significant difference between the groups, while others will not.

A 'No' response to the latter question can be achieved if the 95% confidence intervals in the plots are replaced by 84% confidence intervals, as we explain below.

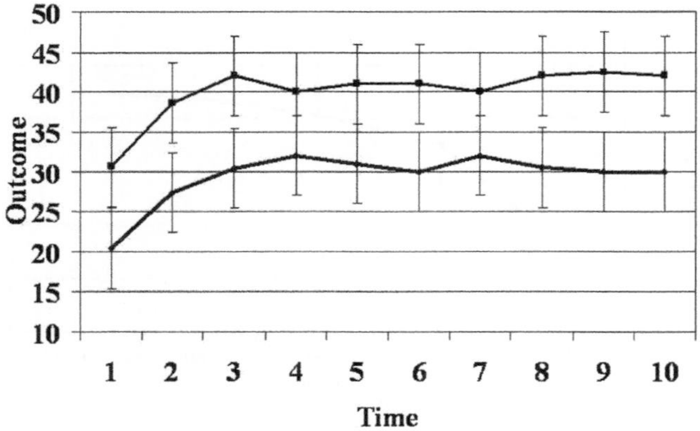

Figure 12.7 Dose response by time for two doses: the means and corresponding 95% intervals for each dose in each group are given.

The probability that two 100(1 − α)% confidence intervals overlap is given by

$$P = 2\left[1 - \Phi\left(\sqrt{2}Z_{1-\alpha/2}\right)\right], \tag{12.1}$$

which is evaluated in Table 12.2, giving the probability of overlap associated with different values of α. This corresponds to the P-value obtained from a test of significance between the two groups (Julious, 2004c).

Note, (12.1) holds if the sample sizes are the same in the two groups. A more general result would be

$$2\left[1 - \Phi\left(\frac{(\sqrt{r}+1)Z_{1-\alpha/2}}{\sqrt{r+1}}\right)\right], \tag{12.2}$$

Table 12.2 Probability of two confidence intervals overlapping for different levels of confidence around individual means.

Level of confidence	Probability of overlap
0.990	0.00027
0.975	0.00153
0.950	0.00557
0.900	0.02009
0.840	0.04691
0.834223	0.05
0.800	0.06993

where r is the allocation ratio between the two groups. For the special case of $r = 1$, (12.2) equals (12.1).

From Table 12.2 it is clear that for the separate 95% confidence intervals around the two means not to overlap, the P-value from the test of significance of the difference between the two groups must be less than or equal to 0.00557. Should the test give a P-value greater than 0.00557 (but less than 0.05) this would be statistically significant using a two-sided test with $\alpha = 0.05$, but the confidence intervals would overlap. This is why overlapping confidence intervals are observed despite significant P-values.

Arising from Table 12.2 is the recommendation for zipper plots that 84% confidence intervals would be appropriate to use. It should be emphasized, however, these 84% confidence intervals are only in this context; for quoting a difference in means it is the 95% confidence interval that should be used.

Note that for Figure 12.7 the variances used in the calculation of the confidence intervals are within group, while the variances used to calculate the P-values are between group. If the two groups are uncorrelated then the use of 84% confidence intervals will hold. If, however, in an analysis covariates are fitted concurrently with treatment such that adjusted means are calculated, a correlation between the groups may be introduced – even if the raw unadjusted comparisons are uncorrelated. A consequence could be that the properties of the 84% confidence intervals will not hold.

12.5 POWERED ON THE SLOPE

Under the assumption of a linear dose response, a formal assessment of the dose response could be one that is powered on the slope of the dose response. This is often termed a model-based approach, and is illustrated in Figure 12.8.

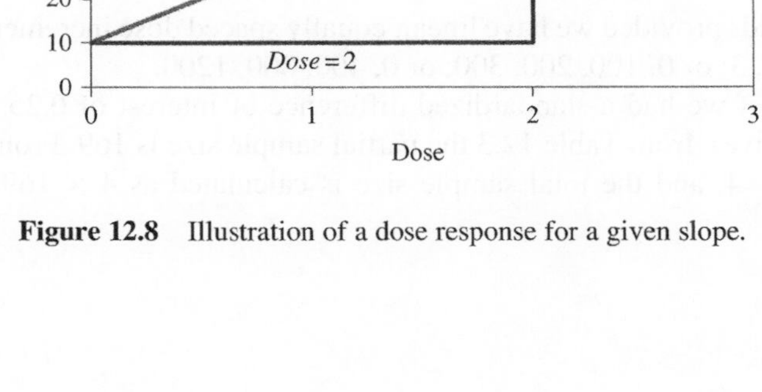

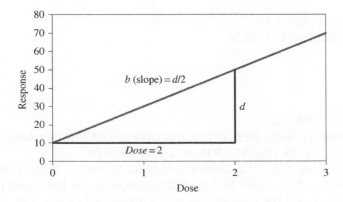

Figure 12.8 Illustration of a dose response for a given slope.

In general, for an anticipated slope of b, the sample size necessary to estimate this is expressed through d, and is

$$n = \frac{\sigma^2 (Z_{1-\beta} + Z_{1-\alpha/2})^2}{d^2} \frac{x_d^2}{\sigma_x^2}. \tag{12.3}$$

Here σ^2 is the variance about the dose response; x_i are the doses to be investigated in the study; d is the clinically meaningful difference, which becomes apparent at a specific dose x_d, and σ_x^2 is the variance of the x-axis (i.e. between doses). For example, in Figure 12.8, d is the treatment effect anticipated at dose, $x_2 = 2$. Thus, the anticipated slope, b, of the dose response is equal to $d / 2$ in this case.

Note, for two doses $x_0 = 0$ and $x_1 = 1$, so that $\sigma_x^2 = ((0 - 0.5)^2 + (1 - 0.5)^2)/2$ and (12.3) becomes

$$n = \frac{4\sigma^2 (Z_{1-\beta} + Z_{1-\alpha/2})^2}{\delta^2}. \tag{12.4}$$

This is the same result as the total sample size for a two-arm trial, from Chapter 3.

As well as dose response, these designs also allow for an investigation of concentration–exposure across a range of exposures.

12.5.1 WORKED EXAMPLE 12.1

It is worth considering how to design a dose–response study through the use of a worked example. First of all let us reconsider (12.3). For just part of (12.3)

$$n_p = \frac{\sigma^2 (Z_{1-\beta} + Z_{1-\alpha/2})^2}{d^2}, \tag{12.5}$$

we can calculate Table 12.3.

For the remaining part of (12.3)

$$\frac{x_d^2}{\sigma_x^2}, \tag{12.6}$$

we can construct Table 12.4.

Table 12.4 holds provided we have linear, equally spaced dose increments, for example 0 (placebo), 1, 2, 3; or 0, 100, 200, 300; or 0, 400, 800, 1200.

For example, if we had a standardized difference of interest of 0.25 with two doses (placebo and active), from Table 12.3 the partial sample size is 169. From Table 12.4 we have that $x_d^2/\sigma_x^2 = 4$, and the total sample size is calculated as $4 \times 169 = 676$, or 338 per arm.

Table 12.3 Partial sample size calculations for a dose–response study, for different standardized differences, for 90% power and two-sided significance level of 5%.

$\delta(=d/\sigma)$	n_p
0.05	4203
0.10	1051
0.15	467
0.20	263
0.25	169
0.30	117
0.35	86
0.40	66
0.45	52
0.50	43
0.55	35
0.60	30
0.65	25
0.70	22
0.75	19
0.80	17
0.85	15
0.90	13
0.95	12
1.00	11
1.05	10
1.10	9
1.15	8
1.20	8
1.25	7
1.30	7
1.35	6
1.40	6
1.45	5
1.50	5

Table 12.4 Squared standardized differences (x_d^2/σ_x^2) on the x-axis scale for different numbers of doses and different doses of interest.

	Number of doses				
Dose of interest	2	3	4	5	6
2	4.00	1.50	0.80	0.50	0.34
3		6.00	3.20	2.00	1.37
4			7.20	4.50	3.09
5				8.00	5.49
6					8.57

Note that here the active dose could have been any value, e.g. 1, 200, 400, 500.

If we had a standardized difference of interest of 0.25 with three doses (0 (placebo), 100, 200) and we expect to see this difference at the highest dose, then from Table 12.3 the partial sample size would again be 169. From Table 12.4 we have that $x_{\mathrm{d}}^2/\sigma_{\mathrm{x}}^2=6$, and the total sample size is calculated as $6 \times 169 = 1014$, or 338 per arm.

If we expect to see this difference at 100, then from Table 12.4 we have that $x_{\mathrm{d}}^2/\sigma_{\mathrm{x}}^2=1.5$, and the total sample size is calculated as $1.5 \times 169 = 253.5$, or 84.5 per arm or 85 in actual subjects.

If we had a standardized difference of interest of 0.25 with 5 doses (0 (placebo), 100, 200, 300 and 400) and we expect to see this difference at 300, then from Table 12.3 the partial sample size remains 169. From Table 12.4 we have that $x_{\mathrm{d}}^2/\sigma_{\mathrm{x}}^2=4.5$, and the total sample size is calculated as $4.5 \times 169 = 760.5$, or 152.1 per arm, or 153 in actual subjects.

If we expect to see this difference at 200, then from Table 12.4 we have that $x_{\mathrm{d}}^2/\sigma_{\mathrm{x}}^2=2$, and the total sample size is calculated as $2 \times 169 = 338$, or 67.6 per arm, or 68 in actual subjects.

12.6 POWERED ASSESSMENT

For late Phase II trials in particular, a powered assessment of the dose response may be undertaken. Such a study would require at least placebo and two active comparator doses to be included (ICH, 1994a) and there may be a need to titrate to each dose.

An active control may also be included in this type of trial. This would be included in order to assess the sensitivity of the study as, if the active comparator shows an effect against placebo but the investigative treatment selected does not, this would indicate we have a failed investigative treatment. In circumstances when both the active control and the investigative treatment fail to show an effect, this would be an indication of a failed study.

The sample size calculation is a conventional one – based on pair-wise comparisons to placebo. The two-group methodology from Chapter 3 could therefore be applied to estimate the sample size for each comparison. Model-based approaches could still be applied as secondary analyses.

12.6.1 MULTIPLE COMPARISONS

With these designs, there would be a need to incorporate methods to control the overall Type I error rate at 5% as there are several pair-wise comparisons to placebo, resulting in multiple comparisons.

12.6.1.1 Bonferroni and Dunnett's Methods

The simplest approach is a method that uses Bonferroni's inequality and consists of dividing the nominal significance level, that is, 5%, by the number of statistical tests to be conducted. Alternatively, it may be preferable instead to multiply the observed

P-values by the number of tests conducted and compare these with the nominal level of 5% significance. The outcome is the same but the latter method 'retains' 5% as the significance level. The Bonferroni approach is a little conservative, especially for correlated outcomes and/or when a relatively large number of comparisons are made.

An alternative approach is to use Dunnett's method, which is specifically used for pair-wise comparisons with a control, and is a little less conservative than the Bonferroni approach. It adjusts the significance level such that although there are multiple comparisons, the nominal level of 5% is retained.

The disadvantage of both the Dunnett and Bonferroni approaches is that they both require greater sample sizes compared to a simple pair-wise test (not allowing for multiplicity) to allow for the adjustment of the significance level. The main advantage, however, is that only one comparison needs to be significant in order to declare statistical significance.

12.6.1.2 Holm or Hochberg Procedures

An alternative is to modify the Bonferroni approach using one of the Hochberg or Holm procedures for k statistical tests. These procedures work as described in Figure 12.9 and the advantage of both is that the sample size does not need to be increased to account for the multiple testing.

The challenge with any statistical multiple testing procedure such as we have described is to get the balance between finding results which are statistically significant versus what is clinically important. A statistically significant result may be of no clinical importance, while conversely a clinically significant result may not be statistically significant. This is particularly important in multiple testing where it may be that the least clinically important endpoints have the greatest chance of statistical significance.

Hochberg procedure

- Order the P-values from smallest to largest.
- If the largest P-value is less than 0.05 then all hypotheses can be rejected.
- If not, if second largest P-value is less than 0.05 / 2, than all bar the largest can be rejected.
- And so on.

Holm procedure

- Order P-values from largest to smallest.
- If smallest is less than $0.05 / k$ then reject this null hypothesis.
- If second smallest is less than $0.05 / (k - 1)$, reject this null hypothesis.
- And so on.

Figure 12.9 Hochberg and Holm procedures for multiple testing involving k comparisons.

Sequential gate keeping

- Order the doses in the order in which you wish to test them (usually from highest to lowest).
- Then undertake hypothesis tests in this predefined order at 5%.

Figure 12.10 Sequential gate keeping.

12.6.2 GATE KEEPING THROUGH SEQUENTIAL TESTING

A sequential gate-keeping approach could also be applied through a testing procedure as described in Figure 12.10

This procedure has the advantage of not inflating the sample size. However, it has the disadvantage that if one test fails at the start of the sequence then you cannot go on to investigate the other tests.

Caution should be exercised when sequential gate keeping. In theory with this approach you can do as many tests as you want: for example once you have been through all the doses on one endpoint, do so for another endpoint; then another, and so on. However, you should avoid compiling a 'laundry list' of different endpoints, and balance *a priori* what is clinically important versus what is most likely (to be statistically significant) when putting together a sequential procedure.

13 Phase II Trials with Toxic Therapies

13.1 INTRODUCTION

Although this chapter is meant to relate to Phase II trials in all disease areas, much of the methodology has been developed and applied in oncology. In that context, the role of a Phase II trial would primarily be to assess whether a new chemotherapeutic (or other) agent has sufficient activity/potential efficacy to warrant further testing, say in a randomized Phase III trial.

More broadly, as indicated in CHMP (2005a), Phase II studies are intended to:

- Determine if significant responses can be achieved with the agent under study in the target tumours at doses and schedules defined in prior Phase I/II studies, or whether to stop investigating that specific tumour type
- To assess the probability of response in the target tumour type and conclude on the need for further studies (investigate earlier stages of the disease, combinations, compare with standard therapy)
- Further characterise the PK profile
- Further characterise dose and schedule dependency, with respect to safety and activity
- Further characterise the side-effects of the medicinal product:

  – detection of less common manifestations of toxicity
  – assessment of cumulative/sub-acute toxicity
  – assess possible measures to manage the toxicity

- When applicable, further characterise the best route of administration.

Many anticancer drugs are cytotoxic, killing a broad range of cells. As a result, the malignant (as well as normal) cells are damaged and hopefully eradicated. Therefore, in the clinical development of cytotoxic drugs, the activity of the treatment drug is often defined by tumour shrinkage ('response'). The objective response rate is then the proportion of patients whose tumours either completely disappear (complete response) or shrink by at least 30% (partial response). Standard criteria are used for this assessment, such as that of the Response Evaluation Criteria in Solid Tumours (Therasse *et al.*, 2000).

An Introduction to Statistics in Early Phase Trials Steven A. Julious, Say Beng Tan and David Machin

However, research in cancer treatment now increasingly focuses on the development of novel therapies that inhibit specific targets that cause malignant disorders. The specific effect of the agents depends on the class of target they inhibit, but in general they modulate and regulate the tumours and/or cellular targets. These new targeting agents inhibit the growth of the tumour and/or the development of metastases without necessarily shrinking the tumour. Thus trial designs which involve the primary endpoint of response rate may not be relevant for measuring the anticancer activity of such new agents. Instead alternative endpoints, including time-to-event endpoints such as progression-free survival, may be more appropriate.

We discuss both Phase II trial designs which involve binary endpoints (such as tumour response rates), as well as those which have time-to-event endpoints. Also described are designs which consider (jointly) acceptable toxicity levels and acceptable response rates, as well as randomized designs. Software to implement all of the designs is available in Machin *et al.* (2008).

In planning such Phase II trials, there are several options to consider, including the number of stages within each design, and alternative designs for essentially the same situation. The options we discuss are summarized in Figure 13.1.

Single stage	*No stopping rules*	*Single endpoint*
Fleming–A'Hern	Sample size fixed	Size determined at the design stage
Randomized	Sample size fixed	Size determined at the design stage and depends on the number of compounds under test
Two stage	*Allow early termination*	*Single endpoint*
Gehan	Maximum sample size unknown	Final sample size depends on the number of responses in Stage 1
Simon – optimal	Maximum sample size fixed	Stage 1 sample size chosen to ensure inactive compound does not go to Stage 2
Simon – minimax	Maximum sample size fixed	Designed for maximum sample size to be a minimum
Tan–Machin	Maximum sample size fixed	Stage 1 sample size chosen to ensure inactive compound does not go to Stage 2
Two stage	*Allow early termination*	*Dual endpoint*
Bryant–Day – optimal	Maximum sample size fixed	Stage 1 sample size chosen to ensure inactive or too toxic compound does not go to Stage 2
Two stage	*Allow early termination*	*Survival endpoint*
Case–Morgan	Maximum sample size fixed	Sample size chosen to minimize either expected duration of accrual or expected total study length for the trial

Figure 13.1 Comparative features of alternative Phase II designs.

13.2 SINGLE-STAGE DESIGNS

A key advantage of single-stage designs is that once the sample size has been determined, this translates directly into the number of patients that need to be recruited. This contrasts with, for example, two-stage designs, in which the total numbers eventually recruited depends on the response rate in those recruited to Stage 1.

In considering the design of a Phase II trial of a new drug, we will usually have some knowledge of the activity of other drugs for the same disease. The anticipated response to the new drug is therefore compared, at the planning stage, with the observed responses to other therapies. This may lead us to prespecify a response probability which, if the new drug fails to achieve results in no further investigation. There might also be some idea of a response probability which, if achieved or exceeded, would certainly imply that the new drug has activity worthy of further investigation.

If a Phase II trial either fails to identify efficacy or overestimates the potential efficacy there will be adverse consequences for the next stage of the drug development process.

13.2.1 FLEMING–A'HERN

The Fleming (1982) single-stage design for Phase II trials recruits a predetermined number of patients to the study, and a decision about activity is obtained from the number of responses amongst these patients.

To use the design, we first set the largest response proportion as π_0 which, if true, would clearly imply that the treatment does not warrant further investigation. We then judge what is the smallest response proportion, π_{New}, that would imply that the treatment certainly warrants further investigation. This means that the one-sided hypotheses to be tested in a Phase II study are

$$H_0 : \pi \leq \pi_0,$$

$$H_1 : \pi \geq \pi_{New},$$

where π is the actual probability of response which is to be estimated at the close of the trial.

In addition to specifying π_0 and π_{New}, it is necessary to specify α, the probability of rejecting the hypothesis H_0: $\pi \leq \pi_0$ when it is in fact true, together with β, the probability of rejecting the hypothesis H_1: $\pi \geq \pi_{New}$ when that is true.

With these inputs, Fleming (1982) details the appropriate sample size to be recruited as

$$N_{Fleming} = \frac{[z_{1-\alpha}\sqrt{\pi_0(1-\pi_0)} + z_{1-\beta}\sqrt{\pi_{New}(1-\pi_{New})}\,]^2}{(\pi_{New}-\pi_0)^2}. \quad (13.1)$$

A'Hern (2001) improved on this by using exact binomial probabilities to calculate the sample size. There is no closed-form expression for this sample size, so it requires the use of a computational search strategy. In general, the more accurate sample sizes from the A'Hern calculations, $N_{\text{A'Hern}}$, are marginally greater than those given by (13.1) and these are recommended for use. The design would reject the null hypothesis, $\pi \leq \pi_0$, if the observed number of responses, R, is $\geq C$. A'Hern determined the critical number of responses as

$$C = N_{\text{A'Hern}} \times \left[\pi_0 + \left(\frac{z_{1-\alpha}}{z_{1-\alpha} + z_{1-\beta}}\right)(\pi_{\text{New}} - \pi_0)\right]. \tag{13.2}$$

To implement the design, the appropriate number of patients is recruited and, once all their responses are observed, the response rate (and corresponding confidence interval) is calculated. A decision with respect to activity is then made.

13.3 TWO-STAGE DESIGNS

In many situations, investigators and sponsors may be reluctant to embark on a single-stage Phase II trial requiring a (relatively) large number of patients exposed to a new and uncertain therapy. In such circumstances, a more cautious approach may be to conduct the study, but in a series of stages, and review progress at the end of each stage. In two-stage designs, patients are recruited to Stage 1 and the move to Stage 2 is consequential on the results observed in the first stage. The main advantage of such a design is that the trial may stop, after relatively few patients have been recruited, should the response rate appear to be (unacceptably) low. The disadvantage is that the final number of patients required is not known until after Stage 1 is complete.

13.3.1 GEHAN

In the approach suggested by Gehan (1961), a minimum requirement of efficacy, π_{New}, is set and patients are recruited in two stages. If no responses are observed in Stage 1, patients are not recruited for Stage 2. On the other hand, if one or more responses are observed then the size of the recruitment to the second stage depends on their number.

To implement the design, the appropriate number of patients is recruited to Stage 1 and once all the responses are observed, a decision on whether or not to proceed to Stage 2 is taken. If Stage 2 is implemented, then once recruitment is complete and all assessments made, the response rate (and corresponding confidence interval) is calculated. A decision with respect to efficacy is then made. If Stage 2 is not activated, the response rate (and confidence interval) can still be calculated for the Stage 1 patients despite failure to demonstrate efficacy. This procedure applies to all the two-stage designs we will discuss.

13.3.2 SIMON OPTIMAL AND MINIMAX

In the approach suggested by Simon (1989), patients are recruited in two stages and there are two alternative designs.

One is *optimal*, in that the expected sample size is minimized if the regimen has low activity. This implies that an important focus is to ensure that as few patients as possible receive what turns out to be an ineffective drug by not continuing to Stage 2 in these circumstances. In this context, 'expected' means, the average sample size that would turn out to have been used had a whole series of studies been conducted with the same design parameters in situations where the true activity is the same.

The other, the *minimax* design, minimizes the maximum sample size for both stages combined, that is, the sum of patients required for Stage 1 and Stage 2 is chosen to minimize the maximum trial size within the parameter constraints as set by the design.

In either case, the designs imply that the one-sided hypotheses to be tested in a Phase II study are as we have described previously. It is also necessary to specify α and β as for the Fleming–A'Hern design.

The trial then proceeds by recruiting n_{S1} patients in Stage 1, from which r_{S1} responses are observed. A decision is then made to recruit n_{S2} patients to Stage 2 if $r_{S1} > R_{S1}$, where R_{S1} is the minimum number of responders required as indicated by the design. Otherwise the trial is closed at the end of Stage 1. At the end of the second stage, the drug is rejected for further use if a predetermined total number of responses is not observed.

The optimal designs have smaller Stage 1 sizes than the minimax designs, and so this smaller Stage 1 reduces the number of patients exposed to an inactive treatment if this turns out to be the case. In cases where the patient population is very heterogeneous, however, a very small Stage 1 may not be desirable because the first patients entered into the study may not be entirely representative of the wider eligible population. In this case, a larger Stage 1 may be preferred and the minimax design chosen.

13.4 TIME-TO-EVENT ENDPOINTS

As already mentioned, a disadvantage of two-stage designs is that the final number of patients required is not known until after recruitment to Stage 1 is complete and response in all these patients has been assessed. This poses a particular difficulty if the endpoint of concern is the time from initiation of treatment to some event (perhaps the death or disease progression of the patient) which is expressed through the corresponding survival time. In this case there will be a variable, and possibly extended, period of follow-up necessary to make the requisite observations. However, estimates of survival at a prechosen fixed point in interval time (say one year post-start of treatment) can be estimated using the Kaplan–Meier (K-M) technique, which takes into account censored observations. Censored survival time observations arise when a patient, although entered on the study and followed for a period of time, has not as yet experienced the 'event' defined as the outcome for the trial. This is illustrated in Figure 13.2, where each horizontal line which ends in a dot indicates that the particular subject has experienced the event, whereas

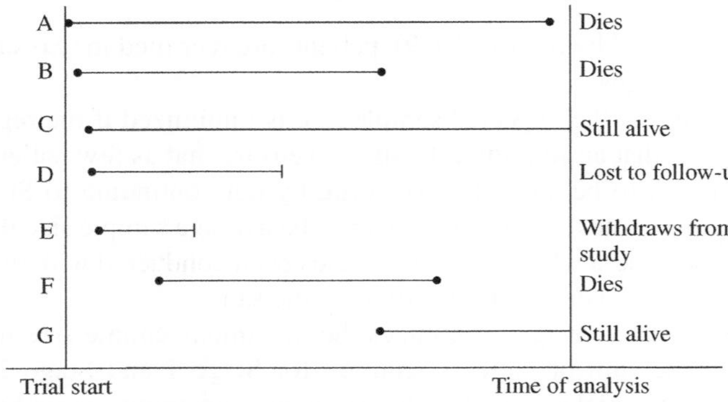

Figure 13.2 Censoring in a time-to-event study.

a short vertical line indicates that censoring has occurred. Note that censoring can occur for a variety of reasons, for example when the subject is lost to follow-up or withdraws from the study, in addition to not having experienced the event of interest at the time of the analysis of the study. So in the figure, subjects C, D, E and G are censored. For survival itself, 'death' will be the 'event' of concern, whereas if event-free survival was of concern, the 'event' may be for example recurrence of the disease.

In this context, when considering the design of a Phase II trial of a new drug, we will usually have some knowledge of the activity of other drugs for the same disease. The anticipated survival rate of the new drug is therefore compared, at the planning stage, with that observed with other therapies. This may lead to us to prespecify a survival probability which, if the new drug does not achieve, results in no further investigation. The planners might also have some idea of a survival probability that, if achieved or exceeded, would certainly imply that the new drug has activity worthy of further investigation.

13.4.1 CASE AND MORGAN

In the Case and Morgan (2003) two-stage designs, 'survival' times usually correspond to the interval between the registration of the patient into the study or the commencement of the Phase II treatment, and the time at which the event of primary concern occurs, for example recurrence of the disease, death, or either of these.

Typically, observing the event takes longer and is more variable in its time of occurrence than, for example, tumour response rate. This implies that any two-stage Phase II design using such an endpoint may require a time window between Stage 1 and (the potential) Stage 2, to allow sufficient events to accumulate for the Stage 1 analysis, so that a decision can be taken on whether or not to continue to Stage 2. The time window is added to the duration of Stage 1 and its necessity may require suspending patient recruitment during this interval. Clearly this will extend the total duration of the study. However, the Case–Morgan designs eliminate the need for this 'time window'.

To implement the design, we need, for a particular interval time, $t = T_{\text{Summary}}$, to set the largest survival proportion as $S_0(T_{\text{Summary}})$ which, if true, would clearly imply that the treatment does not warrant further investigation. We then judge what is the smallest survival proportion, $S_{\text{New}}(T_{\text{Summary}})$, that would imply the treatment warrants further investigation. This implies that the one-sided hypotheses to be tested in the study are

$$H_0 : S(T_{\text{Summary}}) \leq S_0(T_{\text{Summary}}), \qquad H_1 : S(T_{\text{Summary}}) \geq S_{New}(T_{\text{Summary}}),$$

where $S(T_{\text{Summary}})$ is the actual probability of survival which is to be estimated at the close of the trial. In addition to specifying $S_0(T_{\text{Summary}})$ and $S_{\text{New}}(T_{\text{Summary}})$, it is again necessary to specify α and β.

With these inputs, there are then two variants of the Case–Morgan design, depending on whether we wish to minimize the expected duration of accrual (EDA) or the expected total study length (ETSL) for the trial. These are defined as follows

$$\text{EDA} = D_{\text{Stage1}} + (1 - P_{\text{Early}})D_{\text{Stage2}}, \tag{13.3}$$

$$\text{ETSL} = D_{\text{Stage1}} + (1 - P_{\text{Early}})(D_{\text{Stage2}} + T_{\text{Summary}}), \tag{13.4}$$

where D_{Stage1} and D_{Stage2} are the durations of Stage 1 and Stage 2 of the trial respectively, and P_{Early} is the probability of stopping at the end of Stage 1.

With either of these variants, the objective would be to test H_0 at the end of Stage 1. If H_0 is rejected, the trial proceeds to Stage 2. Otherwise, recruitment stops at the end of Stage 1.

13.5 EFFICACY AND TOXICITY

In situations where the toxicity of an agent undergoing Phase II testing is poorly understood, it may be desirable to incorporate toxicity considerations into the trial design. In which case, both a minimum level of activity and a maximum level of (undesirable) toxicity are stipulated in the design. Such designs expand on the Simon two-stage designs discussed earlier.

13.5.1 BRYANT AND DAY

A common situation when considering first-time-into-new-population Phase I (chapter 8) and Phase II trials is that although the former primarily focuses on toxicity and the later on efficacy, each in fact considers both. This provides the rationale for Bryant and Day's (1995) Phase II design in which they combine a design for activity with a similar design for toxicity, thereby simultaneously looking for both *acceptable* toxicity and *high* activity.

As with designs discussed previously, the design implies that two, *one-sided* efficacy hypotheses, are to be tested. These are that the true response rate π_R is either $\leq \pi_{R0}$, the maximum response rate of no interest, or $\geq \pi_{RNew}$, the minimum response rate of interest. Further, the probability of incorrectly rejecting the hypothesis $\pi_R \leq \pi_{R0}$ is set as α_R. Similarly, α_T is set but now for the toxicity hypothesis $\pi_T \leq \pi_{T0}$ where π_{T0} is the maximum nontoxicity rate of no interest. In addition, the hypothesis $\pi_T \geq \pi_{TNew}$ has to be set together with β, the probability of failing to recommend a treatment that is acceptable with respect to both activity and (non)toxicity. (The terminology is a little clumsy here as it is more natural to talk in terms of 'acceptable toxicity' rates rather than 'acceptable non-toxicity' rates. Thus $1 - \pi_{T0}$ is the highest rate of toxicity above which the drug is unacceptable. In contrast, $1 - \pi_{TNew}$ is the lower toxicity level below which the drug would be regarded as acceptable on this basis.)

In the Bryant and Day design, the trial is terminated after Stage 1 if there are an inadequate number of observed responses or an excessive number of observed toxicities. The treatment under investigation is recommended at the end of the Stage 2 *only* if there are a sufficient number of responses *and* an acceptably small number of toxicities in total.

To implement the designs, the appropriate number of patients is recruited to Stage 1, and once all their responses and toxicity experiences are observed, a decision on whether or not to proceed to Stage 2 is taken. If Stage 2 is implemented, then once recruitment is complete and all assessments made the response and toxicity rates, along with their corresponding confidence intervals, are calculated. A decision with respect to efficacy and toxicity is then made. If Stage 2 is not activated, the response and toxicity rates can still be calculated for the Stage 1 patients despite either failure to demonstrate activity, too much toxicity or both.

13.6 BAYESIAN APPROACHES

13.6.1 MOTIVATION FOR BAYESIAN APPROACH

In the frequentist approach for (binary) response designs, the final response rate is estimated by *R*/*N*, where *R* is the total number of responses observed from the total number of patients recruited, *N*, (whether obtained from a single or two-stage design). This response rate, together with the corresponding 95% confidence interval, typically provides the basic information for us to decide if a subsequent Phase III trial is warranted. However, even after the trial is completed, there often remains considerable uncertainty about the true value of π, as characterized by large confidence intervals on π. Moreover, it is often helpful to be able to incorporate external information even at the design stage of a trial. The inevitable uncertainty arising from Phase II trials with small sample sizes, along with the ability to formally incorporate relevant external information at the design stage, suggests that Bayesian approaches may be useful for such Phase II trials.

13.6.2 OVERVIEW OF THE BAYESIAN APPROACH

A general discussion of Bayesian approaches has been given in Chapter 7. In the context of Phase II trials with binary endpoints, the prior distribution is often conveniently assumed to be of the form

$$prior(\pi) \propto \pi^{a-1}(1-\pi)^{b-1}. \qquad (13.5)$$

This is a beta distribution with parameters a and b, which can take any positive value. When a and b are integers, such a distribution corresponds to a prior belief equivalent to having observed a responses out of a hypothetical $T = (a + b)$ patients. This is then similar to the situation modelled by the binomial likelihood distribution, in which we have x as the number of responses from N patients.

Combining the above prior with a binomial likelihood results in a posterior distribution of the form

$$post(\pi|x) \propto \pi^{a+x-1}(1-\pi)^{b+N-x-1}. \tag{13.6}$$

It can be seen that this too is a beta distribution, but of the form beta $(a + x, b + N - x)$.

The posterior distribution represents our overall belief at the close of the trial about the distribution of the population parameter, π. Once we have obtained the posterior distribution, we can calculate the exact probabilities of π being in any region of interest.

The prior distribution summarizes the information on π before the trial commences. In practice, one postulates a prior distribution with a specific mean, M, and variance, V. These values could be obtained from relevant external data, or elicited from subjective clinical opinion or a combination of the two.

Once obtained, these values can then be used to obtain estimates of a and b from

$$a = \frac{M[M(1-M)-V]}{V}, \quad b = \frac{(1-M)[M(1-M)-V]}{V}. \tag{13.7}$$

Chapter 15 gives a detailed example which describes the beta distribution as well as the use of Bayesian methods in the context of Go/No Go criteria.

13.6.3 BAYESIAN SINGLE AND DUAL THRESHOLD

In the Bayesian two-stage single threshold design (STD) the focus is on estimating, for example, the posterior probability that $\pi > \pi_{New}$, so that if this is high, at the end of the Phase II trial, we can be reasonably confident in recommending the compound for testing in a Phase III trial.

The minimum interest response rate, π_{New}, and π_{Prior}, the anticipated response rate of the drug being tested, are set. However, in place of α and β, we specify λ_1, the required threshold probability following Stage 1 that $\pi > \pi_{New}$, and λ_2 ($>\lambda_1$), the required threshold probability after completion of Stage 2 that $\pi > \pi_{New}$. Further, once the first stage of the trial is completed, the estimated value of λ_1 is computed and a decision made on whether or not to proceed to Stage 2. Should the trial continue to Stage 2 then, on trial completion the estimated value of λ_2 is computed. Note that the trial only goes into Stage 2 if the estimate of λ_1, at the end of Stage 1, exceeds the design value. Efficacy is claimed at the end of Stage 2 only if the estimate of λ_2, obtained from all the data, exceeds the design value.

An alternative, two-stage dual threshold design (DTD) is identical to the STD except that the Stage 1 sample size is determined, not on the basis of the probability of exceeding π_{New}, but on the probability that π will be less than the 'no further interest' proportion, π_0. This represents the response rate below which we would have no further interest in the new drug. Thus π_0 functions as a lower threshold on the response rate, as opposed to the upper threshold represented by π_{New}. The rationale behind this aspect of the DTD is that we want our Stage 1 sample size to be large enough so that, if the trial data really does suggest a response rate that is below π_0, we want the posterior probability of π being below π_0 to be at least λ_1. The design determines the smallest Stage 1 sample size that satisfies this criterion. The trial only goes into Stage 2 if the estimate of λ_1 exceeds the design value, and efficacy is claimed at the end of Stage 2 only if the estimate of λ_2 exceeds the design value.

The DTD requires us to set π_{Prior} as the anticipated value of π for the drug being tested. A convenient choice may be $(\pi_0 + \pi_{New})/2$ but this is not a requirement. Further, λ_1 is set as the required threshold probability following Stage 1, that $\pi < \pi_0$, while λ_2 is the required threshold probability that, after completion of Stage 2, $\pi > \pi_{New}$. (Note that unlike in the case of STD, it is no longer a requirement that $\lambda_1 < \lambda_2$.) Once Stage 1 of the trial is completed, the estimated value of λ_1 is computed and should the trial continue to Stage 2 then on its completion, the estimated value of λ_2 is computed. The latter is then used to help make the decision on whether or not a Phase III trial is suggested.

The original design proposed by Tan and Machin (2002) works on the basis of having a 'vague' prior distribution which corresponds to having a prior sample size of three. There are modifications to the original design, including the use of informative priors (Mayo and Gajewski, 2004; Wang *et al*, 2005; Gajewski and Mayo, 2006; and Sambucini, 2008).

13.7 RANDOMIZED PHASE II TRIALS

In the context of this chapter, Phase II trials are of a single-arm, noncomparative design. However, randomized Phase II trials for toxic therapies may also be conducted. Such trials are not an alternative to conducting (large) Phase III randomized controlled trials, and the objective is not to carry out a confirmatory comparison between two treatments. Instead, investigators may wish to obtain an indication of the potential usefulness of the new therapy in comparison with the standard treatment, or perhaps an estimate of efficacy which can then be used in the planning of a Phase III trial.

Or, in another situation, there may be several compounds available for potential Phase III testing in the same type of patients but practicalities imply that only one of these can go forward for this subsequent assessment. Since there are several options, good practice dictates that the eligible patients should be randomized to the alternatives. This can be achieved by using a randomized Phase II selection design in which the objective is to select only one, the 'best', of several agents tested simultaneously.

The randomized designs overcome the difficulties pointed out by Estey and Thall (2003) when discussing single-arm trials, where the actual differences between response rates associated with the treatments (*treatment effects*) are confounded with differences between the trials (*trial effects*), as there is no randomization to treatment. Consequently an apparent treatment effect may in reality only be a trial effect.

The approach to computing the sample sizes for randomized Phase II trials depends critically on the objective of the trial. Should the intention be, for example, to obtain an estimate of the hazard ratio, precision-based approaches such as those discussed in Chapter 3 could be used, where the objective would be to compute a sample size to ensure a certain prespecified width of the confidence interval on the estimate of the hazard ratio. However, for the problem of selecting the most promising treatment, more specialized approaches need to be adopted.

13.7.1 SIMON, WITTES AND ELLENBERG (SWE) DESIGN

The Simon, Wittes and Ellenberg design (Simon *et al.*, 1985) is a randomized (single-stage) Phase II design which selects from several candidate drugs that with the highest level of activity. This approach chooses the observed best treatment for the Phase III trial, however small the advantage over the others. The trial size is determined in such a way that if a treatment exists for which the underlying efficacy is superior to the others by a specified amount, then it will be selected with a high probability.

When the difference in true response rates of the best and next best treatment is δ, the design allows for the computation of sample sizes depending on the desired probability of correct selection, P_{CS}, and the number of treatments being tested, g. P_{CS} is smallest when there is a single best treatment and the other $g - 1$ treatments are of equal but lower efficacy. The response rate of the worst treatment is denoted π_{Worst}.

For a specified response, π, the probability that the best treatment produces the highest observed response rate is

$$\Pr(\text{Highest}) = \sum_{i=0}^{n} f(i)[1 - B(i; \pi_{Worst} + \delta, n)], \qquad (13.8)$$

where $B(R; \pi, n)$is the cumulative binomial distribution and

$$f(i) = [B(i; \pi_{Worst}, n)]^{g-1} - [B(i-1; \pi_{Worst}, n)]^{g-1}.$$

If there is a tie among the treatments for the largest observed response rate, then one of the tied treatments is randomly selected. Hence, in calculating the probability of correct selection, it is necessary to add to expression (13.8) the probability that the best treatment was selected after being tied with one or more of the other treatments for the greatest observed response rate. This is

$$\Pr(\text{Tie}) = \sum_{i=0}^{n} \left[b(i; \pi_{Worst} + \delta, n) \sum_{j=1}^{g-1} \left(\frac{1}{j+1} \right) k(i,j) \right], \qquad (13.9)$$

where

$$k(i,j) = \frac{(g-1)!}{j!(g-1-j)!}[b(i;\pi_{\text{Worst}},n)]^j[B(i-1;\pi_{\text{Worst}},n)]^{g-1-j}$$

The quantity $k(i, j)$ represents the probability that exactly j of the inferior treatments are tied for the largest number of observed responses among the $g - 1$ inferior treatments, and this number of responses is i; $b(i; \pi, n)$ denotes the binomial probability mass function. The factor $[1/(j+1)]$ is the probability that the tie between the best and the j inferior treatments is randomly broken by selecting the best treatment. The sum of expressions (13.8) and (13.9) gives the probability of correct selection, that is $P_{CS} = \Pr(\text{Highest}) + \Pr(\text{Tie})$.

To compute the sample size, a computer search then needs to be carried out for specified values of π_{Worst}, δ, and g, which provides a probability of correct selection equal to the preset value of P_{CS}.

14 Interpreting and Applying Early Phase Trial Results

14.1 INTRODUCTION

After undertaking an early phase trial, a key objective would be to assess whether there are sufficiently encouraging results to proceed to late-phase development. Sufficiently encouraging results would usually be defined in terms of statistical significance. This is appropriate, but in the context of drug development what may be required is some form of prediction of likely outcomes in Phase III.

In effect what we are discussing in this Chapter is replication of results from one study to the next, which although not a straightforward consideration (Senn, 2002) is something we often wish to assess. In early drug development we only initiate certain activities in a development programme (including clinical trials) dependent on observing certain results in trials we have undertaken. From these results we wish to have a degree of 'confidence' as to the ability to see favourable results in prospective trials. Thus, we need to have a degree of replication.

This chapter will describe methods for interpreting and applying early phase trial results in the context of an overall development.

14.2 CONSTRUCTING CONFIDENCE INTERVALS

14.2.1 INFERENCE IN ESTIMATING A POPULATION EFFECT

Confidence intervals are an important way of describing the results of a clinical trial and their utility has been highlighted throughout the book. For early phase trials they are particularly useful as they emphasize the more exploratory nature of these studies. Thus, as highlighted in Chapter 2, we may design a trial during early development to explore possible effects rather than for firmly establishing any effect exists.

An Introduction to Statistics in Early Phase Trials Steven A. Julious, Say Beng Tan and David Machin

For a clinical trial, therefore, a 100(1 − α)% confidence interval can be calculated using the following basic result

$$\overline{x}_A - \overline{x}_B \pm t_{n_A+n_B-2,1-\alpha/2} s_p \sqrt{\frac{1}{n_A} + \frac{1}{n_B}}, \tag{14.1}$$

where $\overline{x}_A$ and $\overline{x}_B$ are sample means for the two treatment groups A and B respectively; n_A and n_B are the sample sizes; s_p is the pooled estimate of the standard deviation; and is the percentage point of the t-distribution with, $n_A + n_B - 2$ degrees of freedom. For a 95% confidence interval $\alpha = 0.05$.

Strictly speaking, a 95% confidence interval is defined in a repeated sampling context. Thus, if we wanted a 95% confidence interval for the treatment effect in a clinical trial we imagine that we undertook a large number of similar trials and for each trial calculated a 95% confidence interval. Then 95% of these confidence intervals would include the true value for the treatment effect. Figure 14.1 illustrates this point giving the results from a

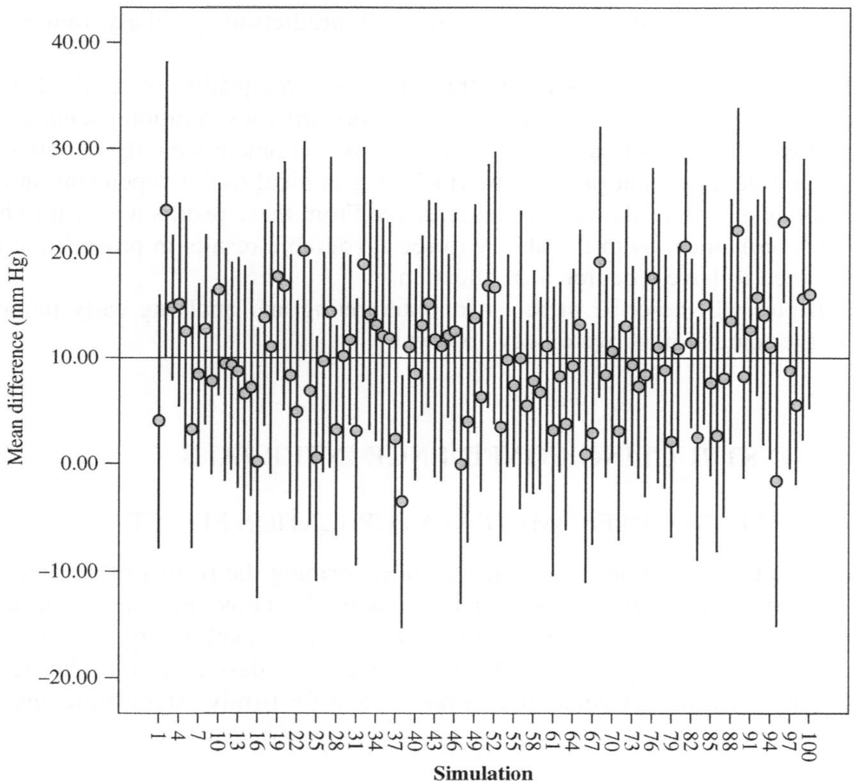

Figure 14.1 Simulation giving mean differences and 95% confidence intervals of 100 two-group studies of 16 subjects per arm sampled from populations with true means 100 and 110 mmHg, each with a common standard deviation of 15 mmHg.

100 simulations. Simply speaking, a confidence interval is an interval within which we are 95% certain that the true value would lie and it therefore provides a range of responses around the mean value to assist in the assessment of the true effect.

14.2.1.1 Worked Example 14.1

A parallel-group trial has been conducted to compare an investigative treatment with control. The trial has 50 subjects (25 on each arm) with the means on the two respective treatments being 110 and 100, with a pooled estimate of the standard deviation of 15. The difference in means is 10, with a corresponding 95% confidence interval of (1.5, 18.5). Hence, we are saying our best estimate of response is 10, but the difference may truly be as low as 1.5 or as high as 18.5.

14.2.2 INFERENCE IN ESTIMATION OF A FUTURE TRIAL EFFECT

An issue with confidence intervals in the context of Phase II trials is that, although they provide estimates of the population mean difference between groups, they do not provide a plausible range of values for any future trial of the same comparison. However, it is this range that will be required when decisions need to be made in the context of progressing or not to Phase III.

Formally the reason can be explained as follows. The confidence interval calculated in Phase II is for the population mean difference, which is a fixed quantity. However, the observed mean difference of the future Phase III trial will have an additional source of variability, namely that of the observed difference obtained from the new data. This is not allowed for in the (Phase II) confidence interval.

What we actually wish to know therefore is the average coverage for a given confidence interval with respect to future trials. In the case of the difference between means this can be estimated from (Julious *et al.*, 2007)

$$\text{Coverage} = 1 - 2\left(t_{n_A+n_B-2,1-\alpha/2}\sqrt{\frac{r}{(r+1)}}, n_A + n_B - 2, 0\right). \qquad (14.2)$$

where r is the ratio of the sample size of the proposed study to the one just conducted, and $(a, b, 0)$ is the cumulative t-distribution with ordinate a and degrees of freedom b.

Table 14.1 is derived from (14.2) and gives the anticipated proportion of future trial mean differences to fall within the 95% confidence interval of the preceding trial as a function of its sample size. With $r = 1$ and a sample size of 100, we would expect 83.6% of future trials to give rise to mean difference estimates which fall within the previous 95% confidence interval.

What is interesting from Table 14.1 is that the greater the ratio of the sample size of any future study to the current study, the greater the probability that the mean response will fall within the confidence interval of the current study. Intuitively, the larger the sample size

Table 14.1 Proportion of mean differences expected to fall within a two-sided 95% confidence interval, for different sample size ratios.

	Ratio of sample size of second study to first						
Sample size	**0.5**	**1**	**2**	**3**	**4**	**5**	**10**
5	0.837	0.890	0.930	0.930	0.935	0.938	0.944
10	0.780	0.858	0.904	0.919	0.927	0.932	0.941
15	0.766	0.849	0.899	0.916	0.925	0.930	0.940
20	0.759	0.845	0.897	0.914	0.923	0.929	0.940
25	0.755	0.843	0.895	0.914	0.923	0.928	0.939
30	0.753	0.841	0.894	0.913	0.922	0.928	0.939
35	0.751	0.840	0.894	0.913	0.922	0.928	0.939
40	0.750	0.840	0.893	0.912	0.922	0.928	0.939
45	0.749	0.839	0.893	0.912	0.922	0.927	0.939
50	0.749	0.838	0.893	0.912	0.922	0.927	0.939
75	0.746	0.837	0.892	0.911	0.921	0.927	0.939
100	0.745	0.836	0.892	0.911	0.921	0.927	0.939
200	0.744	0.835	0.891	0.911	0.921	0.927	0.938
300	0.743	0.835	0.891	0.911	0.921	0.927	0.938
400	0.743	0.835	0.891	0.911	0.921	0.927	0.938
500	0.743	0.835	0.891	0.911	0.921	0.927	0.938

of a future study is, the nearer the mean of this study would be to the true population mean and hence the nearer to 95% the chance that the 95% confidence interval of the current trial will contain this mean response.

Now, (14.2) is the coverage for a given $(1-\alpha)\%$ confidence interval and hence can in turn be rewritten to give α as a function of the appropriate coverage:

$$\alpha = 2\left[1 - \text{Probt}\left(t_{n_A+n_B-2,(1-\text{coverage})/2}\sqrt{\frac{(r+1)}{r}}, n_A+n_B-2, 0\right)\right]. \qquad (14.3)$$

The results from (14.2) and (14.3) converge to

$$1 - 2\Phi\left(\frac{Z_1 - \alpha/2}{\sqrt{2}}\right)$$

and

$$2\left[1 - \Phi\left(\sqrt{2}Z_1 - \alpha/2\right)\right],$$

respectively, as the degrees of freedom increase for (14.3), where $\Phi(\bullet)$ is a cumulative Normal distribution. From (14.2), when $\alpha = 0.05$, the coverage converges to 0.8342 as the sample size becomes large, which is consistent with the probability of the confidence intervals of two means discussed in Chapter 12.

Table 14.2 gives the significance level from (14.3) required to ensure that 95% of the mean responses from the second study fall within the confidence interval of

Table 14.2 Table of α required to ensure that 95% of mean responses are expected to fall within a $100(1-\alpha)\%$ confidence interval, for different sample sizes.

	Ratio of sample size of second study to first						
Sample size	**0.5**	**1**	**2**	**3**	**4**	**5**	**10**
5	0.01186	0.02048	0.02997	0.03488	0.03787	0.03988	0.04446
10	0.00398	0.01151	0.02235	0.02868	0.03271	0.03547	0.04194
15	0.00247	0.00921	0.02017	0.02686	0.03118	0.03415	0.04119
20	0.00188	0.00818	0.01915	0.02600	0.03045	0.03353	0.04083
25	0.00157	0.00761	0.01856	0.02550	0.03003	0.03317	0.04062
30	0.00139	0.00724	0.01818	0.02518	0.02975	0.03293	0.04048
35	0.00127	0.00698	0.01791	0.02495	0.02955	0.03276	0.04038
40	0.00118	0.00679	0.01771	0.02478	0.02941	0.03264	0.04031
45	0.00112	0.00665	0.01756	0.02465	0.02930	0.03254	0.04025
50	0.00107	0.00654	0.01744	0.02454	0.02921	0.03246	0.04021
75	0.00093	0.00621	0.01708	0.02423	0.02895	0.03224	0.04008
100	0.00086	0.00604	0.01690	0.02408	0.02882	0.03212	0.04001
200	0.00077	0.00581	0.01663	0.02385	0.02862	0.03196	0.03991
300	0.00074	0.00573	0.01655	0.02378	0.02856	0.03190	0.03988
400	0.00073	0.00569	0.01650	0.02374	0.02853	0.03187	0.03987
500	0.00072	0.00567	0.01648	0.02372	0.02851	0.03186	0.03986

the first. Using this table we can obtain values for α to ensure a confidence interval estimate from (14.1) will have appropriate coverage for a 95% confidence interval.

Note, for the special case $r = 1$ the corresponding result to the 95% confidence interval of (14.1) is to increase the width of the confidence interval by a factor of $\sqrt{2}$, to give

$$\overline{x}_{\mathrm{A}} - \overline{x}_{\mathrm{B}} \pm t_{n_{\mathrm{A}}+n_{\mathrm{B}}-2,1-\alpha/2}\sqrt{2}s_{\mathrm{p}}\sqrt{\frac{1}{n_{\mathrm{A}}}+\frac{1}{n_{\mathrm{B}}}}. \tag{14.4}$$

This ensures that the 95% confidence of the future Phase III trial will indeed have 95% coverage of this (modified) interval.

Note that the equivalent results to (14.2) and (14.3) for a two-period crossover trial, assuming the total sample size is n subjects, are

$$\text{Coverage} = 1 - 2\text{Probt}\left(t_{n-2,1-\alpha/2}\sqrt{\frac{r}{(r+1)}}, n-2, 0\right), \tag{14.5}$$

$$\alpha = 2\left[1 - \text{Probt}\left(t_{n-2,(1-\text{coverage})/2}\sqrt{\frac{(r+1)}{r}}, n-2, 0\right)\right]. \tag{14.6}$$

While for a single arm in a parallel-group trial, they are

$$\text{Coverage}=1-2\text{Probt}\left(t_{n_A-1,1-\alpha/2}\sqrt{\frac{r}{(r+1)}},n_A-1,0\right), \quad (14.7)$$

$$\alpha=2\left[1-\text{Probt}\left(t_{n_A-1,(1-\text{coverage})/2}\sqrt{\frac{(r+1)}{r}},n_A-1,0\right)\right]. \quad (14.8)$$

14.2.2.1 Worked Example 14.2

A Phase III parallel-group trial is being planned based on the results of an earlier Phase II investigation with sample size of 25. With the information from the Phase II trial we wish to have an estimate of the response we are likely to see in the Phase III trial. The difference in means observed was 10 and we plan the Phase III trial to have sample size r 5-times larger. From Table 14.2, to ensure the confidence interval has 95% coverage we need to set the level of $\alpha = 0.03317$ in (14.1) to ensure we are 95% confident that the revised confidence interval is likely to contain the new trial response.

The confidence interval is now (0.7, 19.2). Hence, we are saying our best estimate of response is 10 but the difference we may see in the future trial may be as low as 0.7 or as high as 19.2.

14.3 SELECTING AN EFFECT SIZE FOR A FUTURE TRIAL

Suppose we have designed a clinical trial and for the sample size calculation we have assumed values for the standard deviation, s, and the treatment difference of interest, d. The sample size in each group is calculated to be n_A ($n_A = n_B$), which we have estimated with 90% power and two-sided significance level of 5%.

We then conduct the trial and see exactly the same treatment difference, d, and standard deviation, s, which we used for design purposes. Our P-value would then be $P < 0.002$ and not $P = 0.05$ as might have been expected. The reason for this is attributable to the distribution under the alternative hypothesis. Suppose the alternative hypothesis is true as illustrated in Figure 14.2.

Under this alternative hypothesis the treatment differences are distributed about d such that there is a 50 : 50 chance of being above or below this response. Also, under the alternative hypothesis we have the chance of declaring there is no statistical difference, which from Chapter 3 we know to be the Type II error.

If the P-value is less than 0.002 if we see the anticipated response used for powering the study, d, then, therefore, logically we can see some fraction of d and still have a statistically significant response. In fact, for a P-value less than 0.05, if d is the true effect, then we would be observing a response at a level of $0.6 \times d$.

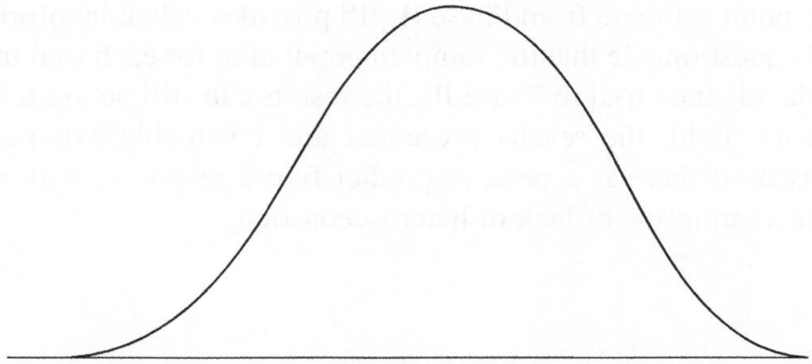

Figure 14.2 Distribution of treatment response under the alternative hypothesis.

Where this is important is in the selection of the response to design the Phase III trial. If we had $P = 0.05$ exactly, then this could be evidence that the true effect is actually $0.6 \times d$. Hence, if we still chose a response that is d as an effect size, then the Phase III study would only have power of 50%.

Conversely if we are to use the point estimate from Phase IIb to design the Phase III trial then it could be argued that we would need a P-value of at least 0.002 to ensure we have 90% power.

14.4 APPLICATION OF THE RESULTS

For the purpose of predicting the response of a future trial we should not use a straightforward 95% confidence interval for the current trial but instead adjust the significance level to ensure we have an appropriate coverage. Also if the power of a planned trial is based solely on the effect size observed in Phase II, then this new trial may subsequently have lower power than anticipated.

A major consideration, though, is that what we have discussed so far assumes that there is no heteroscedasticity between trials. This may not be the case, as different trials have different inclusion and exclusion criteria and different concomitant care, particularly over time. Particularly within a drug development programme, a trial conducted in Phase II may be in a different trial population compared to a trial conducted in Phase III. The former, for example, may involve more specialist centres being used or have narrower inclusion criteria. In addition they may have different primary endpoints – for example the Phase II trial may be a shorter-duration study.

A further consideration when interpreting Phase II studies is an effect known as 'regression to the mean'. In practice, we will usually only proceed to Phase III if Phase II is successful. Hence, Phase III will only be initiated if sufficiently encouraging results had previously been observed. Thus, for Phase II we may only have positive (and encouraging) results, while in Phase III we may have a range of observed response. This would have the effect of reducing cumulative effect. Hence, caution should be exercised in using a point estimate from Phase II to design a Phase III trial.

Of course, the point estimate from Phase II still provides valuable information. Even if the assumption is questionable that the sampled population for each trial in Phase II is the same as that in the planned trial in Phase III, the results can still be used. Even where the assumptions do not hold, the results presented are a valuable extension to standard confidence intervals if there is a need to predict future response, with the appropriate caveats about the assumption of lack of heteroscedasticity.

15 Go/No-Go Criteria

15.1 INTRODUCTION

A Go/No-Go decision is a hurdle in a clinical development path to necessitate further progression or otherwise of an asset. The hurdles can be set low or high depending on the stage of development of the compound. For example, a very early trial may have a relatively low 'Go' hurdle as these trials may provide little information on which to make a definitive decision. The converse of this would be a late-stage early trial (Phase IIb) which may have a relatively high hurdle for a 'Go', as a decision based on these results may initiate expensive late-phase activities.

When setting a Go/No-Go decision criterion, it is best to make it as objective as possible, preferably based on quantified results from trial information. For example, working Go/No-Go criteria for a new formulation may take the form

We wish the pharmacokinetic profile to look like Ayer's Rock (Uluru) for the new formulations.

Which when quantified may become

We wish C_{max} to be reached within 4 hours, and 90% of C_{max} to be maintained for 12 hours

When designing the study, a development team would have a number of choices on the setting of which Go/No-Go criteria to use. With an early phase trial a Go/No-Go criterion could be set to minimize the probability of a false positive (progressing a drug that will fail in Phase III). Thus, a high 'Go' hurdle could be set for this study. However, this would have the impact of increasing the probability of a false negative (terminating a drug that works), such that a 'No-Go' might actually terminate a valuable therapy.

An individual study, therefore, and its Go/No-Go criteria must be evaluated within the context of the overall development plan and on the whole portfolio. For a given compound, for example, there may be a wish for a 'fast-fail' decision to avoid launching a late-phase development while also allowing resources to be concentrated on better assets which may reach the market quicker as a result.

In this chapter we discuss how Go/No-Go criteria can be constructed within a simple Bayesian framework. We introduce the Bayesian approaches through a single case study with a binary endpoint. It should be noted though that the methodologies described in this

An Introduction to Statistics in Early Phase Trials Steven A. Julious, Say Beng Tan and David Machin

chapter are a solution and not *the* solution to making informed decisions in drug development (Burman and Senn, 2003; Julious and Swank, 2005).

15.2 BINARY DATA

For the construction of 'Go/No-Go' criteria for binary data we must first revisit the construction of confidence intervals for binary data, particularly exact confidence intervals.

15.2.1 EXACT CONFIDENCE INTERVALS

Exact confidence intervals, also known as Clopper–Pearson confidence intervals, are calculated by summing each of the tail probabilities from the binomial distribution, given the observed number of cases (k) for the sample size (n).

Defining the individual cell probabilities as

$$Pr(X=k) = \binom{n}{k} p^k (1-p)^{(n-k)}, \tag{15.1}$$

the lower limit of the confidence interval is defined as the lowest cumulative value of $Pr(X=k)$ such that the lower tail area of the distribution is no more than $\alpha / 2$. Likewise, the upper limit is calculated as the point where the cumulative distribution exceeds $1 - \alpha / 2$. Formally, the lower point of a confidence interval is defined as

$$\sum_{i=0}^{k} \binom{n}{i} p_{\mathrm{L}}^{i} (1 - p_{\mathrm{L}})^{(n-i)} < \alpha/2, \tag{15.2}$$

whilst the upper point is defined as,

$$\sum_{k=0}^{k} \binom{n}{i} p_{\mathrm{U}}^{i} (1 - p_{\mathrm{U}})^{(n-i)} / 1 - \alpha/2. \tag{15.3}$$

The link between the F-distribution and the binomial distribution can also be used to calculate exact confidence intervals such that the lower limit is

$$\frac{k}{k + (n-k+1)F_{1-\alpha/2,\,2n-2k+2,\,2k}}, \tag{15.4}$$

and the upper limit is

$$\frac{k+1}{k+1+(n-k)/F_{1-\alpha/2,\,2k+2,\,2n-2k}}. \tag{15.5}$$

The beta distribution can also be used for confidence intervals, as the probability density function of the F-distribution

$$p_F(x;a,b) = \frac{a^{a/2}b^{b/2}\Gamma(a/2+b/2)}{\Gamma(a/2)\Gamma(b/2)}\int_0^x \frac{t^{(a-2)/2}}{(at+b)^{(a+b)/2}}\mathrm{d}t. \qquad (15.6)$$

is related to the beta distribution

$$\mathit{BETAINV}(x;a,b) = \frac{\Gamma(a+b)}{\Gamma(a)\Gamma(b)}\int_0^x t^{a-1}(1-t)^{b-1}\mathrm{d}t, \qquad (15.7)$$

such that (Daly, 1992; Julious, 2005b)

$$F_{P,a,b} = \frac{b\mathit{BETAINV}(P,a/2,b/2)}{a(1-\mathit{BETAINV}(P,a/2,b/2))}. \qquad (15.8)$$

Use of this relationship gives, from (15.4), the lower confidence limit as

$$1-\mathit{BETAINV}(1-\alpha/2, n-k+1, k), \qquad (15.9)$$

and the upper limit as

$$\mathit{BETAINV}(1-\alpha/2, k+1, n-k). \qquad (15.10)$$

This gives more straightforward expressions for the confidence interval than (15.4) and (15.5). There is a beta function in most statistical packages, for example *BETAINV* in SAS (from which the notation in (15.9) and (15.10) is taken), so the confidence interval calculation is operationally straightforward.

Finally, the Normal approximation result for a confidence interval is

$$p \pm Z_{1-\alpha/2}\sqrt{\frac{\pi(1-\pi)}{\nu}}. \qquad (15.11)$$

15.2.1.1 Worked Example 15.1: Calculating Confidence Intervals for a Single Proportion

Table 15.1 illustrates how confidence intervals are calculated from (15.2) and (15.3). In the example, the sample size was 20, with 12 responders, giving a prevalence of 0.6. From the column of cumulative probabilities (the shaded areas), the 95% confidence interval is thus estimated as (0.35, 0.80).

Table 15.1 Frequency and cumulative frequency of the binomial distribution for a sample size of 20 and response rate of 0.6.

n	Probability	Cumulative probability
0	0.00000	0.00000
1	0.00000	0.00000
2	0.00000	0.00001
3	0.00004	0.00005
4	0.00027	0.00032
5	0.00129	0.00161
6	0.00485	0.00647
7	0.01456	0.02103
8	0.03550	0.05653
9	0.07099	0.12752
10	0.11714	0.24466
11	0.15974	0.40440
12	0.17971	0.58411
13	0.16588	0.74999
14	0.12441	0.87440
15	0.07465	0.94905
16	0.03499	0.98404
17	0.01235	0.99639
18	0.00309	0.99948
19	0.00049	0.99996
20	0.00004	1.00000

Using the corresponding F-distribution, and (15.4) and (15.5), the confidence interval is estimated to be (0.36, 0.81).

To calculate the confidence intervals using the beta distribution, SAS code for the example is given in Figure 15.1 (using (15.9) and (15.10)).

As it should, this approach gives the same result, that is (0.36, 0.81), as that using the F-distribution given earlier. Exact confidence intervals are quite conservative, such that a 95% confidence interval will contain the true value greater than 95% of the time. However, as *n* gets large, exact methods and Normal approximation tend to give similar results.

Finally, the Normal approximation result calculates the confidence interval to be (0.39, 0.81).

```
DATA ci;
n = 20;
k = 12;
lci = 1-betainv(0.975,n-k+1,k);
uci = betainv(0.975,k+1,n-k);
RUN;
PROC print;RUN;
```

Figure 15.1 SAS code to calculate the 95% confidence interval for a proportion.

15.2.2 BAYESIAN APPROACHES

For inference about an unknown binary parameter, θ, what we are interested in is how would our belief about the true value of θ change once a trial is complete. If the prior distribution on θ is expressed in the density $p(\theta)$ and if subsequently data x are observed, then the posterior distribution is, $p(\theta \mid x)$, where Bayes rule states

$$p(\theta/x) \propto \lambda(x/\overline{\theta})p(\theta), \tag{15.12}$$

where $\lambda(x \mid \theta)$ is the likelihood function. Note the constant of proportionality is chosen so that it integrates to 1, and the likelihood function is considered defined for the whole range (though may be zero for parts of it).

For binary data, the beta distribution form can be used for the prior responses, such that

$$Prior(p, a, b) \propto p^{a-1}(1-p)^{b-1}. \tag{15.3}$$

Using a beta prior in the context of binary data results in a posterior distribution which is also of the beta form. Such a property is known as conjugacy in that both the prior and posterior have the same distributional form.

15.2.2.1 Prior Response

Prior values for $PROBBETA(p_{percentile}, a_0, b_0)$ (and the corresponding $p_{percentile}$=$BETAINV(percentile, a_0, b_0)$) could be derived as follows. For an informative prior we could use the mode (or most likely value) and a percentile to build a prior. For a beta distribution the mode is defined by

$$m = \frac{a_0 - 1}{a_0 + b_0 - 2}. \tag{15.14}$$

Hence, a_0 (and consequently b_0) could be derived from

$$p_{percentile} = BETAINV\left(percentile, a_0, \frac{(a_0 - 1)}{m} - a_0 + 2\right) \tag{15.15}$$

if a percentile for the control response can be postulated.

If we wished to use a noninformative prior, then a Jeffrey's prior could be used, such that

$$p_{percentile} = BETAINV(percentile, 0.5, 0.5). \tag{15.16}$$

This Jeffrey's prior has the advantage of being invariant with respect to transformations.

15.2.2.2 Worked Example 15.2: Constructing a Prior Response

As a preliminary to a clinical trial, we need to anticipate what is the most likely response, that is, suggest a plausible modal value and also a higher value, for which we are (say) 80% sure that the response is less than it.

```
DATA priors;
DO a = 1 to 100 by 0.001 until (flag = 1);
prob = probbeta(0.12,a,(a-1)/0.06+2-a);
     IF prob > 0.8 then DO;
     flag = 1;
     END;
END;
b = (a-1)/0.06+2-a;
RUN;
TITLE "Print of Priors";
PROC print;
RUN;
```

Figure 15.2 SAS code for generating a beta prior.

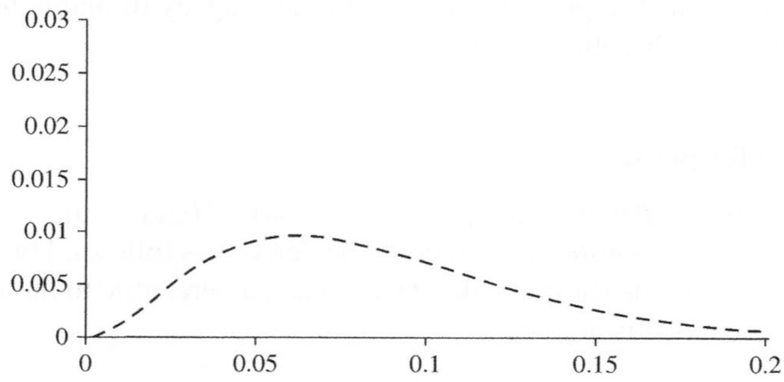

Figure 15.3 Prior response.

For example, *a priori* suppose we think the most likely response is 6%, and we are 80% certain it is less than 12%. Using (15.14) and (15.15) leads to $a_0 = 3.026$ and $b_0 = 32.7407$. We can thus estimate the percentiles for the prior distribution from

$$p_{percentile} = BETAINV(percentile, 3.026, 32.7407). \quad (15.17)$$

Example SAS code for doing this is given in Figure 15.2.

Figure 15.3 gives an illustration of the prior response for the worked example.

15.2.2.3 Anticipated Response

The anticipated control response, p, and the consequent variance term $p(1 - p)$ is taken from the data from a previous clinical trial. In that trial, the observed number of successes was a_1 and failures b_1, giving $p = a_1 / (a_1 + b_1)$.

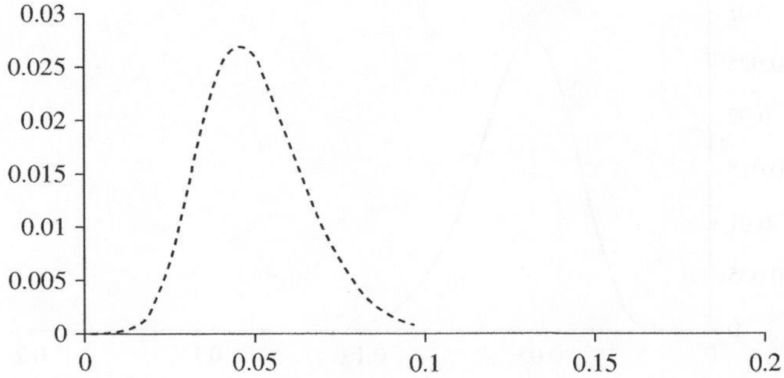

Figure 15.4 Observed response.

15.2.2.4 Worked Example 15.3: Constructing an Observed Response

Suppose we observed a situation where 10 subjects out of 200 experienced the event of interest. For this, $a_1 = 10$ and $b_1 = 190$. Hence we would have

$$p_{percentile} = BETAINV(percentile, 10, 190). \quad (15.18)$$

Figure 15.4 gives an illustration of the observed response for the worked example.

15.2.2.5 Posterior Response

With the anticipated and prior responses, the posterior distribution can be calculated from the following result

$$p_{percentile} = BETAINV(percentile, a_1 + a_0, b_1 + b_0). \quad (15.19)$$

15.2.2.6 Worked Example 15.4: Constructing a Posterior Response

For this worked example we have $a_0 = 3.026$ and $b_0 = 32.7407$, and $a_1 = 10$ and $b_1 = 190$. Hence we would have

$$p_{percentile} = BETAINV(percentile, 13.026, 222.7407). \quad (15.20)$$

Figure 15.5 gives a posterior response.

Figure 15.6 gives an illustration of the prior, observed and posterior distribution together. Note how here the prior distribution, which was quite vague, has had very little impact, with the observed distribution not too far away from the posterior.

15.2.2.7 Effect of Sample Size on Posterior Distribution

In Worked Example 15.3 and Worked Example 15.4 we had a 5% response rate in a sample size of 200. For the same response rate and prior distribution (most likely response

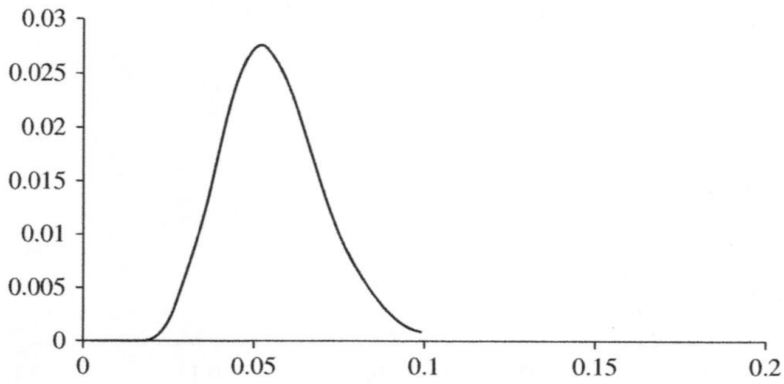

Figure 15.5 Posterior response.

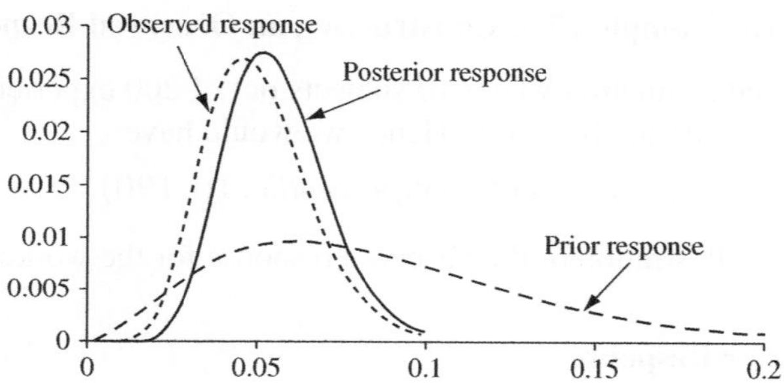

Figure 15.6 Prior, observed and posterior response.

to be 6%, and we are 80% certain it is less than 12%), Figure 15.7 gives an illustration of how the sample size of the observed response affects the posterior distribution.

From Figure 15.7 it is clear that for small sample sizes the posterior distribution is pulled towards the prior, but as the sample size increases it moves away from the prior and to the observed data. We have previously observed a similar feature in Chapter 7 in the discussion on Bayesian methods for first-into-man studies.

The result is intuitive for, clearly, if we have no data, then all the information present will be in the prior. Likewise for very little data the prior is still important, but as we collect more and more data its importance diminishes.

15.2.2.8 Effect of Prior on Posterior Distribution

Now if we fix the response rate at 5% and sample size at 200 but change the prior distribution, then Figure 15.8 illustrates how these different priors affect the resulting posterior distributions.

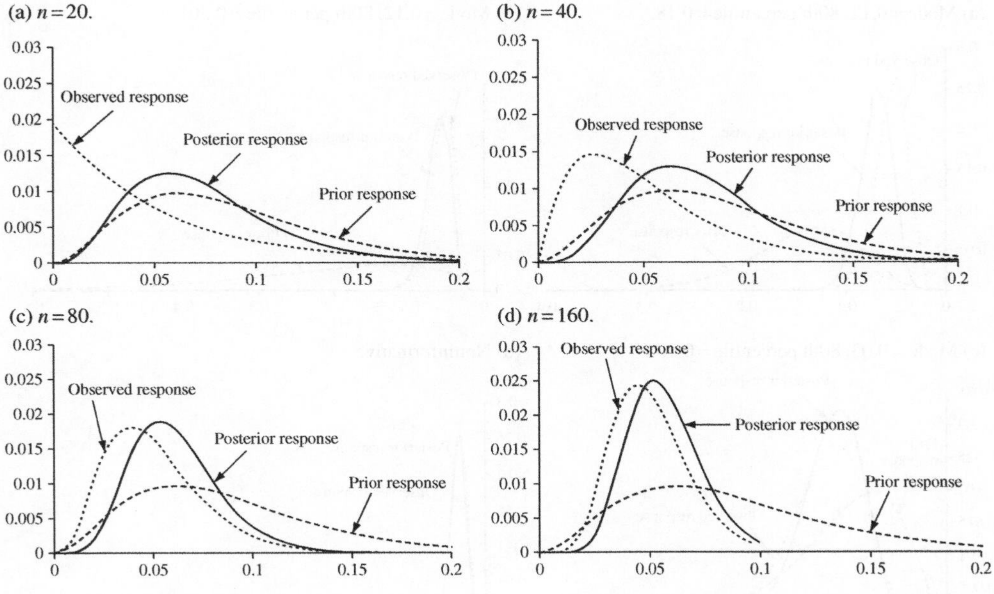

Figure 15.7 The effect of sample size, *n*, on the posterior distribution for the same observed response and prior.

We can see from Figure 15.8 that the different priors for these data have some effect, but due to the relatively large sample size the effect is not great. For the noninformative prior, Figure 15.8d, we can see that the observed and posterior distributions are virtually identical.

There are two sceptical priors, in Figure 15.8a and Figure 15.8b, with Figure 15.8b being a little wide (and hence vague) and we can see these have the effect of producing a posterior response a little higher than that observed.

The last prior in Figure 15.8c is a little optimistic and has pulled the posterior a little towards it, such that it is lower than the observed.

Table 15.2 gives a summary of the results from the worked example, but now for illustration with a number of priors (and not just mode = 6%, 80% sure less it is than 12%). For the frequentist approach we have that the point estimate is 0.05 with a 95% confidence interval of (0.024, 0.084). For the Bayesian approach the point estimate is taken as the 50th percentile of the posterior distribution, and the credibility interval from the 2.5th and 97.5th percentiles. These results confirm Figure 15.8 and illustrate how different priors affect estimation.

15.2.3 Go/No-Go Criteria

What we have demonstrated so far is how Bayesian approaches are a useful way of combining prior beliefs with observed data to form posterior responses for the outcome of interest. As we have seen, with very little observed data, the prior dominates the posterior response, while with a relatively large sample size, the observed data will dominate the posterior distribution.

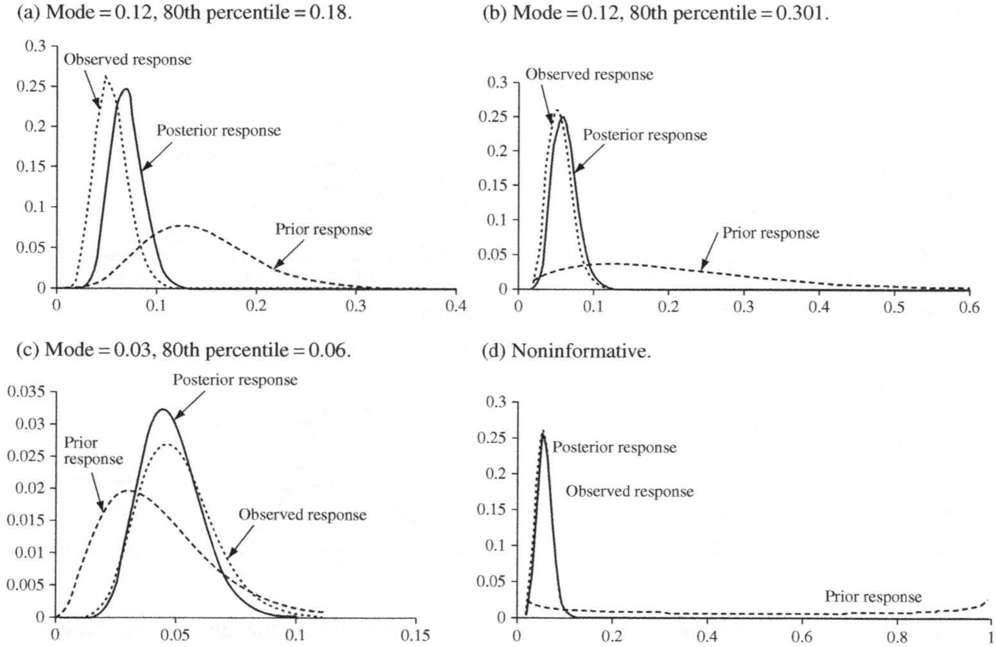

Figure 15.8 Influence of different priors on the posterior distributions for a fixed sample size of 200 and observed response rate of 5%.

Thus far we have been discussing Bayesian approaches for a single binary response, but the work can be extended to trials of two treatments, A and B. In this context, the Go/No-Go criteria can be based on the probability that A is better than B. Hence a Go criterion at the

Table 15.2 Point estimates and confidence (frequentist) or credibility (Bayesian) intervals.

	Frequentist	
	Point estimate	95% Confidence interval
	0.050	0.024 to 0.084
	Bayesian	
Priors	Point estimate	95% Credibility intervals
Noninformative	0.051	0.026 to 0.087
Mode = 0.12, 80th = 0.30	0.055	0.030 to 0.092
Mode = 0.12, 80th = 0.18	0.064	0.038 to 0.100
Mode = 0.06, 80th = 0.12	0.053	0.030 to 0.088
Mode = 0.03, 80th = 0.06	0.046	0.026 to 0.075

end of the Phase II stages could be written in terms of a probability of an asset having a required profile.

As with many things it is best to illustrate this with an example.

15.2.3.1 Worked Example 15.5: Construction of a Go/No-Go Criterion

The Go criterion decided upon for a new compound in development prior to the start of Phase III is as follows:

We need to be 90% certain that the experimental drug has an adverse-event response within 5% of placebo.

From previous experience in the therapeutic area, suppose we have a reasonable idea of the adverse-event rate with placebo. We believe it is most likely to be 0.015 (the mode), with the 80th percentile being 0.13. Hence, from (15.14) and (15.15) we have that $a_0 = 1.19$ and $b_0 = 13.4767$ for placebo, while the percentiles for the distribution would be estimated from

$$p_{percentile_A} = BETAINV(percentile, 1.19, 13.4767). \quad (15.21)$$

For the investigative drug we are not sure what the adverse event response would be. Due to the class effects and experience with other compounds, we anticipate the number of adverse events to be higher. The most likely response which we expect is therefore 0.12, with the 80th percentile being less than 0.301. Hence, we have $a_1 = 1.893$ and $b_1 = 7.54867$ for the investigative treatment and the percentiles for the distribution would be estimated from

$$p_{percentile_B} = BETAINV(percentile, 1.893, 7.54867). \quad (15.22)$$

Note here that the prior is quite vague and it is also a sceptical one, as the belief is that the new treatment has a worse adverse event profile than placebo.

Figure 15.9 gives an illustration of the priors for both placebo and active.

In planning the randomized trial, suppose the sample size is first set to be 200 on each arm, and a range of alternative outcomes for the treatments are considered, from which a range of possible differences need to be derived.

Suppose for example there were no adverse events on placebo, that is $a_1 = 0$ and $b_1 = 200$, then the posterior distribution would be

$$p_{percentile_A} = BETAINV(percentile, 1.19, 213.4767). \quad (15.23)$$

What we need to imagine now is how many adverse events we could see on the investigative treatment to be 90% sure we are within 5% of placebo. For this we need a degree of iteration. For active we need to first set $a_1 = 1$ and $b_1 = 199$ and then calculate the probability of active being within 5% of placebo from the posterior responses; then $a_1 = 2$ and $b_1 = 198$, and so on.

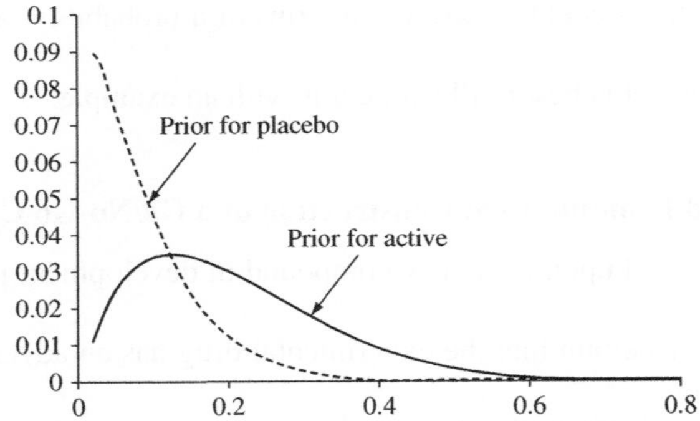

Figure 15.9 Two prior distributions for the anticipated adverse event rates for placebo and active drug.

Table 15.3 gives a summary of the iterations. From the table we see that, so long as we see five or less adverse events, the investigative treatment would be within 5% of the placebo.

The process could be repeated with the scenario of one adverse event with placebo, then two adverse events on placebo, and so on. This is a computationally intensive thing to do and could be implemented with the SAS code given in Figure 15.10

A range of scenarios for placebo are summarized in Table 15.4 with the corresponding number of adverse events allowed for the investigative treatment so as to be able to satisfy the Go criteria.

Table 15.3 Probability of being within 5% of placebo for different investigative adverse-event rates for a fixed placebo rate of 0%.

Placebo		Active		
a_0	b_0	a_1	b_1	P
0	200	1	199	0.99940
0	200	2	198	0.99690
0	200	3	197	0.99053
0	200	4	196	0.97384
0	200	5	195	0.94572
0	200	6	194	0.89515
0	200	7	193	0.82129
0	200	8	192	0.72547
0	200	9	191	0.61428
0	200	10	190	0.49848
0	200	11	189	0.38482
0	200	12	188	0.28878
0	200	13	187	0.19998
0	200	14	186	0.13627
0	200	15	185	0.08835

```
OPTIONS nodate nonumber;
TITLE "Table for Go/No Go";
DATA data;
DO placebo_k = 0 to 8;
DO active_k = 1 to 15;
   iter = 100000;
   ****Anticipated Responses***;
   placebo_a1 = placebo_k;
   placebo_b1 = 200-placebo_k;
   active_a1 = active_k;
   active_b1 = 200-active_k;
   ****************************;
   ***Difference of Interest***;
   delta = 0.05;
   ****************************;

   ****Prior Responses***;
   placebo_a0 = 1.19;
   placebo_b0 = 13.4767;
   active_a0 = 1.893;
   active_b0 = 7.54867;
   ********************;

  ****Posterior Responses*********;
  placebo_a = placebo_a0+placebo_a1;
   placebo_b = placebo_b0+placebo_b1;
  active_a = active_a0+active_a1;
   active_b = active_b0+active_b1;
  *********************************;

 ****Permutations to Work out the Probability***;
 sum = 0;
 DO i = 0 to iter;
 u1 = ranuni(0);
 p0 = BETAINV(u1,placebo_a,placebo_b);
 u2 = ranuni(0);
 p1 = BETAINV(u2,active_a,active_b);
 diff = p0-p1+delta;
 IF diff > 0 THEN flag = 1;
 ELSE flag = 0;
 sum = sum+flag;
 probdiff = sum/iter;
 END; OUTPUT; END; END; RUN;
 *******************************************;

 PROC print data = data;
 VAR placebo_a1 placebo_b1 active_a1 active_b1 probdiff; RUN;
```

Figure 15.10 SAS code for the iterative procedure for a binary response.

Table 15.4 Maximum number of adverse events that could be observed on a test compound to ensure with 90% certainty that the rate in excess of that for placebo is less than 5% with a sample size of 200 in each arm.

	Given number of adverse events on placebo								
	0	1	2	3	4	5	6	7	8
Active	5	6	7	7	8	9	9	10	11

This table assists greatly in the interpretation of the 'Go/No-Go' criterion for, although the calculations may be complex, this table is easy to understand and follow.

15.2.3.2 Worked Example 15.6: Reconstruction of a Go/No-Go Criterion

Suppose that there was a reconsideration of the study design in Worked Example 15.5 such that the sample size has been halved to just 100 per arm in the trial. This has an impact on the certainty that could be obtained in the Go/No-Go criterion. The prior remained the same, but Table 15.4 was recalculated in Table 15.5.

In light of the change in the study design, the Go criterion decided upon for a new compound in development prior to the start of Phase III has changed as follows:

We need to be 80% certain that the experimental drug has an adverse event response within 5% of placebo.

In point of fact this change is not a trivial one, for what we have actually done is lowered the hurdle to pass into late-phase development. There is thus now an increased chance of a drug, which should have had its development stopped, proceeding. The impact of the decision would need to be considered seriously.

Table 15.5 Maximum number of adverse events that could be observed on a test compound to ensure with 90, 80 and 75% certainty that the rate in excess of that for placebo is less than 5% with a sample size of 100 in each arm.

		Given number of adverse events on placebo								
	Certainty (%)	0	1	2	3	4	5	6	7	8
Active	**90**	1	2	3	3	4	5	5	6	7
	80	2	3	4	5	5	6	7	8	8
	75	3	3	4	5	6	7	7	8	9

Appendix

All the tables produced in this appendix were calculated using Excel.

Table A.1 One-sided Normal probability values.

z	0.00	0.01	0.02	0.03	0.04	0.05	0.06	0.07	0.08	0.09
0.00	0.50000	0.49601	0.49202	0.48803	0.48405	0.48006	0.47608	0.47210	0.46812	0.46414
0.10	0.46017	0.45620	0.45224	0.44828	0.44433	0.44038	0.43644	0.43251	0.42858	0.42465
0.20	0.42074	0.41683	0.41294	0.40905	0.40517	0.40129	0.39743	0.39358	0.38974	0.38591
0.30	0.38209	0.37828	0.37448	0.37070	0.36693	0.36317	0.35942	0.35569	0.35197	0.34827
0.40	0.34458	0.34090	0.33724	0.33360	0.32997	0.32636	0.32276	0.31918	0.31561	0.31207
0.50	0.30854	0.30503	0.30153	0.29806	0.29460	0.29116	0.28774	0.28434	0.28096	0.27760
0.60	0.27425	0.27093	0.26763	0.26435	0.26109	0.25785	0.25463	0.25143	0.24825	0.24510
0.70	0.24196	0.23885	0.23576	0.23270	0.22965	0.22663	0.22363	0.22065	0.21770	0.21476
0.80	0.21186	0.20897	0.20611	0.20327	0.20045	0.19766	0.19489	0.19215	0.18943	0.18673
0.90	0.18406	0.18141	0.17879	0.17619	0.17361	0.17106	0.16853	0.16602	0.16354	0.16109
1.00	0.15866	0.15625	0.15386	0.15151	0.14917	0.14686	0.14457	0.14231	0.14007	0.13786
1.10	0.13567	0.13350	0.13136	0.12924	0.12714	0.12507	0.12302	0.12100	0.11900	0.11702
1.20	0.11507	0.11314	0.11123	0.10935	0.10749	0.10565	0.10383	0.10204	0.10027	0.09853
1.30	0.09680	0.09510	0.09342	0.09176	0.09012	0.08851	0.08691	0.08534	0.08379	0.08226
1.40	0.08076	0.07927	0.07780	0.07636	0.07493	0.07353	0.07215	0.07078	0.06944	0.06811
1.50	0.06681	0.06552	0.06426	0.06301	0.06178	0.06057	0.05938	0.05821	0.05705	0.05592
1.60	0.05480	0.05370	0.05262	0.05155	0.05050	0.04947	0.04846	0.04746	0.04648	0.04551
1.70	0.04457	0.04363	0.04272	0.04182	0.04093	0.04006	0.03920	0.03836	0.03754	0.03673
1.80	0.03593	0.03515	0.03438	0.03362	0.03288	0.03216	0.03144	0.03074	0.03005	0.02938
1.90	0.02872	0.02807	0.02743	0.02680	0.02619	0.02559	0.02500	0.02442	0.02385	0.02330
2.00	0.02275	0.02222	0.02169	0.02118	0.02068	0.02018	0.01970	0.01923	0.01876	0.01831
2.10	0.01786	0.01743	0.01700	0.01659	0.01618	0.01578	0.01539	0.01500	0.01463	0.01426
2.20	0.01390	0.01355	0.01321	0.01287	0.01255	0.01222	0.01191	0.01160	0.01130	0.01101
2.30	0.01072	0.01044	0.01017	0.00990	0.00964	0.00939	0.00914	0.00889	0.00866	0.00842
2.40	0.00820	0.00798	0.00776	0.00755	0.00734	0.00714	0.00695	0.00676	0.00657	0.00639
2.50	0.00621	0.00604	0.00587	0.00570	0.00554	0.00539	0.00523	0.00508	0.00494	0.00480
2.60	0.00466	0.00453	0.00440	0.00427	0.00415	0.00402	0.00391	0.00379	0.00368	0.00357
2.70	0.00347	0.00336	0.00326	0.00317	0.00307	0.00298	0.00289	0.00280	0.00272	0.00264
2.80	0.00256	0.00248	0.00240	0.00233	0.00226	0.00219	0.00212	0.00205	0.00199	0.00193
2.90	0.00187	0.00181	0.00175	0.00169	0.00164	0.00159	0.00154	0.00149	0.00144	0.00139
3.00	0.00135	0.00131	0.00126	0.00122	0.00118	0.00114	0.00111	0.00107	0.00104	0.00100
3.10	0.00097	0.00094	0.00090	0.00087	0.00084	0.00082	0.00079	0.00076	0.00074	0.00071
3.20	0.00069	0.00066	0.00064	0.00062	0.00060	0.00058	0.00056	0.00054	0.00052	0.00050
3.30	0.00048	0.00047	0.00045	0.00043	0.00042	0.00040	0.00039	0.00038	0.00036	0.00035
3.40	0.00034	0.00032	0.00031	0.00030	0.00029	0.00028	0.00027	0.00026	0.00025	0.00024
3.50	0.00023	0.00022	0.00022	0.00021	0.00020	0.00019	0.00019	0.00018	0.00017	0.00017
3.60	0.00016	0.00015	0.00015	0.00014	0.00014	0.00013	0.00013	0.00012	0.00012	0.00011
3.70	0.00011	0.00010	0.00010	0.00010	0.00009	0.00009	0.00008	0.00008	0.00008	0.00008
3.80	0.00007	0.00007	0.00007	0.00006	0.00006	0.00006	0.00006	0.00005	0.00005	0.00005
3.90	0.00005	0.00005	0.00004	0.00004	0.00004	0.00004	0.00004	0.00004	0.00003	0.00003
4.00	0.00003	0.00003	0.00003	0.00003	0.00003	0.00003	0.00002	0.00002	0.00002	0.00002

An Introduction to Statistics in Early Phase Trials Steven A. Julious, Say Beng Tan and David Machin

Table A.2 Two-sided Normal probability values.

z	0.00	0.01	0.02	0.03	0.04	0.05	0.06	0.07	0.08	0.09
0.00	1.00000	0.99202	0.98404	0.97607	0.96809	0.96012	0.95216	0.94419	0.93624	0.92829
0.10	0.92034	0.91241	0.90448	0.89657	0.88866	0.88076	0.87288	0.86501	0.85715	0.84931
0.20	0.84148	0.83367	0.82587	0.81809	0.81033	0.80259	0.79486	0.78716	0.77948	0.77182
0.30	0.76418	0.75656	0.74897	0.74140	0.73386	0.72634	0.71885	0.71138	0.70395	0.69654
0.40	0.68916	0.68181	0.67449	0.66720	0.65994	0.65271	0.64552	0.63836	0.63123	0.62413
0.50	0.61708	0.61005	0.60306	0.59611	0.58920	0.58232	0.57548	0.56868	0.56191	0.55519
0.60	0.54851	0.54186	0.53526	0.52869	0.52217	0.51569	0.50925	0.50286	0.49650	0.49019
0.70	0.48393	0.47770	0.47152	0.46539	0.45930	0.45325	0.44725	0.44130	0.43539	0.42953
0.80	0.42371	0.41794	0.41222	0.40654	0.40091	0.39533	0.38979	0.38430	0.37886	0.37347
0.90	0.36812	0.36282	0.35757	0.35237	0.34722	0.34211	0.33706	0.33205	0.32709	0.32217
1.00	0.31731	0.31250	0.30773	0.30301	0.29834	0.29372	0.28914	0.28462	0.28014	0.27571
1.10	0.27133	0.26700	0.26271	0.25848	0.25429	0.25014	0.24605	0.24200	0.23800	0.23405
1.20	0.23014	0.22628	0.22246	0.21870	0.21498	0.21130	0.20767	0.20408	0.20055	0.19705
1.30	0.19360	0.19020	0.18684	0.18352	0.18025	0.17702	0.17383	0.17069	0.16759	0.16453
1.40	0.16151	0.15854	0.15561	0.15272	0.14987	0.14706	0.14429	0.14156	0.13887	0.13622
1.50	0.13361	0.13104	0.12851	0.12602	0.12356	0.12114	0.11876	0.11642	0.11411	0.11183
1.60	0.10960	0.10740	0.10523	0.10310	0.10101	0.09894	0.09691	0.09492	0.09296	0.09103
1.70	0.08913	0.08727	0.08543	0.08363	0.08186	0.08012	0.07841	0.07673	0.07508	0.07345
1.80	0.07186	0.07030	0.06876	0.06725	0.06577	0.06431	0.06289	0.06148	0.06011	0.05876
1.90	0.05743	0.05613	0.05486	0.05361	0.05238	0.05118	0.05000	0.04884	0.04770	0.04659
2.00	0.04550	0.04443	0.04338	0.04236	0.04135	0.04036	0.03940	0.03845	0.03753	0.03662
2.10	0.03573	0.03486	0.03401	0.03317	0.03235	0.03156	0.03077	0.03001	0.02926	0.02852
2.20	0.02781	0.02711	0.02642	0.02575	0.02509	0.02445	0.02382	0.02321	0.02261	0.02202
2.30	0.02145	0.02089	0.02034	0.01981	0.01928	0.01877	0.01827	0.01779	0.01731	0.01685
2.40	0.01640	0.01595	0.01552	0.01510	0.01469	0.01429	0.01389	0.01351	0.01314	0.01277
2.50	0.01242	0.01207	0.01174	0.01141	0.01109	0.01077	0.01047	0.01017	0.00988	0.00960
2.60	0.00932	0.00905	0.00879	0.00854	0.00829	0.00805	0.00781	0.00759	0.00736	0.00715
2.70	0.00693	0.00673	0.00653	0.00633	0.00614	0.00596	0.00578	0.00561	0.00544	0.00527
2.80	0.00511	0.00495	0.00480	0.00465	0.00451	0.00437	0.00424	0.00410	0.00398	0.00385
2.90	0.00373	0.00361	0.00350	0.00339	0.00328	0.00318	0.00308	0.00298	0.00288	0.00279
3.00	0.00270	0.00261	0.00253	0.00245	0.00237	0.00229	0.00221	0.00214	0.00207	0.00200
3.10	0.00194	0.00187	0.00181	0.00175	0.00169	0.00163	0.00158	0.00152	0.00147	0.00142
3.20	0.00137	0.00133	0.00128	0.00124	0.00120	0.00115	0.00111	0.00108	0.00104	0.00100
3.30	0.00097	0.00093	0.00090	0.00087	0.00084	0.00081	0.00078	0.00075	0.00072	0.00070
3.40	0.00067	0.00065	0.00063	0.00060	0.00058	0.00056	0.00054	0.00052	0.00050	0.00048
3.50	0.00047	0.00045	0.00043	0.00042	0.00040	0.00039	0.00037	0.00036	0.00034	0.00033
3.60	0.00032	0.00031	0.00029	0.00028	0.00027	0.00026	0.00025	0.00024	0.00023	0.00022
3.70	0.00022	0.00021	0.00020	0.00019	0.00018	0.00018	0.00017	0.00016	0.00016	0.00015
3.80	0.00014	0.00014	0.00013	0.00013	0.00012	0.00012	0.00011	0.00011	0.00010	0.00010
3.90	0.00010	0.00009	0.00009	0.00008	0.00008	0.00008	0.00007	0.00007	0.00007	0.00007
4.00	0.00006	0.00006	0.00006	0.00006	0.00005	0.00005	0.00005	0.00005	0.00005	0.00004

Table A.3 Critical values of a t-distribution: one-tailed test.

	Significance level									
df	0.400	0.300	0.250	0.200	0.150	0.100	0.050	0.025	0.010	0.001
1	0.325	0.727	1.000	1.376	1.963	3.078	6.314	12.706	31.821	318.309
2	0.289	0.617	0.816	1.061	1.386	1.886	2.920	4.303	6.965	22.327
3	0.277	0.584	0.765	0.978	1.250	1.638	2.353	3.182	4.541	10.215
4	0.271	0.569	0.741	0.941	1.190	1.533	2.132	2.776	3.747	7.173
5	0.267	0.559	0.727	0.920	1.156	1.476	2.015	2.571	3.365	5.893
6	0.265	0.553	0.718	0.906	1.134	1.440	1.943	2.447	3.143	5.208
7	0.263	0.549	0.711	0.896	1.119	1.415	1.895	2.365	2.998	4.785
8	0.262	0.546	0.706	0.889	1.108	1.397	1.860	2.306	2.896	4.501
9	0.261	0.543	0.703	0.883	1.100	1.383	1.833	2.262	2.821	4.297
10	0.260	0.542	0.700	0.879	1.093	1.372	1.812	2.228	2.764	4.144
11	0.260	0.540	0.697	0.876	1.088	1.363	1.796	2.201	2.718	4.025
12	0.259	0.539	0.695	0.873	1.083	1.356	1.782	2.179	2.681	3.930
13	0.259	0.538	0.694	0.870	1.079	1.350	1.771	2.160	2.650	3.852
14	0.258	0.537	0.692	0.868	1.076	1.345	1.761	2.145	2.624	3.787
15	0.258	0.536	0.691	0.866	1.074	1.341	1.753	2.131	2.602	3.733
16	0.258	0.535	0.690	0.865	1.071	1.337	1.746	2.120	2.583	3.686
17	0.257	0.534	0.689	0.863	1.069	1.333	1.740	2.110	2.567	3.646
18	0.257	0.534	0.688	0.862	1.067	1.330	1.734	2.101	2.552	3.610
19	0.257	0.533	0.688	0.861	1.066	1.328	1.729	2.093	2.539	3.579
20	0.257	0.533	0.687	0.860	1.064	1.325	1.725	2.086	2.528	3.552
21	0.257	0.532	0.686	0.859	1.063	1.323	1.721	2.080	2.518	3.527
22	0.256	0.532	0.686	0.858	1.061	1.321	1.717	2.074	2.508	3.505
23	0.256	0.532	0.685	0.858	1.060	1.319	1.714	2.069	2.500	3.485
24	0.256	0.531	0.685	0.857	1.059	1.318	1.711	2.064	2.492	3.467
25	0.256	0.531	0.684	0.856	1.058	1.316	1.708	2.060	2.485	3.450
26	0.256	0.531	0.684	0.856	1.058	1.315	1.706	2.056	2.479	3.435
27	0.256	0.531	0.684	0.855	1.057	1.314	1.703	2.052	2.473	3.421
28	0.256	0.530	0.683	0.855	1.056	1.313	1.701	2.048	2.467	3.408
29	0.256	0.530	0.683	0.854	1.055	1.311	1.699	2.045	2.462	3.396
30	0.256	0.530	0.683	0.854	1.055	1.310	1.697	2.042	2.457	3.385
35	0.255	0.529	0.682	0.852	1.052	1.306	1.690	2.030	2.438	3.340
40	0.255	0.529	0.681	0.851	1.050	1.303	1.684	2.021	2.423	3.307
45	0.255	0.528	0.680	0.850	1.049	1.301	1.679	2.014	2.412	3.281
50	0.255	0.528	0.679	0.849	1.047	1.299	1.676	2.009	2.403	3.261
60	0.254	0.527	0.679	0.848	1.045	1.296	1.671	2.000	2.390	3.232
70	0.254	0.527	0.678	0.847	1.044	1.294	1.667	1.994	2.381	3.211
80	0.254	0.526	0.678	0.846	1.043	1.292	1.664	1.990	2.374	3.195
90	0.254	0.526	0.677	0.846	1.042	1.291	1.662	1.987	2.368	3.183
100	0.254	0.526	0.677	0.845	1.042	1.290	1.660	1.984	2.364	3.174
125	0.254	0.526	0.676	0.845	1.041	1.288	1.657	1.979	2.357	3.157
150	0.254	0.526	0.676	0.844	1.040	1.287	1.655	1.976	2.351	3.145
175	0.254	0.525	0.676	0.844	1.040	1.286	1.654	1.974	2.348	3.137
200	0.254	0.525	0.676	0.843	1.039	1.286	1.653	1.972	2.345	3.131
225	0.254	0.525	0.676	0.843	1.039	1.285	1.652	1.971	2.343	3.127
250	0.254	0.525	0.675	0.843	1.039	1.285	1.651	1.969	2.341	3.123
300	0.254	0.525	0.675	0.843	1.038	1.284	1.650	1.968	2.339	3.118
350	0.254	0.525	0.675	0.843	1.038	1.284	1.649	1.967	2.337	3.114
400	0.254	0.525	0.675	0.843	1.038	1.284	1.649	1.966	2.336	3.111
450	0.253	0.525	0.675	0.842	1.038	1.283	1.648	1.965	2.335	3.108
500	0.253	0.525	0.675	0.842	1.038	1.283	1.648	1.965	2.334	3.107
750	0.253	0.525	0.675	0.842	1.037	1.283	1.647	1.963	2.331	3.101
1000	0.253	0.525	0.675	0.843	1.037	1.282	1.646	1.962	2.330	3.098

Table A.4 Critical values of a t-distribution: two-tailed test.

	Significance level										
df	0.500	0.400	0.300	0.250	0.200	0.150	0.100	0.050	0.025	0.010	0.001
1	1.000	1.376	1.963	2.414	3.078	4.165	6.314	12.706	25.452	63.657	636.619
2	0.816	1.061	1.386	1.604	1.886	2.282	2.920	4.303	6.205	9.925	31.599
3	0.765	0.978	1.250	1.423	1.638	1.924	2.353	3.182	4.177	5.841	12.924
4	0.741	0.941	1.190	1.344	1.533	1.778	2.132	2.776	3.495	4.604	8.610
5	0.727	0.920	1.156	1.301	1.476	1.699	2.015	2.571	3.163	4.032	6.869
6	0.718	0.906	1.134	1.273	1.440	1.650	1.943	2.447	2.969	3.707	5.959
7	0.711	0.896	1.119	1.254	1.415	1.617	1.895	2.365	2.841	3.499	5.408
8	0.706	0.889	1.108	1.240	1.397	1.592	1.860	2.306	2.752	3.355	5.041
9	0.703	0.883	1.100	1.230	1.383	1.574	1.833	2.262	2.685	3.250	4.781
10	0.700	0.879	1.093	1.221	1.372	1.559	1.812	2.228	2.634	3.169	4.587
11	0.697	0.876	1.088	1.214	1.363	1.548	1.796	2.201	2.593	3.106	4.437
12	0.695	0.873	1.083	1.209	1.356	1.538	1.782	2.179	2.560	3.055	4.318
13	0.694	0.870	1.079	1.204	1.350	1.530	1.771	2.160	2.533	3.012	4.221
14	0.692	0.868	1.076	1.200	1.345	1.523	1.761	2.145	2.510	2.977	4.140
15	0.691	0.866	1.074	1.197	1.341	1.517	1.753	2.131	2.490	2.947	4.073
16	0.690	0.865	1.071	1.194	1.337	1.512	1.746	2.120	2.473	2.921	4.015
17	0.689	0.863	1.069	1.191	1.333	1.508	1.740	2.110	2.458	2.898	3.965
18	0.688	0.862	1.067	1.189	1.330	1.504	1.734	2.101	2.445	2.878	3.922
19	0.688	0.861	1.066	1.187	1.328	1.500	1.729	2.093	2.433	2.861	3.883
20	0.687	0.860	1.064	1.185	1.325	1.497	1.725	2.086	2.423	2.845	3.850
21	0.686	0.859	1.063	1.183	1.323	1.494	1.721	2.080	2.414	2.831	3.819
22	0.686	0.858	1.061	1.182	1.321	1.492	1.717	2.074	2.405	2.819	3.792
23	0.685	0.858	1.060	1.180	1.319	1.489	1.714	2.069	2.398	2.807	3.768
24	0.685	0.857	1.059	1.179	1.318	1.487	1.711	2.064	2.391	2.797	3.745
25	0.684	0.856	1.058	1.178	1.316	1.485	1.708	2.060	2.385	2.787	3.725
26	0.684	0.856	1.058	1.177	1.315	1.483	1.706	2.056	2.379	2.779	3.707
27	0.684	0.855	1.057	1.176	1.314	1.482	1.703	2.052	2.373	2.771	3.690
28	0.683	0.855	1.056	1.175	1.313	1.480	1.701	2.048	2.368	2.763	3.674
29	0.683	0.854	1.055	1.174	1.311	1.479	1.699	2.045	2.364	2.756	3.659
30	0.683	0.854	1.055	1.173	1.310	1.477	1.697	2.042	2.360	2.750	3.646
35	0.682	0.852	1.052	1.170	1.306	1.472	1.690	2.030	2.342	2.724	3.591
40	0.681	0.851	1.050	1.167	1.303	1.468	1.684	2.021	2.329	2.704	3.551
45	0.680	0.850	1.049	1.165	1.301	1.465	1.679	2.014	2.319	2.690	3.520
50	0.679	0.849	1.047	1.164	1.299	1.462	1.676	2.009	2.311	2.678	3.496
60	0.679	0.848	1.045	1.162	1.296	1.458	1.671	2.000	2.299	2.660	3.460
70	0.678	0.847	1.044	1.160	1.294	1.456	1.667	1.994	2.291	2.648	3.435
80	0.678	0.846	1.043	1.159	1.292	1.453	1.664	1.990	2.284	2.639	3.416
90	0.677	0.846	1.042	1.158	1.291	1.452	1.662	1.987	2.280	2.632	3.402
100	0.677	0.845	1.042	1.157	1.290	1.451	1.660	1.984	2.276	2.626	3.390
125	0.676	0.845	1.041	1.156	1.288	1.448	1.657	1.979	2.269	2.616	3.370
150	0.676	0.844	1.040	1.155	1.287	1.447	1.655	1.976	2.264	2.609	3.357
175	0.676	0.844	1.040	1.154	1.286	1.446	1.654	1.974	2.261	2.604	3.347
200	0.676	0.843	1.039	1.154	1.286	1.445	1.653	1.972	2.258	2.601	3.340
225	0.676	0.843	1.039	1.153	1.285	1.444	1.652	1.971	2.257	2.598	3.334
250	0.675	0.843	1.039	1.153	1.285	1.444	1.651	1.969	2.255	2.596	3.330
300	0.675	0.843	1.038	1.153	1.284	1.443	1.650	1.968	2.253	2.592	3.323
350	0.675	0.843	1.038	1.152	1.284	1.443	1.649	1.967	2.251	2.590	3.319
400	0.675	0.843	1.038	1.152	1.284	1.442	1.649	1.966	2.250	2.588	3.315
450	0.675	0.842	1.038	1.152	1.283	1.442	1.648	1.965	2.249	2.587	3.312
500	0.675	0.842	1.038	1.152	1.283	1.442	1.648	1.965	2.248	2.586	3.310
750	0.675	0.842	1.037	1.151	1.283	1.441	1.647	1.963	2.246	2.582	3.304
1000	0.675	0.842	1.037	1.151	1.282	1.441	1.646	1.962	2.245	2.581	3.300

Table A.5 Critical values of a chi-squared distribution.

	Significance level												
df	0.999	0.990	0.975	0.950	0.900	0.750	0.500	0.250	0.100	0.050	0.025	0.010	0.001
1	0.000002	0.0002	0.001	0.004	0.02	0.10	0.45	1.32	2.71	3.84	5.02	6.63	10.83
2	0.002	0.020	0.05	0.10	0.21	0.58	1.39	2.77	4.61	5.99	7.38	9.21	13.82
3	0.02	0.11	0.22	0.35	0.58	1.21	2.37	4.11	6.25	7.81	9.35	11.34	16.27
4	0.09	0.30	0.48	0.71	1.06	1.92	3.36	5.39	7.78	9.49	11.14	13.28	18.47
5	0.21	0.55	0.83	1.15	1.61	2.67	4.35	6.63	9.24	11.07	12.83	15.09	20.52
6	0.38	0.87	1.24	1.64	2.20	3.45	5.35	7.84	10.64	12.59	14.45	16.81	22.46
7	0.60	1.24	1.69	2.17	2.83	4.25	6.35	9.04	12.02	14.07	16.01	18.48	24.32
8	0.86	1.65	2.18	2.73	3.49	5.07	7.34	10.22	13.36	15.51	17.53	20.09	26.12
9	1.15	2.09	2.70	3.33	4.17	5.90	8.34	11.39	14.68	16.92	19.02	21.67	27.88
10	1.48	2.56	3.25	3.94	4.87	6.74	9.34	12.55	15.99	18.31	20.48	23.21	29.59
11	1.83	3.05	3.82	4.57	5.58	7.58	10.34	13.70	17.28	19.68	21.92	24.72	31.26
12	2.21	3.57	4.40	5.23	6.30	8.44	11.34	14.85	18.55	21.03	23.34	26.22	32.91
13	2.62	4.11	5.01	5.89	7.04	9.30	12.34	15.98	19.81	22.36	24.74	27.69	34.53
14	3.04	4.66	5.63	6.57	7.79	10.17	13.34	17.12	21.06	23.68	26.12	29.14	36.12
15	3.48	5.23	6.26	7.26	8.55	11.04	14.34	18.25	22.31	25.00	27.49	30.58	37.70
16	3.94	5.81	6.91	7.96	9.31	11.91	15.34	19.37	23.54	26.30	28.85	32.00	39.25
17	4.42	6.41	7.56	8.67	10.09	12.79	16.34	20.49	24.77	27.59	30.19	33.41	40.79
18	4.90	7.01	8.23	9.39	10.86	13.68	17.34	21.60	25.99	28.87	31.53	34.81	42.31
19	5.41	7.63	8.91	10.12	11.65	14.56	18.34	22.72	27.20	30.14	32.85	36.19	43.82
20	5.92	8.26	9.59	10.85	12.44	15.45	19.34	23.83	28.41	31.41	34.17	37.57	45.31
21	6.45	8.90	10.28	11.59	13.24	16.34	20.34	24.93	29.62	32.67	35.48	38.93	46.80
22	6.98	9.54	10.98	12.34	14.04	17.24	21.34	26.04	30.81	33.92	36.78	40.29	48.27
23	7.53	10.20	11.69	13.09	14.85	18.14	22.34	27.14	32.01	35.17	38.08	41.64	49.73
24	8.08	10.86	12.40	13.85	15.66	19.04	23.34	28.24	33.20	36.42	39.36	42.98	51.18
25	8.65	11.52	13.12	14.61	16.47	19.94	24.34	29.34	34.38	37.65	40.65	44.31	52.62
26	9.22	12.20	13.84	15.38	17.29	20.84	25.34	30.43	35.56	38.89	41.92	45.64	54.05
27	9.80	12.88	14.57	16.15	18.11	21.75	26.34	31.53	36.74	40.11	43.19	46.96	55.48
28	10.39	13.56	15.31	16.93	18.94	22.66	27.34	32.62	37.92	41.34	44.46	48.28	56.89
29	10.99	14.26	16.05	17.71	19.77	23.57	28.34	33.71	39.09	42.56	45.72	49.59	58.30
30	11.59	14.95	16.79	18.49	20.60	24.48	29.34	34.80	40.26	43.77	46.98	50.89	59.70
35	14.69	18.51	20.57	22.47	24.80	29.05	34.34	40.22	46.06	49.80	53.20	57.34	66.62
40	17.92	22.16	24.43	26.51	29.05	33.66	39.34	45.62	51.81	55.76	59.34	63.69	73.40
45	21.25	25.90	28.37	30.61	33.35	38.29	44.34	50.98	57.51	61.66	65.41	69.96	80.08
50	24.67	29.71	32.36	34.76	37.69	42.94	49.33	56.33	63.17	67.50	71.42	76.15	86.66
60	31.74	37.48	40.48	43.19	46.46	52.29	59.33	66.98	74.40	79.08	83.30	88.38	99.61
70	39.04	45.44	48.76	51.74	55.33	61.70	69.33	77.58	85.53	90.53	95.02	100.43	112.32
80	46.52	53.54	57.15	60.39	64.28	71.14	79.33	88.13	96.58	101.88	106.63	112.33	124.84
90	54.16	61.75	65.65	69.13	73.29	80.62	89.33	98.65	107.57	113.15	118.14	124.12	137.21
100	61.92	70.06	74.22	77.93	82.36	90.13	99.33	109.14	118.50	124.34	129.56	135.81	149.45
125	81.77	91.18	95.95	100.18	105.21	114.00	124.33	135.27	145.64	152.09	157.84	164.69	179.60
150	102.11	112.67	117.98	122.69	128.28	137.98	149.33	161.29	172.58	179.58	185.80	193.21	209.26
175	122.83	134.44	140.26	145.41	151.49	162.04	174.33	187.23	199.36	206.87	213.52	221.44	238.55
200	143.84	156.43	162.73	168.28	174.84	186.17	199.33	213.10	226.02	233.99	241.06	249.45	267.54
225	165.10	178.61	185.35	191.28	198.28	210.35	224.33	238.92	252.58	260.99	268.44	277.27	296.29
250	186.55	200.94	208.10	214.39	221.81	234.58	249.33	264.70	279.05	287.88	295.69	304.94	324.83
300	229.96	245.97	253.91	260.88	269.07	283.14	299.33	316.14	331.79	341.40	349.87	359.91	381.43
350	273.90	291.41	300.06	307.65	316.55	331.81	349.33	367.46	384.31	394.63	403.72	414.47	437.49
400	318.26	337.16	346.48	354.64	364.21	380.58	399.33	418.70	436.65	447.63	457.31	468.72	493.13
450	362.96	383.16	393.12	401.82	412.01	429.42	449.33	469.86	488.85	500.46	510.67	522.72	548.43
500	407.95	429.39	439.94	449.15	459.93	478.32	499.33	520.95	540.93	553.13	563.85	576.49	603.45

References

ABPI (2007) *Guidelines for Phase 1 Clinical Trials:* 2007 Edition. The Association of the British Pharmaceutical Industry, London.

ABPI/BIA (2006) *Early Stage Clinical Trial Task Force. Joint ABPI/BIA Report*. ABPI, London.

A'Hern,R.P. (2001) Sample size tables for exact single stage phase II designs. *Statistics in Medicine*, **20**, 859–866.

Begg, C., Cho, M., Eastwood, S. *et al.* (1996) Improving the quality of reporting randomized controlled trials: the CONSORT statement. *Journal of the American Medical Association*, **276**, 637–639.

Bryant, J. and Day, R. (1995) Incorporating toxicity considerations into the design of two-stage Phase II clinical trials. *Biometrics*, **51**, 1372–1383.

Burman,C.-F. and Senn, S.J. (2003) Examples of option value in drug development, *Pharmaceutical Statistics*. **2**, 113–125.

Case, L.D. and Morgan, T.M. (2003) Design of Phase II cancer trials evaluating survival probabilities. *BMC Medical Research Methodology*, **3**, 6.

Cheung, Y.K. and Chappel, R. (2000) Sequential designs for phase I clinical trials with late-onset toxicities. *Biometrics*, **56**, 1177–1182.

Chevret, S. (1993) The continual reassessment method for phase I clinical trials: a simulation study. *Statistics in Medicine*, **12**, 1093–1108.

CHMP (2004) *Note for Guidance on the Evaluation of the Pharmacokinetics of Medicinal Products in Patients with Impaired Renal Function.* EMEA, London.

CHMP (2005a) *Guideline for the Evaluation of Anticancer Medicinal Products in Man.* EMEA, London.

CHMP (2005b) *Guideline for the Evaluation of the Pharmacokinetics of Medicinal Products in Patients with Impaired Hepatic Function.* EMEA, London.

CHMP (2006a) *Draft Guideline on Reporting the Results of Population Pharmacokinetic Analyses.* EMEA, London.

CHMP (2006b) *Concept Paper for an Addendum to the Note for Guidance on the Investigation of Bioavailability and Bioequivalence: Evaluation of Bioequivalence of Highly Variable Drugs and Drug Products.* EMEA, London.

CHMP (2006c) *Guideline on the Role of Pharmacokinetics in the Development of Products in the Paediatric Population.* EMEA, London.

CHMP (2006d) *Guideline on Clinical Trials in Small Populations.* EMEA, London.

CHMP (2007a) *Guideline on Strategies to Identify and Mitigate Risks for First in Human Clinical Trials with Investigational Medicinal Products.* EMEA, London.

CHMP (2007b) *Guideline on the Investigation of Medicinal Products in the Term and Preterm Neonate.* EMEA, London.

CHMP (2008) *Draft Guideline on the Investigation of Bioequivalence*. EMEA, London.

CPMP (1997) *Notes for Guidance on the Investigation of Drug Interactions.* EMEA, London.

An Introduction to Statistics in Early Phase Trials Steven A. Julious, Say Beng Tan and David Machin

CPMP (1998a) *Notes for Guidance on the Investigation of Bioavailability and Bioequivalence.* EMEA, London.

CPMP (1998b) *Note for Guidance on the Pre-Clinical Evaluation of Anticancer Medicinal Products.* CPMP/SWP/997/96. EMEA, London.

CPMP (2002) *Points to Consider on Multiplicity Issues in Clinical Trials.* EMEA, London.

CPMP (2003) *Note for Guidance on Evaluation of Anticancer Medicinal Products in Man. Addendum on Paediatric Oncology.* EMEA, London.

Daly, L. (1992) Simple SAS macros for the calculation of exact binomial and Poisson confidence limits. *Computational and Biological Medicine*, **22**, 351–361.

EMEA (2007) *European Medicines Agency Decision of 3 December 2007 on a Class Waiver on Conditions in Accordance with Regulations (EC) No. 1901/2006 of the European Parliament and of the Council as Amended.* EMEA/551894/2007. EMEA, London.

Estey, E.H. and Thall, P. (2003) New designs for phase 2 clinical trials. *Blood*, **102**, 442–448.

European Commission (2006) *Ethical Considerations for Clinical Trials Performed in Children: Recommendations of the Ad Hoc Group for the Development of Implementing Guidelines for Directive 2001/20/EC Relating to Good Clinical Practice in the Conduct of Clinical Trials on Medicinal Products for Human Use.* (Draft guideline.) EMEA, London.

FDA (1998a) *Guidance for Industry. Pharmacokinetics in Patients with Impaired Renal Function – Study Design, Data Analysis and Impact on Dosing and Labeling.* Food and Drug Administration, Rockville, MD.

FDA (1998b) *Guidance for Industry. General Considerations for Pediatric Pharmacokinetic Studies for Drugs and Biological Products. Draft Guidance.* Food and Drug Administration, Rockville, MD.

FDA (1998c) Guidance for Industry. Submission of Abbreviated Reports and Synopses in Support of Marketing Applications. Draft Guidance. Food and Drug Administration, Rockville, MD.

FDA (1999a) *Guidance for Industry. In Vivo Drug Metabolism/Drug Interaction Studies – Study Design, Data Analysis, and Recommendations for Dosing and Labeling.* Food and Drug Administration, Rockville, MD.

FDA (1999b) *Draft Guidance for Industry. Pharmacokinetics in Patients with Impaired Hepatic Function: Study Design, Data Analysis and Impact on Dosing and Labeling.* Food and Drug Administration, Rockville, MD.

FDA (1999c) *Guidance for Industry. Population Pharmacokinetics.* Food and Drug Administration, Rockville, MD.

FDA (2000) *Guidance for Industry. Bioavailability and Bioequivalence Studies for Orally Administered Drug Products – General Considerations.* Food and Drug Administration, Rockville, MD.

FDA (2001) *Statistical Approaches to Establishing Bioequivalence.* Food and Drug Administration, Rockville, MD.

FDA (2002a) *Guidance for Industry. Food-Effect Bioavailability and Fed Bioequivalence Studies.* Food and Drug Administration, Rockville, MD.

FDA (2002b) *Draft Guidance for Industry and Reviewers: Estimating the Safe Starting Dose in Clinical Trials for Therapeutics in Adult Healthy Volunteers.* Food and Drug Administration, Rockville, MD.

FDA (2003a) *Concept Paper on End-Of-Phase-2A Meeting with Sponsors Regarding Exposure Response of IND and NDA Products.* Draft 16 October 2003. Food and Drug Administration, Silver Spring, MD.

FDA (2003b) *Guidance for Industry. Bioavailability and Bioequivalence Studies for Orally Administered Drug Products – General Considerations.* Food and Drug Administration, Rockville, MD.

FDA (2003c) *Guidance for Industry. Guideline for the Study and Evaluation of Gender Differences in the Clinical Evaluation of Drugs.* Food and Drug Administration, Rockville, MD.

FDA (2005a) CFR Title 21 – Food and Drugs (320): Bioavailability and Bioequivalence Requirements. 21CFR320.

FDA (2005b) CFR Title 21 – Food and Drugs (320): Bioavailability and Bioequivalence Requirements. Section 33: Criteria and Evidence to Assess Actual or Potential Bioequivalence Problems. 21CFR320.33.

FDA (2006a) *Critical Path Opportunities Report*. March 2006. Food and Drug Administration, Silver Spring, MD.

FDA (2006b) *Approved Drug Products with Therapeutic Equivalence Evaluations*, 26th edn. Food and Drug Administration, Silver Spring, MD.

Fleming, T.R. (1982) One-sample multiple testing procedure for Phase II clinical trial. *Biometrics*, **38**, 143–151.

Gajewski, B.J. and Mayo, M.S. (2006) Bayesian sample size calculations in phase II clinical trials using a mixture of informative priors. *Statistics in Medicine*, **25**, 2554–2566.

Gehan, E.A. (1961) The determination of the number of patients required in a preliminary and follow-up trial of a new chemotherapeutic agent. *Journal of Chronic Diseases*, **13**, 346–353.

Goodman, S.N., Zahurak, M.L. and Piantadosi, S. (1995) Some practical improvements in the continual reassessment method for phase I studies. *Statistics in Medicine*, **14**, 1149–1161.

Gough, K., Hutchinson, M., Keene, O. *et al.* (1995) Assessment of dose proportionality: report from the Statisticians in the Pharmaceutical Industry/Pharmacokinetics UK Joint Working Party. *Drug Information Journal*, **29**, 1039–1048.

Gould, A.L. (1995) Group sequential extensions of a standard bioequivalence testing procedure. *Journal of Pharmacokinetics and Biopharmaceutics*, **23**, 5–86.

Haidar, S.H. (2004) Bioequivalence of highly variable drugs: regulatory perspectives. Presentation at Food and Drug Administration Advisory Committee for Pharmaceutical Science meeting, 14 April 2004.

Haidar, S.H., Nwakama, P.E., Yang, Y.S. *et al.* (2006) A review of ANDAs approved 1996–2005 reveals small differences in bioavailability for BCS Class I and other generic drug products relative to the brand name equivalents. Presented at the American Association of Pharmaceutical Scientists (AAPS) National Biotechnology Conference June 18–21, 2006, Boston, MA.

Health Canada (1992) *Guidance for Industry. Conduct and Analysis of Bioavailability and Bioequivalence Studies - Part A: Oral Dosage Formulations Used for Systemic Effects*. Health Canada, Ontario.

Health Canada (1996) *Guidance for Industry. Conduct and Analysis of Bioavailability and Bioequivalence Studies - Part B: Oral Modified Release Formulations*. Health Canada, Ontario.

Health Canada (2003) *Discussion Paper. Bioequivalence Requirements: Highly Variable Drugs and Highly Variable Drug Products: Issues and Options*. Health Canada, Ontario.

Health Canada (2006) *Guidance for Industry. Bioequivalence Requirements: Critical Dose Drugs*. Health Canada, Ontario.

Health Canada Expert Advisory Committee on Bioavailability and Bioequivalence (2003) *Record of Proceedings: March 13 & 14, 2003*. Health Canada, Ontario.

Heyd, J.M. and Carlin, B.P. (1999) Adaptive design improvements in the continual reassessment method for phase I studies. *Statistics in Medicine*, **18**, 1307–1321.

ICH (1994a) *ICH Topic E4: Dose Response Information to Support Drug Registration*. EMEA, London.

ICH (1994b) *ICH Topic E7: Note for Guidance on Studies in Support of Special Populations: Geriatrics*. EMEA, London.

ICH (1996a) *ICH Topic E6: Guideline for Good Clinical Practice*. EMEA, London.

ICH (1996b) *ICH Topic E3: Structure and Content of Clinical Study Reports*. EMEA, London.

ICH (1998a) *ICH Topic E8: Note for Guidance on General Considerations for Clinical Trials*. EMEA, London.

ICH (1998b) *ICH Topic E9: Statistical Principles for Clinical Trials*. September 1998. EMEA, London.

ICH (1998c) *ICH Topic E5: Ethnic Factors in the Acceptability of Foreign Clinical Data*. EMEA, London.

ICH (2001) *ICH Topic E11: Note for Guidance on Clinical Investigation of Medicinal Products in the Paediatric Population*. EMEA, London.

Julious, S.A. (2004a) Designing early phase trials with uncertain estimates of variability. *Pharmaceutical Statistics*, **3**, 261–268.

Julious, S.A. (2004b) Tutorial in biostatistics: sample sizes for clinical trials with Normal data. *Statistics in Medicine*, **23**, 1921–1986.

Julious, S.A. (2004c) Using confidence intervals around individual means to assess statistical significance between two means. *Pharmaceutical Statistics*, **3**, 217–222.

Julious, S.A. (2005a) Sample size of 12 per group rule of thumb for a pilot study. *Pharmaceutical Statistics*, **4**(4), 287–291.

Julious, S.A. (2005b) Two-sided confidence intervals for the single proportion: comparison of seven methods. (Letter.) *Statistics in Medicine*, **24**, 3383–3384.

Julious, S.A. (2005c) Why do we use pooled variance analysis of variance? *Pharmaceutical Statistics*, **4**, 3–5.

Julious, S.A. (2007) A personal perspective on the Royal Statistical Society report of the working party on statistical issues in first-in-man studies. *Pharmaceutical Statistics*, **6**, 75–78.

Julious, S.A., Campbell, M.J. and Walters, S.J. (2007) Predicting where future means will lie based on the results of the current trial. *Contemporary Clinical Trials*, **28**, 352–357.

Julious, S.A. and Debarnot, C.A.M. (2000) Why are pharmacokinetic data summarised by arithmetic means? *Journal of Biopharmaceutical Statistics*, **10**(1), 55–71.

Julious, S.A. and Paterson, S.D. (2004) Sample sizes for estimation in clinical research. *Pharmaceutical Statistics*, **3**, 213–215.

Julious, S.A. and Swank, D. (2005) Moving statistics beyond the individual clinical trial: applying decision science to optimise a clinical development plan. *Pharmaceutical Statistics*, **4**, 37–46.

Keene, O.N. (1995) The log transformation is special. *Statistics in Medicine*, **14**, 811–819.

Korn, E.L., Midthune, D., Chen, T.T. *et al.* (1994) A comparison of two Phase I trial designs. *Statistics in Medicine*, **13**, 1799–1806.

Lacey, F.N., Keene, O.N., Pritchard, J.F. and Bye, A. (1997) Common non-compartmental pharmacokinetic variables: are they Normally or log-Normally distributed? *Journal of Biopharmaceutical Statistics*, **7**(1), 171–178.

Machin, D., Campbell, M.J., Tan, S.B. and Tan, S.H. (2008) *Sample Size Tables for Clinical Studies*. John Wiley & Sons, Ltd, Chichester.

Mayo, M.S. and Gajewski, B.J. (2004) Bayesian sample size calculations in phase II clinical trials using informative conjugate priors. *Controlled Clinical Trials*, **25**, 157–167.

Mizuta, E. and Tsubotani, A. (1985) Preparation of mean drug concentration-time curves in plasma. A study on the frequency distribution of pharmacokinetic parameters. *Chemical & Pharmaceutical Bulletin*, **33**(4), 1620–1632.

Moher, D., Schultz, K.F. and Altman, D.G., for the CONSORT Group (2001) The CONSORT statement: revised recommendations for improving the quality of reports of parallel-group randomised trials. *Lancet*, **357**, 1191–1194.

Newcombe, R.G. (1998) Two-sided confidence intervals for the single proportion: comparison of seven methods. *Statistics in Medicine*, **17**, 857–872.

NIHS, Japan (1997) Guideline for Bioequivalence Studies of Generic Products. National Institute of Health Sciences, Japan.

O'Quigley, J. (2001) Dose-finding designs using continual reassessment method, in *Handbook of Statistics in Clinical Oncology* (ed. J. Crowley), Marcel Dekker Inc., New York, pp. 35–72.

O'Quigley, J., Pepe, M. and Fisher, L. (1990) Continual reassessment method: a practical design for phase I clinical trials in cancer. *Biometrics*, **46**, 33–48.

Patterson, S. and Jones, B. (2006) *Bioequivalence and Statistics in Clinical Pharmacology*. Chapman and Hall, London.

Peace, K. (1988) *Biopharmaceutical Statistics for Drug Development*. Marcel Dekker, New York.

Rowland, M. and Tozer, T.N. (1995) *Clinical Pharmacokinetics, Concepts and Applications*. Lea & Febiger, London.

Sambucini, V. (2008) A Bayesian predictive two-stage design for Phase II clinical trials. *Statistics in Medicine*, **27**, 1199–1224.

Senn, S.J. (2002) *Cross-over Trials in Clinical Research*. John Wiley & Sons, Ltd, Chichester.

Senn, S.J. (2007) *Statistical Issues in Drug Development*, 2nd edn. John Wiley & Sons, Inc., Hoboken.

Senn, S., Amin, D., Bailey, R.A. *et al.* (2007) Statistical issues in first-in-man studies, *Journal of the Royal Statistical Society Series A – Statistics in Society*, **170**, 517–579.

Sethuraman, V.S., Leonov, S., Squassante, L., Mitchell, T.R. and Hale, M.D. (2007) Sample size calculation for the Power Model for dose proportionality studies. *Pharmaceutical Statistics*, **6**(1), 35–41.

Simon, R. (1989) Optimal two-stage designs for phase II clinical trials. *Controlled Clinical Trials*, **10**, 1–10.

Simon, R., Wittes, R.E. and Ellenberg, S.S. (1985) Randomized phase II clinical trials. *Cancer Treatment Reports*, **69**, 1375–1381.

Storer, B.E. (2001) Choosing a Phase I design, in *Handbook of Statistics in Clinical Oncology* (ed. J. Crowley), Marcel Dekker Inc., New York, pp. 73–91.

Tan, S.B. and Machin, D. (2002) Bayesian two-stage designs for phase II clinical trials. *Statistics in Medicine*, **21**, 1991–2012.

Therasse, P., Arbuck, S.G., Eisenhauer, E.A. *et al.* (2000) New guidelines to evaluate the response to treatment in solid tumors. *Journal of the National Cancer Institute*, **92**(3), 205–216.

Wang, Y.G., Leung, D.H.Y., Li, M. and Tan, S.B. (2005) Bayesian designs with frequentist and Bayesian error rate considerations. *Statistical Methods in Medical Research*, **14**, 445–456.

Whitehead, J., Zhou, Y., Patterson, S., Webber, D. and Francis, S. (2001) Easy to implement Bayesian methods for dose escalation studies in healthy volunteers. *Biostatistics*, **2**, 47–61.

Zohar, S. and O'Quigley,J. (2006) Identifying the most successful dose (MSD) in dose-finding studies in cancer. *Pharmaceutical Statistics*, **5**, 187–199.

Index

Note: Page numbers in italics and bold refer to figures and tables respectively.

An Introduction to Statistics in Early Phase Trials Steven A. Julious, Say Beng Tan and David Machin

Printed and bound by CPI Group (UK) Ltd, Croydon, CR0 4YY
16/04/2025
14658551-0001